Adult Day Care
A Practical Guide

Carole Lium O'Brien, RN, MS

Wadsworth Health Sciences Division
Monterey, California

Wadsworth Health Sciences Division
A Division of Wadsworth, Inc.

© 1982 by Wadsworth, Inc., Belmont, California 94002
All rights reserved. No part of this book may be reproduced,
stored in a retrieval system, or transcribed, in any form or by
any means—electronic, mechanical, photocopying, recording,
or otherwise—without the prior written permission of the
publisher. Wadsworth Health Sciences Division, Monterey,
California 93940, a division of Wadsworth, Inc.

Printed in the United States of America

10 9 8 7 6 5 4 3 2 1

Library of Congress Cataloging in Publication Data

O'Brien, Carole Lium.
   Adult day care.

   Bibliography: p.
   Includes index.
   1. Day care centers for the aged—United States.
2. Aged—Services for—United States. I. Title.
[DNLM: 1. Day care—In old age. 2. Long term care
—In old age. WT 29.1 013a]
HV1465.025   362.6'3   81-16212
ISBN 0-8185-0506-0   AACR2

Sponsoring Editors: Edward Murphy/James Keating
Production: Ron Newcomer & Associates, San Francisco, California
Manuscript Editor: Mary Anne Stewart
Interior Design: Ron Newcomer
Cover Design: Albert Burkhardt
Illustrations: Irene Imfeld
Typesetting: Graphic Typesetting Service, Los Angeles, California

*This book is dedicated in memory to my very special parents,
Mr. and Mrs. Hans Lium*

Foreword

by Congressman Robert F. Drinan, House Select Committee on Aging

The graying of America . . . spiraling health-care costs . . . institutionalization! We in the Congress stagger under the weight of statistical reports and testimony clearly attesting to the need for a coherent long-term health-care policy for our elderly citizens that does not rely on institutionalization. While Congress and the administration consider changes in our major health care policy, especially as regards the allocation of Medicare and Medicaid funds, professionals in the field are already experimenting with innovative ways to meet the health needs of our growing elderly population.

Adequate care for chronic illness represents one of the most pressing needs of the elderly. Traditional approaches to the treatment and care of chronic illness have focused primarily on institutionalization as the long-term-care solution. With a growing elderly population placing heavier demands on the health-care system and with the growing recognition that the elderly are entitled as a matter of right to a dignified and independent old age, attention must begin to focus on a greater array of health-care services and more nontraditional approaches to the complex health needs of the aging.

This book tells us about one of these new approaches, adult day-care services.

Day-care centers for the elderly represent a much needed alternative to institutionalization. In the majority of communities where no day health services are available, the frail elderly often are forced into institutions for lack of any other alternative. In the few communities that do have such services, however, the frail elderly are provided with the opportunity of remaining with their families and friends and sustaining ties to their communities. Certainly, we do not mean to suggest that the care provided by health professionals in day-care centers could ever substitute for 24-hour institutional care when no other alternative is medically desirable. Nevertheless, it is an excellent alternative for those frail elderly who do not require full-time care.

The aim of adult day-care services is twofold: to encourage the elderly to maintain their physical level of functioning and to promote a renewed interest in life through a variety of social and emotional support services. This approach has been tremendously successful, for, in the end, a program's real worth can be measured only in terms of its human value. By preventing premature institutionalization, day-care services enable the elderly to continue to lead full and satisfying lives. Adult day-care centers, along with other alternatives to long-term care, will be one of the major issues facing Congress in this decade.

Preface

The effective fulfillment of the health- and human-service needs of our elderly, aged, and disadvantaged groups will depend in no small measure on the problem-solving capabilities and skills of health- and human-services professionals. Until recently, professionals desiring to improve their understanding of adult day-care services, and their skills in determining the need for such services, could find little of direct relevance in the literature. One reason for the lack of literature on adult day care is the multiple and diverse physical, biological, sociopolitical, and economic factors that must be taken into account in such programs. Another difficulty is that adult day-care programs are not well established as a service component in this country, but rather have just begun to evolve.

The aim of the present volume is to formulate, within a unified systems framework, the concepts of assessment, planning, implementation, and evaluation relevant to the development of adult day-care programs and to apply these concepts directly to the circumstances encountered by professionals involved in planning or delivering such services to the elderly disabled population.

The systems approach provides a framework that is both practical and timely, with a common basic language that can enhance communication among disciplines and professionals. The problem-solving models and visualizations will facilitate comprehension, synthesis, and application of content.

The book considers the establishing of adult day-care centers within a community perspective and long-term continuum-of-care options. The proposed adult day center thus becomes part of the community's health-care and social-service system and not merely an additional program in an already too-fragmented community system of services.

This book is addressed primarily to graduate students, health and human-service professionals, multidisciplinary groups, and those concerned with the health and human welfare of our elderly citizens. It is hoped that it will fill the need, to which more than one Senate Investigative Committee on Aging has drawn attention, for an exposition of the methodology and theoretical concepts suitable for use by health- and human-service program planners at the community level.

Acknowledgments

It is impossible for me to name all my colleagues who contributed to the thinking expressed in this text. In the area of adult day services, the largest credit is due to Gretchen Dix of the Weston Manor Adult Day Health Program. The case material, forms, procedures, and many examples were arrived at in close collaboration with her and her staff at Weston Manor. In addition, special recognition is given to Anne Klapfish of the Massachusetts Department of Public Welfare, who was more than cooperative in sharing her information and knowledge about adult day services.

Special thanks go to Margaret B. Connolly, Administrator of Weston Manor Nursing Home, who from the very inception of my idea has been dedicated to, and has helped in, the implementation of the Weston Manor Adult Day Health Program. In addition, much appreciation is given to Congressman Robert F. Drinan for his continuous encouragement and support from the beginning of this project. For the inspiration and enthusiasm I received from Ann Burgess, as a mentor and friend, I am deeply indebted. And, above all, I owe a special debt to Betty Perrault for her suggestions and encouragement throughout the writing.

In developing this text, I received much assistance and support from the contributing authors. Their professional competence and perceptiveness aided greatly in the development of the final draft of this manuscript. Moreover, there is one specific person who contributed to the development of all chapters and to whom I am grateful: Sarah French Schiermeyer.

Mary L. Pekarski and Anne F. Lippman, librarians at the Boston College School of Nursing, were very helpful in assisting me with reference sources. There is no way to describe adequately the contributions of the superb secretarial support given by Mary E. Robinson and Judy Sweeney, who helped in the typing of the manuscript. I particularly express gratitude to Edward Murphy for his assistance with the publication of this book.

Finally, my warmest thanks to my family: Megan, Heather, and Deirdre

O'Brien, my children; John Lium, my brother; Lenore Pennaccllia, my aunt; and Ann Bonica, a dear friend. Without their continued interest and patience through all phases of the manuscript development, the book wouldn't be a reality today.

Chestnut Hill, Massachusetts   Carole Lium O'Brien, RN, MS

Contributors

Ana Morgan Clark RN, MS
*Administrator Walpole Visiting Nurse
   Association*
Walpole, Massachusetts

Elizabeth Ballas Daly RN, MSN, DNSc
*Coordinator, Division of Graduate
   Community Health*
Boston College, School of Nursing
Chestnut Hill, Massachusetts

Gretchen V. Dix RN, MS
*Director, Weston Manor Adult Day
   Health Center*
Weston, Massachusetts

*Former Director, East Village Nursing
   Home*
Lexington, Massachusetts

JoAnne Gerr MSW
Research Assistant
Harvard School of Public Health
Boston, Massachusetts

Vera Teyrovsky Goupille MSc
Senior Administrative Assistant
*Coordinated Care Sector Brent Health
   District*
London, England

Carl U. Granger MD
*Professor of Family Medicine and
   Community Health*
Brown University
Providence, Rhode Island

*Former Frederick Henry Prince Scholar
Distinguished Scholar in Physical
   Medicine and Rehabilitation*

John N. Morris PhD
Assistant Director
*Department of Social Gerontological
   Research*
Hebrew Rehabilitation Center for Aged
Boston, Massachusetts

*Recipient of Polaroid Teger Fellowship
   in Social Gerontology*

Carole Lium O'Brien RN, MS
Assistant Professor
Boston College School of Nursing
Chestnut Hill, Massachusetts

*Consultant: Women's Educational and
   Industrial Union*
*Weston Manor Adult Day Health
   Center and Nursing Home*

Sarah June Schiermeyer, RN
*Free Lance Writer and Editorial
   Consultant*
Weston, Massachusetts

Trudy B. White MS
*Director, Adult Day Health Center,
   Multipurpose Senior Center*
Fort Lauderdale, Florida

Contents

I The Conceptual Frame of Reference — 1

1 Introduction — 3
Carole Lium O'Brien, RN, MS

    Adult Day Care as Part of the Long-Term-Care Continuum, 3
    Hypotheses of Adult Day Care, 4
    Disability Impacts on the Elderly, 4
    Health-Care Expenditures and the Elderly, 5
    Population Shifts, 6
    Needs and Demands, 6
    Health-Insurance Reimbursement Policies and Long-Term Care, 13
    Residential Long-Term Care, 13
    Planning for Long-Term Care, 13
    Purpose of This Book, 14
    References, 14

2 General Systems Theory and Planning   16
Elizabeth Ballas Daly, RN, MSN, DNSc

    Introduction, 16
    Defining the System for Study, 17
    Characteristics of a System, 18
    Planning, 22
    Parts of the Long-Term-Care Planning System, 25
    Process, 26
    Summary, 34
    References, 35

3 Planning for Adult Day Care Within a Continuum of Long-Term-Care Services   36
Ann Clark, RN, MS

    Introduction, 36
    Model of Continuum of Community Services for the Elderly, 38
    Model Components, 40
    Outreach, 52
    Planning Organization, 54
    Model Coordination Projects, 61
    Summary, 67
    References, 67

4 Needs Assessment: Methods and Data Sources   69
Elizabeth Ballas Daly, RN, MSN, DNSc

    Introduction, 69
    Basic Concepts, 71
    Baseline-Data Guide, 73
    Data Sources, 76
    Data-Collection Methods and Techniques, 82
    Application of the Questioning Method, 90
    Application of Assessment Data, 99
    Summary, 101
    References, 102

5 Assessing and Meeting the Needs of the Long-Term-Care Person — 104
John N. Morris, PhD and *Carl U. Granger,* MD

    Population at Risk, 104
    Service Support Systems, 108
    Functional Assessment of Disability, 111
    Purposes and Analyses Served Through Functional Assessment, 112
    Methods of Functional Assessment, 113
    Spectrum of Long-Term-Care Services and the Need for Knowledge, 124
    Summary, 133
    References, 136

II The Adult Day-Care Experience — 143

6 The History of Adult Day-Care Programs — 145
Carole Lium O'Brien, RN, MS

    Introduction, 145
    Historical Review of the Psychiatric Day Hospital, 146
    Overview of the British Day-Hospital Movement, 146
    Day Hospitals in Israel, 148
    Canadian Adult Day Care, 148
    European Adult Day Health Programs, 150
    The Adult Day-Care Movement in the United States, 151
    Summary, 173
    References, 179

7 British Geriatric Day Hospitals: Implications for America — 181
Vera Teyrovsky Goupille, MSC

    Introduction, 181
    Background, 183

Service Characteristics, 184
Policies and Trends, 188
Method of Funding, 189
Within a System, 190
Summary, 192
References, 193

8 Community-Based Adult Day-Care Programs in Florida   195
Trudy B. White, MS

Introduction, 195
Funding/Administration, 196
Fees, 196
Licenses, 196
Models and Goals, 197
Participants, 197
Facilities, 198
Staffing, 198
Participant Assessment, 199
Indirect Services, 201
Summary, 201
References, 201

9 Funding   202
Carole Lium O'Brien, RN, MS and *Sarah J. Schiermeyer*, RN

Introduction, 202
Government Funding Sources, 206
Private Funding Sources, 224
Summary, 228
References, 228

III Setting Up a Day-Care Program   231

10 Program Development   233
Carole Lium O'Brien, RN, MS

Introduction, 233

Definition of Philosophy, 233
Relationship of Various Groups in Philosophy Development, 235
Program Definition Stems from the Scope of the Philosophy, 238
Four Models of Adult Day Care, 239
Psychiatric Day-Treatment Programs, 242
Consideration of Various Adult Day-Care Choices, 243
Program Objectives Stem from the Focus of the Philosophy, 244
Evaluation as an Integral Part of Objective Development, 246
Summary, 249
References, 249

11 Adult Day-Care Staffing 251
Carole Lium O'Brien, RN, MS

Introduction, 251
Major Staffing Categories, 252
Professional Staff Members, 256
Support Personnel, 263
Summary, 264
References, 265

12 Implementation 266
Gretchen Dix, RN, MS

Introduction, 266
Medical-Rehabilitative Model of Adult Day Care, 267
Budget, 268
Facility Requirements, 270
Staffing Patterns, 272
Volunteers, 273
Policies and Procedures, 277
Community Outreach, 282
Admission Process, 284
Transportation System, 288

Family Involvement, 295
Program Activities, 296
Role of the State Association, 302
Summary, 304

13 Records and the Problem-Oriented Record System 305
Carole Lium O'Brien, RN, MS

Functions of a Record System, 305
Criteria for a Record System, 307
The Computer, 307
The Annual Report, 307
Overview of the Problem-Oriented Record System, 308
The Problem-Oriented Record, 316
The Problem-Oriented Record Format, 318
Audit of the Record, 319
Composition of the Problem-Oriented Record, 322
Advantages of the Problem-Oriented Record System, 339
Summary, 341
References, 341

14 Evaluation 342
Carole Lium O'Brien, RN, MS and *Sarah J. Schiermeyer*, RN

Introduction, 342
Definition, 342
Relationship of Evaluation to Objectives and Assessment, 345
Uses of Evaluation, 348
Planning for Evaluation, 351
Evaluative Tools, 352
Evaluation Flow Sheet, 358
Choice of Method, 359
Methodology, 362
Current Evaluation Reports, 367

Implications for Research, 374
Summary, 376
References, 377

Readings 379
General, 379
Planning, 382
Implementation, 384
Records and the Problem-Oriented Record
  System, 384
Evaluation, 384

APPENDIX A   Medicaid Community Care Act (HR6194)   387

APPENDIX B   State Agencies Giving Population Estimates   391

APPENDIX C   Systematic Functional Assessment Tool   397

APPENDIX D   A Community Needs Survey for Adult Day Care   408

Index   419

I

The Conceptual Frame of Reference

1

Introduction

Carole Lium O'Brien, RN, MS

Adult Day Care as Part of the Long-Term-Care Continuum

Adult day care is a blend of psychosocial and health services that may exist in a variety of balances. What is essential is that the two services exist together, for the two needs cannot be separated.

The National Conference on Aging in April 1980 chose adult day care as the preferred title for these services, which may also be called *day hospital,* as in England, or *adult day health care,* as in Massachusetts and California. The latter title carries the connotation of a medical model, but the author believes that, if the term *health* is used in its broadest sense, *adult day health care* provides a better description of the services. The author also feels that the connotation of childhood in the words *day care* should be further examined and remedied.

The services provided in adult day care are part of a continuum of long-term-care services, an idea that was part of our society before hospitals became commonplace. We are just now returning to this concept, and the development of a long-term-care model (which is traced in Chapter 3) has been slow and unmethodical. The need for long-term-care planning, with adult day care as part of it, is substantial. Each planner must first conceive of adult day care as part of a system with interacting parts and then deliberately and methodically plan the adult daycare center as part of the total system. Without this concept, the adult day care center may contain features that are uncoordinated, duplicative, and ineffective.

Adult day care as part of a community network of long-term-care services can serve people with limited capacity to function, provide health supervision and essential support in activities of daily living, and enable disadvantaged and disabled older adults to move freely in and out of various community-service settings. Within this context, adult day care is part of the long-term-care system; it is not conceived of as an alternative to institutionalization.

Hypotheses of Adult Day Care

Most adult day-care programs have in common the following hypotheses:

1. Psychosocial functioning is maintained at a healthy level when individuals remain in the community and are not isolated from it.
2. Physical health benefits from psychosocial health.
3. Many needs, even those requiring sophisticated therapy, can be adequately met without 24-hour care.
4. Given a choice, older people prefer to remain in their communities.
5. Given a choice, older people would prefer adult day care to institutionalization.
6. Adult day care can be cheaper than institutionalization.
7. Adult day care meets needs not provided for in other long-term-care options.

The above statements represent a belief in the positive outcomes of adult day care. However, coordinated data collection and evaluation are needed to give the program direction. For adult day care to be adequately funded and to become an accepted mode of long-term care, these hypotheses must be documented. It is the belief of the author that these hypotheses will be supported by research and that the elderly, who comprise most of the population receiving adult day care, will be the most notable beneficiaries.

Disability Impacts on the Elderly

Disability and chronic disease in any age group present problems for both the affected individuals and those involved in their welfare. During 1972, an estimated 12.7% of the noninstitutionalized civilian population were reported to be limited to some extent in their activity due to chronic disease or physical impairment; an additional 6.6% were limited in their ability to carry out major activities because of health-related disabilities.[1] (p6) Of these, more than 4 million were over age 65 and limited in the amount or kind of major activity they were able to carry out;

an additional 3 million over age 65 were unable to carry out their major activity, such as working and keeping house.[1(p7)]

Disability is more common among people above age 65. Hospital and nursing-home stays lengthen as the person ages and are predictably longest for the frail elderly—those age 85 and over.[1(p9)] One out of five people over the age 65 is institutionalized, and their average yearly nursing-home stay (1976) is 86.4 days.[1(p9)] For lack of a social life, these elderly frequently lose social skills and resultant social support; for lack of a community support system, they are sometimes prematurely institutionalized; for lack of consistent health intervention, they frequently develop greater disability and deteriorate faster than they would have had they had the necessary health care. To be disabled is painful, but to be deprived of what independence one retains because of the lack of a comprehensive network of services allowing one to remain in the community is itself disabling.

Health-Care Expenditures and the Elderly

The elderly represent 11% of the population but account for 29% of all personal health-care expenditures.[1(p7)] Two-thirds of these expenses are paid for by public programs.[1(p7)]

In 1977, the average health-care costs of an individual aged 65 or over was $1,745,[1(p7)] three times the amount spent by a younger person. Hospital care accounted for 44% of these costs; nursing-home care, 26%; physicians, 17%; drugs, 7%; dentists, 3%; and all other items 3%.[1(p7)] Adult day care was not mentioned. Medicare paid 44.3% of these costs; Medicaid, 16.4%; and smaller public programs, 6%.[1(p7)] Few older persons are covered by private insurance, as was reflected in private insurances' 5.8% share of the costs.[1(p8)] Out-of-pocket payment for the elderly averaged $462.[1(p8)]

Income Changes

1978 data show that the income of the elderly was only half that of people under 65.[1(p2)] Incomes of $195 per week were reported for families with over-65 heads of household.[1(p3)] For the elderly living alone or with unrelated people, the average income was $83 per week.[1(p3)] 1979 data indicate a sex element in this discrepancy: older women were three times as likely as older men to live alone or with unrelated people.[1(p15)] This statistic is due, in part, to the better work and economic status of men. Older men also remarry eight times as often as older women.[1(p15)] In addition, women have a longer life expectancy than men (see Table 1-1), resulting in a ratio of 130 women to 100 men between ages 65 and 74, 178 women to 100 men between ages 75 and 84, and 224 women to 100 men after age 85.[1(p15)]

Fourteen percent (3.2 million) of the aged had incomes below the poverty line.[1(p3)] Raising the poverty line by 25% increases the number of aged poor to 5.4 million (23.4%).[1(p4)]

Table 1-1
Life expectancy based on death rates in 1977, by sex and color (United States)

	Both Sexes *Years*	Male *Years*	Female *Years*
At birth:			
Total	73.2	69.3	77.1
White	73.8	70.0	77.7
All other	68.8	64.6	73.1
At age 65:			
Total	16.3	13.9	18.3
White	16.3	13.9	18.4
All other	16.0	14.0	17.8

From *Every Ninth American*, by H. B. Brotman. Washington, D.C.: U.S. Government Printing Office, 1980.

The correlation between poverty and disability is significant. The implications for adult day care are that a majority of participants will be moderately to severely impoverished and that a majority of these will be women. Adult day-care advocates and funding planners for adult day care need to anticipate these facts as part of long-term-care planning.

Population Shifts

Long-term care is being affected by the growth of the aged population. As the baby-boom population shown in Figure 1-1 moves toward retirement, work practices, taxation levels, health-care-consumption patterns, leisure-time activities, federal interventions and expenditures, business marketing practices, personal-income profiles, and even the Gross National Product are bound to experience tremendous upheavals and change. Each of these will in turn affect long-term-care needs and the adult day-care movement in the United States.

Needs and Demands

Due in part to the rapid increase in both actual numbers of elderly and in their proportion of the total population, the needs and demands for long-term care for the elderly have become a major concern. This concern has been reflected in public and political response, but it has not always been understood that needs and demands are separate issues and require differing satisfactions.

Needs are perceived discrepancies, deficiencies, or conditions limiting individuals, families, groups, or communities in meeting their full potential. A need is a gap between what is and what is desired or desirable. People with elevated blood pressure, for example, have a definable need, even though the condition may at

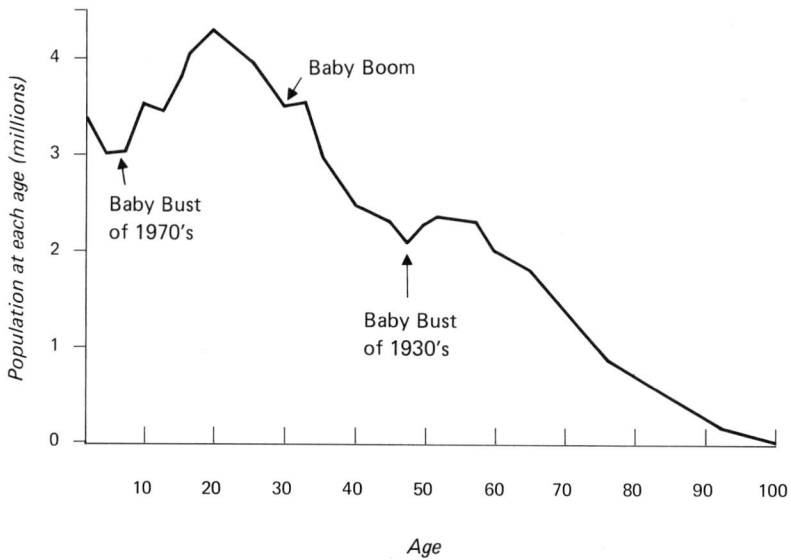

Figure 1-1. Age Distribution of U.S. Population, 1980 (From *The Proposed Fiscal 1981 Budget: What It Means for Older Americans*. Special Committee on Aging, United States Senate, February, 1980.)

a particular point in time be asymptomatic and nondebilitating. What constitutes a need is often strongly affected by the values of the perceiver.

A demand, on the other hand, is that which a population desires. When a need becomes severe enough that a person seeks long-term-care services and professional help, the need becomes a demand. The person who reduces his weight or uses home remedies to treat an illness does not translate a need into a demand. Similarly, the need for health-care and human services frequently is greater than the effective demand being made upon the long-term-care system and its services. The capacity to purchase or obtain health-care and human services is also an important factor influencing the effective demand. Factors such as continuity of care, accessibility, cost of care, and availability and acceptability of services also determine the degree to which needs may be translated into demands. As a result, many more elderly people need health-care and human services than actually receive them.

Long-Term-Care Needs of an Aging Population

A perusal of demographic trends may help clarify the magnitude of the present and potential long-term-care needs of the elderly. From a historical perspective, trends indicate that not only is the total population increasing, but the elderly portion will continue to increase. Advancing life expectancy, primarily due to reduced infant-mortality rates, has swollen the over-65 age segment of the population. Between 1900 and 1970, the total population tripled, but the older segment grew sevenfold.[1(p2)] Between 1960 and 1970, the older segment increased by 21%, while the rest of the population grew by only 13%.[1(p2)] The difference in the last decade is the most dramatic. A birthrate below that needed for zero population growth has resulted in a 23.5% increase in the number of elderly and only a 6.3% increase in the rest of the population.[1(p2)] Figure 1-2 and Table 1-2 show the results of this trend projected to the year 2050.

State variations. The percentage of the elderly population over 65 varies considerably from state to state, as is shown in Table 1-3. As a result,

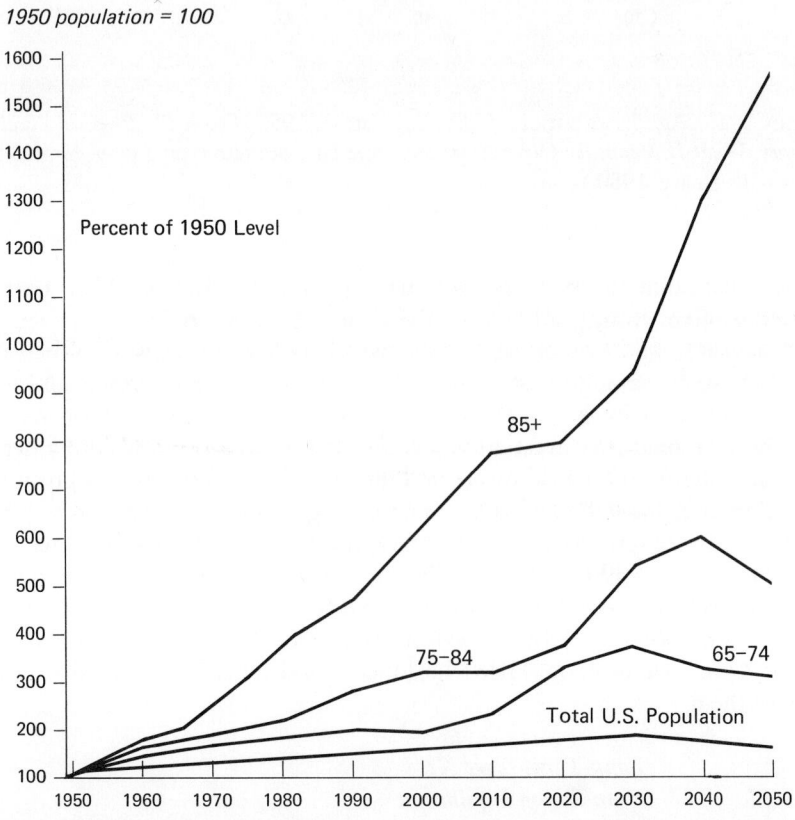

Figure 1-2. Growth of U.S. Population Age Groups, 1950–2050 (From *The Proposed Fiscal 1981 Budget: What It Means for Older Americans.* Special Committee on Aging, United States Senate, February, 1980.)

Table 1-2
United States population projections (series II), total and aged 65-plus, 1980–2050 (numbers in thousands)

Year	All ages Number	65-plus Both Sexes Number	65-plus Both Sexes *Percent of All Ages*	65-plus Male Number	65-plus Female Number	65-plus Female *Per 100 Men*
1980	222,159	24,927	11.2	10.108	14,819	147
1985	232,880	27,305	11.7	11,012	16,293	148
1990	243,513	29,824	12.3	11,999	17,824	149
1995	252,750	31,401	12.4	12,602	18,799	149
2000	260,378	31,822	12.2	12,717	19,105	150
2005	267,603	32,436	12.1	12,924	19,512	151
2010	275,335	34,837	12.7	13,978	20,858	149
2015	283,164	39,519	14.0	16,063	23,456	146
2020	290,115	45,102	15.6	18,468	26,634	144
2025	295,742	50,920	17.2	20,861	30,059	144
2030	300,349	55,024	18.3	22,399	32,624	146
2035	304,486	55,805	18.3	22,434	33,371	149
2040	308,400	54,925	17.8	21,816	33,108	152
2045	312,054	54,009	17.3	21,335	32,674	153
2050	315,622	55,494	17.6	22,055	33,439	152

From *Every Ninth American*, by H. B. Brotman. Washington, D.C.: U.S. Government Printing Office, 1980.

the size and the nature of the needs of the elderly and their demands for long-term care can differ markedly from one area to another. In 1979, 15 states had an unusually high percentage of the elderly—12% or more—in their total populations: Florida (18.1%); Arkansas (13.7%); Rhode Island (13.2%); Iowa (13.1%); South Dakota (13.1%); Missouri and Nebraska (13.0%); Kansas (12.7%); Pennsylvania (12.7%); Oklahoma (12.5%); Massachusetts and Maine (12.3%); North Dakota (12.1%); and West Virginia and New York (12.0%). In 1974, only 8 states had this high a percentage. While variations occur from state to state and from one part of the country to another, variations in the elderly population can also occur from town to town in greater proportions than in either the state or parts of the country, thus placing an even greater burden on local communities concerned with the welfare and quality of life of the elderly.

*Demands of the Elderly
on the Long-Term-Care System*

Changes in the demographic composition of the population and the trends towards an older population are not only pointing in the direction of changes in the needs of the elderly, but are affecting the demand for long-term care in a number of ways.

Table 1-3
Resident population aged 65-plus, by state, 1970 and 1979*

State	Number (in Thousands) 1970[1]	Number (in Thousands) 1979	Percent Increase 1960–70	Percent Increase 1970–79	Percent of All Ages 1970	Percent of All Ages 1979	State Rank[2] Number 1970	State Rank[2] Number 1979	State Rank[2] Percent Increase 1960–70	State Rank[2] Percent Increase 1970–79	State Rank[2] Percent of All Ages 1970	State Rank[2] Percent of All Ages 1979
Total, 51 States	19,972	24,658	21.1	23.5	9.8	11.2	[3]	[3]	[3]	[3]	[3]	[3]
Alabama	324	421	24.7	29.7	9.4	11.2	21	19	16	16	30	25
Alaska	7	10	27.9	54.2	2.3	2.6	51	51	11	6	51	51
Arizona	161	289	79.0	79.5	9.1	11.8	35	30	1	2	34	16
Arkansas	237	300	22.0	26.6	12.3	13.7	28	28	21	22	3	2
California	1,792	2,316	30.9	29.3	9.0	10.2	2	1	9	18	36	34
Colorado	187	239	18.8	27.8	8.5	8.6	33	33	24	20	38	47
Connecticut	288	356	19.1	24.0	9.5	11.4	26	26	23	26	27	21
Delaware	44	57	22.6	30.0	8.0	9.7	48	48	20	15	42	37
District of Columbia	70	73	2.4	3.2	9.3	11.1	41	45	51	51	32	28
Florida	985	1,603	78.2	62.7	14.5	18.1	7	3	2	3	1	1
Georgia	365	488	26.4	33.6	8.0	9.5	17	16	15	11	42	40
Hawaii	44	70	51.3	59.9	5.7	7.7	47	46	4	4	50	50
Idaho	67	91	16.3	34.4	9.5	10.0	44	41	29	10	27	36
Illinois	1,089	1,220	12.2	12.0	9.8	10.9	4	6	40	47	24	29
Indiana	492	570	10.8	16.0	9.5	10.6	12	13	45	40	27	32
Iowa	349	381	6.9	9.2	12.4	13.1	19	22	49	49	2	4
Kansas	265	301	10.8	13.6	11.8	12.7	27	27	45	44	7	8
Kentucky	336	393	15.1	17.1	10.4	11.2	20	21	35	38	21	26
Louisiana	305	379	27.0	24.1	8.4	9.4	23	24	12	25	39	41
Maine	114	135	7.6	18.6	11.5	12.3	36	36	48	32	9	11
Maryland	298	380	32.3	27.3	7.6	9.2	25	23	8	21	45	44
Massachusetts	633	711	11.3	12.3	11.1	12.3	10	10	43	46	10	12
Michigan	749	887	18.0	18.4	8.4	9.6	8	8	25	34	39	39
Minnesota	407	470	15.4	15.4	10.7	11.6	15	18	33	41	14	19

10

Mississippi	221	276	17.0	24.8	10.0	11.4	30	31	27	24	22	22
Missouri	558	635	11.4	13.7	11.9	13.0	11	11	42	43	6	6
Montana	68	83	5.1	21.1	9.9	10.6	43	43	50	29	23	33
Nebraska	183	204	11.8	11.6	12.3	13.0	34	35	41	48	3	7
Nevada	31	61	70.4	96.6	6.3	8.6	49	47	3	1	49	46
New Hampshire	78	98	15.8	25.9	10.6	11.1	39	40	31	23	19	27
New Jersey	694	843	24.4	21.6	9.7	11.5	9	9	17	27	25	20
New Mexico	70	109	37.7	54.8	6.9	8.8	42	38	5	5	48	45
New York	1,951	2,115	15.8	8.4	10.7	12.0	1	2	31	50	14	15
North Carolina	412	571	32.7	38.6	8.1	10.2	14	12	7	8	41	35
North Dakota	66	80	13.3	20.5	10.7	12.1	45	44	36	31	14	13
Ohio	993	1,142	11.2	15.0	9.3	10.6	5	7	44	42	32	30
Oklahoma	299	363	20.1	21.5	11.7	12.5	24	25	22	28	8	10
Oregon	226	294	23.5	30.3	10.8	11.6	29	29	19	14	13	18
Pennsylvania	1,267	1,491	12.7	17.7	10.7	12.7	3	4	37	37	14	9
Rhode Island	104	123	16.1	18.6	10.9	13.2	37	37	30	33	12	3
South Carolina	190	269	26.8	41.6	7.3	9.2	32	32	13	7	46	43
South Dakota	80	90	12.5	12.4	12.1	13.1	38	42	38	45	5	5
Tennessee	382	492	24.0	28.8	9.7	11.2	15	15	18	19	25	24
Texas	988	1,302	32.9	31.9	8.8	9.7	6	5	6	13	37	38
Utah	77	106	29.4	37.3	7.3	7.7	40	39	10	9	46	49
Vermont	47	56	8.6	17.9	10.6	11.3	46	49	47	36	19	23
Virginia	364	483	26.6	32.7	7.8	9.3	18	17	14	12	44	42
Washington	320	415	15.4	29.5	9.4	10.6	22	20	33	17	30	31
West Virginia	194	226	12.5	16.6	11.1	12.0	31	34	38	39	10	14
Wisconsin	471	556	17.4	18.1	10.7	11.8	13	14	26	35	14	17
Wyoming	30	36	16.6	20.6	9.1	8.1	50	50	28	30	34	48

[1]Corrected for errors in number of centenarians.
[2]States ranked in decreasing order; State with largest quantity is ranked 1.
[3]Not applicable.
*From *Every Ninth American*, by H. B. Brotman. Washington, D.C.: U.S. Government Printing Office, 1980.

Medical attention. Older persons on a per capita basis suffer more from health deficiencies than do younger people. As a result, older people require more medical attention at all levels of care. The prevalence of chronic conditions, such as ischemic heart disease, arthritis, respiratory disease, and various orthopedic, visual, and hearing impairments, sharply increases with age. Limitations of the ability to carry out activities of daily living and self-care can and do frequently occur.

Physician visits. Physician visits per person per year increase considerably with age. Persons age 75 and over visit physicians on the average of 7.4 times a year compared with younger people, ages 17–24, who on the average visit a physician fewer than 5 times a year.[2(p26)]

Hospital admission rates. Hospital admission rates are greater for older people as a result of the greater prevalence of health deficiencies and limitations. During 1972, nearly 17% of the population over 65 was hospitalized in short-stay hospitals at least once during the year, compared with less than 12% of the population in the 17–24-year-old category.[2(p21)] According to a study done by Anderson in 1973, age represented the third most influential factor in the use of short-term hospitals and was surpassed in importance only by economic factors, such as hospital- and health-insurance coverage and family income, and demographic factors of sex and marital status.[3] Karafiath claimed in a study done in 1976 that 20%–30% of inpatient admissions were due to social rather than medical reasons, leading to an improper utilization of high-cost facilities and escalation of costs of health care.[4] With increasing absolute numbers of an aging population, needless institutionalization of many older adults, and a projected greater prevalence of health deficiencies due to more elderly, the trend could conceivably be toward a greater demand for health-care and human services in the future.

Hospital stays. The length of stay of older adults in hospitals is a serious factor affecting the demand for health services. Older people, when hospitalized, tend to require a longer hospital stay than those who are younger with the same illness, thus placing a great demand on hospital beds. Elderly people hospitalized for fractures, for example, stay an average of 27.5 days, compared with 5.4 days for people age 17 and under.[5] For all conditions requiring hospitalization, older adults stay in the hospital more than twice as long as those between ages 15 and 44.[6] If the demographic trends and disease, illness, and disability patterns continue into the future, probably even more older adults will be hospitalized, for longer periods, and utilizing a greater percentage of hospital resources than at present.

Rehabilitation. Older adults are more likely to require longer time periods for rehabilitation and more medical and health-care supervision than younger people, especially following hospital episodes.

Health-Insurance Reimbursement Policies and Long-Term Care

If the current mode of hospital and health-insurance reimbursement policies continues into the future, the traditional models of care used for rehabilitation, health-care promotion, maintenance, and supervision, such as nursing homes and hospital care, will also continue into the future, and the demand for their services will probably increase. Adult day-care services under present reimbursement policies could very well be retarded in growth.

Medicare and Medicaid have long favored payment only for institutional care, and Medicaid has become the principal public mechanism for funding nursing-home care. National Health Insurance offers poor prospects for remedying the situation. Catastrophic health insurance is still measured in terms of major episodes, with little regard for long-term care for the elderly. When economic and social pressures and the needs of other family members become critical, the residential institution is frequently seen as the only alternative option.

Residential Long-Term Care

Many older adults, following hospitalization or an illness, are unable to care for themselves and carry out activities of daily living. Their capacity to function is limited. In addition, many older people live alone, either by choice, or because their spouse has died, or because they are unable to live with younger relatives. Therefore, when they become seriously ill and disabled, they do not have someone living with them who can care for them. Because they need long-term-care services, of necessity they become residents of nursing homes.

In 1960, 3.4% of the elderly resided in nursing homes; by 1970, the number had increased to 5%.[7] At the end of 1973, most of the elderly residing in institutions were in nursing homes—according to Kovar, about 962,000 people.[7] Future projections indicate that these trends are very likely to continue to increase unless new and different organizational structures and processes for the care of the elderly are developed. Although many residents of nursing homes suffer from multiple chronic conditions requiring 24-hour care, many who could live outside such an institution could remain at home if care were available on a regular basis. The lives of those living with and caring for elderly individuals could be eased considerably if such services as adult day care were readily available as an option.

Planning for Long-Term Care

Planning for the long-term care of a large population of elderly people is of major importance and a need that will remain with us in the foreseeable future. Using fragmented and isolated approaches, muddling through, or not planning at all could easily result in a loss to the elderly of their dignity and opportunity to function as independently as possible. Only when the needs of the elderly are clearly identified, options creatively generated and analyzed, decisions systematically made, and programs implemented and evaluated can we hope to humanize the existence of older adults who are limited in their capacity for self-care, disabled, disadvantaged, ignored, or treated as outcasts. All people are interdependent and have a right to achieve maximum self-fulfillment and biopsychosocial functioning. A system of services to meet their needs is a sine qua non to dignity.

The philosophical basis of long-term-care planning is the belief that objectives can best be attained by a systematic approach and that long-term-care planners, practitioners, and various health-related organizations can influence the future by such an approach.

Purpose of This Book

Adult day care is a desirable option for the elderly population that long-term-care professionals have long been seeking. This book introduces an approach to adult day-care planning that is designed to help achieve the human dignity and optimal well-being of this population group when it does not exist and to increase it when it only partially exists. This approach places the elderly in the center of a dynamic system composed of many surrounding interacting systems and assures that the uniqueness of the elderly population is brought to the forefront as the basic referent for long-term-care planning and achievement.

The organizing framework of this book is systems and planning theory. After a discussion of this theory in Chapter 2 and a presentation of a model for adult day-care services in Chapter 3, the chapters follow in the order of the planning process: assessment, planning, implementation, and evaluation.

The systems framework is presented early in the book so that the reader will have the systems approach firmly understood before reading on in the text. Without the systems framework, bits and pieces of this book can be used in just as uncoordinated a manner as any information. The book is designed to be comprehensive, with systems and planning theory as its basic referents, because the author firmly believes that adult day care can be approached as a logical process within this framework. Finally, the author's intent is to give the reader not simply a compendium of information, but rather a working tool.

References

1. Brotman HB: *Every Ninth American*. Prepared for the Special Committee on Aging, United States Senate, 1980.

2. U.S. Department of Health, Education and Welfare, National Center for Health Statistics: *Current Estimates from the Health Interview Survey, U.S., 1972*, publication (HRA) 74-1512. Rockland, Md, U.S. Dept of Health, Education and Welfare, September 1973.

3. Anderson J: Demographic factors affecting health service utilization: A causal model. *Medical Care* **42:** 107, 1973.

4. Karafiath D: Home care makes sense today. *J Nursing Admin* **25:** 32–38, 1976.

5. U.S. Dept of Health, Education and Welfare, National Center for Health Statistics: *Age Patterns in Medical Care, Illness and Disability, United States, 1968–1969,* publication (HSM) 72-1026. U.S. Dept of Health, Education and Welfare, April 1972, p 29.

6. U.S. Dept of Health, Education and Welfare, National Center for Health Statistics: *Utilization of Short Stay Hospitalization: Summary of Non-Medical Statistics, United States, 1972,* publication (HRA) 75-1768. U.S. Dept of Health, Education and Welfare, August 1974, p 27.

7. Kovar, MG: Health of the elderly and use of health services. *Public Health Reports* **92(1):** 18.

2

General Systems Theory and Planning

Elizabeth Ballas Daly, RN, MS, DNSc

Introduction

General systems theory contends that nothing can be studied as a lone entity and that general concepts can describe systems and the reaction between systems irrespective of the nature of the systems and their components.[1] The term *system* covers a broad spectrum of our physical, biological, and social world. Although it is not easy to make a neat division of the components of a system, varying degrees of systems do exist. The system model provides a useful overall conceptual framework within which otherwise-unconnected parts may be integrated. It enables a planner to take a holistic view of the interactions of adult day-care participants with their environments and is a valuable method for considering outcomes and effectiveness in meeting community needs.

Many systems theorists do not consider any entity a system unless perceived elements of parts of the system are found to interact with other elements. Von-Bertalanffy refers to a system as a complex of elements in interaction.[1] Elements are parts specific to a system. Hall and Fagan conceive of a system as a set of parts or components together with relationships between the parts and between properties of the parts.[2] Thus, a system becomes a group of related structures, processes, or substances that together perform certain functions designed to achieve particular goals. Concepts and principles of systems theory are not limited to biological systems but can be applied to any "whole" consisting of interacting or interrelated "elements."

Long-Term-Care Planning

Long-term-care planning can also be considered a system because it is composed of a number of related processes and methods that together perform certain functions designed to achieve various goals. The long-term-care planning system consists of four subsystems: assessment, planning, implementation, and evaluation. Each subsystem is constrained by, conditioned by, or dependent on the state of the other subsystems. Charges leveled against the long-term-care system have included lack of coordination and fragmentation of health-care and human services. To the extent that health-care and human services are not interacting with each other or with individuals, they constitute an array of services, not an integrated system. General systems theory can serve to organize diverse elements of the long-term-care system and can be helpful in understanding and identifying desirable relationships and outcomes.

The purpose of this chapter is to discuss systems theory as a basis for developing adult day-care programs within a planning framework. One advantage of systems theory when applied to long-term-care planning for the elderly population is that the focus is on the whole rather than on the individual parts of the long-term-care system. Systems theory is particularly valuable in developing new adult day-care programs because it is only through such an organized approach that the successful growth pattern of these programs within the United States will continue.

Defining the System for Study

Several factors must be considered in defining a system. First, planners must identify *what* they wish to deal with. This information enables them to limit the scope of the system to be studied, since there are many sizes of systems from which to choose. Some long-term-care planners may wish to study a target population residing in one community; others may be more interested in a target population within several communities.

Second, the reasons *why* the planner wants to study a particular system must be identified. The reasons for studying an elderly population group located in a specific local community might be requests for increased services or some perception of need for alternative models of long-term-care. *Why* the planner wants to study the system indicates the planner's value-based goals. These goals can then be communicated to other professionals and community people currently involved with the system or who could become so at some future time.

Characteristics of a System

Certain characteristics are common to all systems. A given entity is not regarded as a system unless the following characteristics are present.

Parts

The parts of a system, or its elements, are interdependent and interacting units. A change in one part of the system affects not only the other parts or its elements, but the entire system and its relationship to other systems. A family as a whole system, for example, is made up of individuals with physical, emotional, mental, spiritual, and social aspects. A change in the state of one part of a family, such as the biological dysfunctioning of one of its members, induces changes, minor or major, in the states of its other members.

Environment

Every system works in an environment that affects it. The environment is defined as factors that surround or affect the elements or parts of a system.

In defining a system for study, one must include identification of all the possible environmental factors that are related to the system or that have an impact on the system. Because the planner is mainly concerned with the health and social aspects of elderly human systems, factors related to elderly systems need to be identified. Various environmental factors impacting on an elderly target population group might include: the delays for nursing-home beds; local health-care agencies' referral policies; the amount of travel time to nearest health-care agencies; the availability and accessibility of human services; and the income levels required for eligibility for these services.

Boundary

A demarcation line, parameter, or barrier that isolates the system or its elements from its environment and within which information is exchanged is conceived of as a boundary. Boundaries also define degrees of openness for admission of members into the system and for other inputs into the system. An open system is one whose boundaries are partially permeable and permit sizable magnitudes of certain sorts of matter/energy or information transmissions to cross them, allowing for the building up and breaking down of the system's material and informational components. In open systems, boundary transactions must occur in order for the system to survive. Not only do open systems depend on the environment for inputs, they also frequently exist to produce outputs for consumers or target populations in the environment. Thus, system-environmental interaction can occur on both the input and the output sides of a system.

Information/Communication

Information is the sending and receiving of data concerning behaviors, activities, and decisions and varies with the system and its elements. Not only must living systems have specific forms of matter/energy, but they must also have specific patterns of information. Some systems do not develop normally unless they have appropriate information during infancy. Information in the form of *feedback* is also an essential ingredient for correcting, improving, or supplementing future decisions, behaviors, or activities.

An information/communication control system is applicable to long-term-care planning because it provides both direction and guidance to the planner in following a systematic course. Such a system should be an integral part of each of the four planning subsystems (assessment, planning, implementation, and evaluation) of the total long-term-care planning-system model described later in this chapter.

An information/communication control system not only has a feedback mechanism, but also includes *inputs, throughputs,* and *outputs.* Figure 2-1 illustrates schematically how these components are related to each other.

Inputs. Inputs are defined as those elements that are transformed by the system into outputs. Informational inputs in a long-term-care planning system may include the following data: departures from optimal health functioning, numbers of elderly and their characteristics, available long-term-care

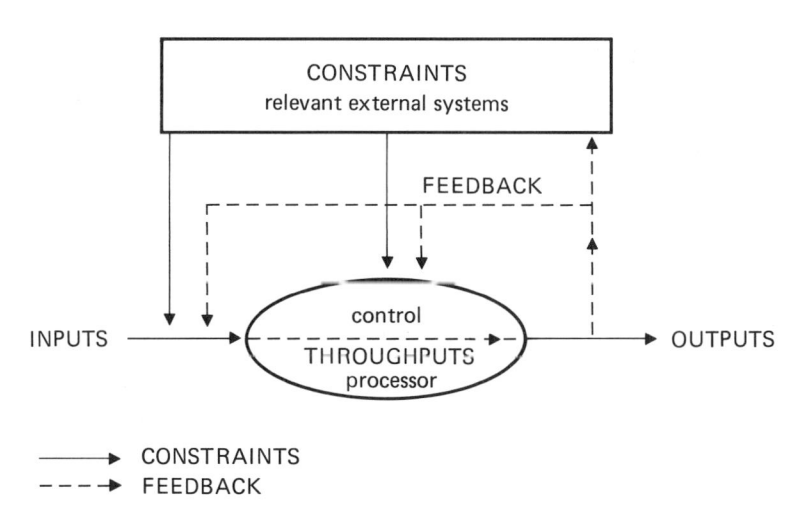

Figure 2-1. Components of an Information/Communication System in Health-Care Planning

resources, utilization of health and social services by the elderly, unmet needs and demands, publicly voiced apprehensions related to the well-being of an elderly population in a community, and anticipated long-term-care problems.

Throughputs. Throughputs are the mechanisms and processes of activities within a planning phase that act upon or transform inputs in some way into outputs. Transformations can be induced in persons, materials, and information. In planning, the mechanism commonly transforming inputs into outputs is the processor—the planner or practitioner.

Outputs. Outputs are the products, results, outcomes, or effects of the process of activities occurring in each system of planning. Outputs frequently encompass the purposes and goals for which the particular long-term-care system functions. The outputs from the assessment system should become inputs for the planning system. For example, problem identification as an output of the assessment system becomes input for the planning system.

Feedback. In any planning system that is concerned with information, communication, and outcomes, feedback is of vital importance. Feedback is information about the consequences of action taken and decisions made and is necessary in order to correct, improve, or supplement future decisions, behaviors, and activities. In riding a bicycle, for example, individuals receive feedback in regard to direction and balance that causes them to take corrective action. In planning, feedback has a control function because it is received by planners and practitioners, who process it and decide on corrective actions or appropriate behaviors. Many types of feedback systems can be designed to facilitate control. (*Control* is used here in terms of cybernetics and is not meant to imply coercive control.)

Constraints

Constraints refer to conditions, forces, or expectations that impact on a system. Conditions or forces can be determinants of health, both physical and social, that arise within the system itself or can be of an external nature arising from the environment. Illness—chronic or acute—is a condition arising within a system and can affect or limit the functioning of biological systems. External forces that can affect individual systems include various political, environmental, socioeconomic and long-term-care delivery conditions and trends. These same external forces can also affect, either individually or together, the long-term-care planning system and its various subsystems.

As shown in Figure 2-1, inputs flow through the processor—the long-term-care planner or practitioner—to become outputs. As the model indicates, control is a function of the processor. External constraints are important because, as the model indicates, they have a direct relationship to the general components of the system—mainly to the inputs and the processor.

External constraints are emphasized because they are those conditions, forces, or expectations that can have an impact on the input of various phases of planning as well as on the control function of the processor. External forces having an impact on the planning inputs may include the type of data available, funding, and eligibility requirements for participants in adult day-care programs. External forces having an impact on the processor may include state and local mandates, policies, technology, and requirements for special workers to carry out specific program activities.

Constraints can also be of an internal nature and arise within the planning process itself. Internal constraints may include such forces as the ability of a processor, long-term-care planner, practitioner, or others to collect, process, and analyze data; implement a plan of action; operationalize policies; perform budgeting activities; or establish criteria for the measurement of behavior and health outcomes.

Constraints of an external or internal nature should not be given positive or negative values. Rather they should be looked upon as forces to be identified "whose significance is to be measured in terms of how they condition the system and set its parameters . . ."[3(p43)] Once constraints are recognized, some may need to be accepted, whereas others may be modified over time, if not immediately. Some constraints may even change in character over time because of changing environments, changing beliefs and values, and increasing knowledge and skills of long-term-care planners and practitioners.

Organization

The organization of a system is the formal or informal arrangement of its parts, elements subsystems, components, or activities at a given moment of time. The particular arrangement has a working order that results in the attainment of desirable goals, established customs, strategies, guidance, or rules. Long-term-care planning may be organized into assessment, planning, implementation, and evaluation as a way of differentiating activities. The organization of a system can change over time, from moment to moment, or it may remain relatively stable for long periods of time, depending upon the state of the environment and processes occurring within and between its parts.

In the open-system approach, consideration must be given to each target-population system as if it were a separate entity. This approach is based on the assumption that each system is unique and can differ from other similar systems in that some of the elements characterizing it can differ. Each locality, for example, finds a group of elderly living in an environment with different external constraints and having different environmental relationships. Therefore, the long-term-care needs of each elderly population group are highly individual. These needs and constraints are important and relevant environmental elements. Clearly, problem identification and definition and strategies for intervention must all be considered and addressed anew for each group in a community, as they would be for each individual in a family.

Planning

No apparent agreement exists on how planning should be defined,[4] largely because of the lack of planning theory in general. Whether planning should be identified as a conceptual process or as an activity is uncertain. Consequently, planners tend to be content with a pragmatic approach emphasizing techniques and procedures. The lack of planning theory, however, does allow each planner to conceive a personal definition that best expresses the planner's idea of what is done and how it is done. Thus, planning can have quite different meanings, each correct in terms of what it attempts to describe.

Planning Defined

Planning is a thinking ahead, determining what shall be done. Broadly viewed, planning is a process through which a planner strives to move a system from one state of affairs to another; it generally involves a number of steps or related parts. Long-term-care planning as a process with related and interdependent parts is also a system having *subsystems*. These subsystems are influenced by all other subsystems within the planning system.

It is through planning that long-term-care planners determine the *what, when, who,* and *where* of possible courses of action to cope with the present and desirable future states of systems and their environment. Long-term-care planning is devoted to directing and attaining deliberate and desirable change and involves people in activities that bring about change in desired ways. All members involved in planning adult day-care services therefore require a clear understanding of the planning function, requirements, techniques, and skills.

Planning Characteristics, Techniques, and Skills

A number of factors are characteristic of the planning function. These basic characteristics, which are frequently thought of as requirements, are inherent in long-term-care planning, whether described as a two- or ten-step process. Long-term-care planning is characterized as being goal directed, future oriented, and purposive. These requirements frequently characterize each phase of planning and reflect the nature of long-term-care planning functions and activities.

Goals. Goals are descriptions of aspirations that represent desirable ends or outcomes that may be the change or maintenance of a given situation or condition. Goals may be unattainable, as well as practical and attainable. Systems may have external goals, such as developing relationships with other systems in the environment. Some systems may have several goals operating simultaneously. A system's external goals may change over time while its internal purpose remains the same. Because goals are generally broadly stated, they must be further broken down into more tangible and specific objectives if they are to be measured and evaluated (see Chapter 10).

Long-term-care planning begins with overall goals. Overall goals, sometimes referred to as precursor goals, are those goals or values that exert influence on all of our activities and channel and define our desires. Precursor goals are descriptions of aspirations representing the fruition of ideals established by values.[5(p24)] Values originate from some idea, belief, or aspiration about how things or conditions should or could be and are frequently used as criteria or preference items for goals, as well as being the origin of goals.[6]

Goals originating out of values, however, can give rise to very different priorities, from which flow very different planning emphases, objectives, and evaluation criteria. For example, values such as "promoting the optimal level of functioning, potential, and ability of disabled elderly via comprehensive systems of health and human services" and "all people have a right to health care" are based on different beliefs and value systems than are values such as "long-term care for the elderly requires institutionalization" and "long-term care is a privilege for the wealthy." We need to understand our own value systems and those of others concerned with the welfare of the elderly because they influence the way we perceive things.

Different value systems may be encountered at the community level. This diversity can have great utility for guidance when the greatest numbers of people and viewpoints are involved, for it helps ensure that deleterious options do not go uninvestigated. Disagreements are bound to occur, and some negotiating is necessary if the needs of the elderly are to be met and desirable goals attained.

Some value problems that arise for long-term-care planners and practitioners may in fact be solved by decisions beyond their control. Planning goals can be set by public demands, legal constraints, official guidelines, regulatory bodies, and various agencies. Some communities may demand that certain health-care and human services be provided for their elderly. Others may value the health and well-being of other population groups over the elderly. When value systems conflict, creating internal tension, some means of resolution must be found. Some long-term-care planners and practitioners who believe that the long-term care system requires alterations, modification, or additional long-term-care structures in order to change the present and future quality of life (a value) to more desirable state of affairs might set about campaigning for adoption of these new and desirable values much the same way politicians campaign for adoption of their specific proposals for national health insurance. In both instances, the ultimate goal originating from such values is that all people have access to care.

Future Orientation. Long-term-care planning that is future oriented can predict what will happen in a future time frame if alternatives are in fact carried out. Because long-term-care planning deals with the future, inputs from the system impacting on elderly population groups at the present time, and anticipated to continue into the future if something is not done, are necessary information for planning activities. The nature of current resources, their capabilities, and input from various long-term-care professionals and community members are also important ingredients for planning desired futures. Community input is most important since it is frequently from members of the community and target population groups themselves that current or anticipated conditions not readily disclosed by other customary data-collection procedures are brought to light.

Together, the statistical data plus the perceptions and apprehensions of community members and professionals can in the hands of skilled planners and practitioners suggest or point to some of the present problems that are on their way to becoming first-class problems for a target population. Long-term-care planners and practitioners can then begin to act and seek innovative and creative options that can prevent anticipated future problems and provide desired futures.

Purposes. Long-term-care planning is characterized as being purposive. A number of purposes have been prescribed for planning: few planning theorists speak to a single purpose; some combine half a dozen or more. The author subscribes to one particular set of long-term-care planning purposes, from which a planning system has been developed and the steps of the planning process identified. Their practical application is the main thrust of the remaining chapters of this book.

The four major purposes of long-term-care planning, modified from some of the ideas suggested by Blum,[7(pp51-53)] are the following:

1. Defining desired improvements
2. Defining the necessary plans to carry out what have been identified as necessary improvements
3. Implementing the necessary plans
4. Measuring the attainment of the desired improvements

Each of the four purposes represents the "why" of four major elements or parts of planning that the author has identified as *assessment, planning, implementation,* and *evaluation.*

Parts of the Long-Term-Care Planning System

Assessment, planning, implementation, and evaluation make up a total planning system. Each part of the planning system is considered a separate subsystem having characteristics of interdependency and interrelatedness. Thus, each part of the planning system influences and is influenced by its other parts. Long-term-care planners and practitioners should be prepared, therefore, to expect that the activities and functions carried out by any part of the long-term-care planning system are subject to change as a result of feedback from the activities and functions of other parts of the system. Thus, each subsystem is neither static or instant, but a continuous, evolving process. Figure 2-2 shows the four subsystems of assessment, planning, implementation, and evaluation and their dynamic relationship.

Assessment

Assessment is a means by which the long-term-care planner and practitioner, by examining past trends, present realities, and desired futures, is able to predict a plan for the future. Assessment is the planning undertaken to define or delineate need and desired improvements.

Planning

Planning as a separate but related subsystem is planning for action to meet the defined need and desired improvement. Planning utilizes the data and information generated by the activities of the assessment system, which include data collection,

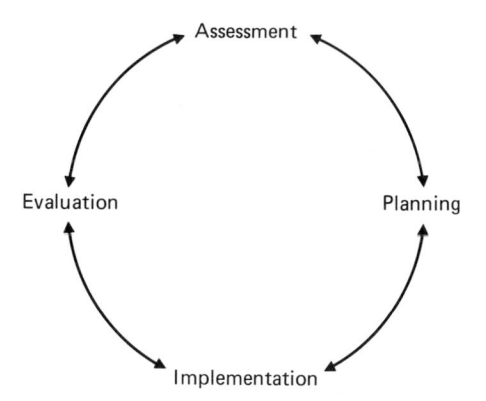

Figure 2-2. Interrelation of Long-Term-Care Planning Subsystems

analysis, and interpretation. The planning subsystem also sets into motion activities designed to harness all available resources into the most appropriate and effective channels for implementation. Thus, the planning subsystem is concerned with what we are going to do, who is going to do it, and when it is to be completed. It is future-oriented in that it lays out a systematic and orderly design for reaching some desired prospective destination—a desired future state.

Implementation

Implementation is the means employed by planners and professionals to achieve a given end, a prospective destination, a desired improvement, or a desired future state. Implementation is the initiation and completion of the actions necessary to accomplish an objective. Because implementation implies taking action, it is the part of the planning system that can make a significant change in the delivery of health-care and human services. Conscious and deliberate attention needs to be given to objectives during the implementation part of the planning process.

Evaluation

To evaluate means to examine and judge, to ascertain the value of, to appraise. Inherent in evaluation is the process of assigning value to some objective and then determining the degree of success in attaining the valued objective. Evaluation may be thought of in terms of comparing and contrasting. Whereas assessment should be nonjudgmental, evaluation measures the worth or value of action and answers such questions as "What effect is the program or intervention having?"; "Is the program working as we expected?" Evaluation is the process of judging the worthwhileness of a program or activity, regardless of the method employed.

Evaluation also has an intrinsic relationship to planning, development, and implementation. Evaluation provides the basic information for designing and redesigning action programs and participant intervention. Thus, evaluation involves not only the ascertaining of success or value but also encompasses understanding and redefinition of objectives, techniques, and various actions that have been undertaken during the entire planning process.

Process

Long-term-care planning is generally conceived of as a process. A *process* is a method of doing something that involves a number of steps or related parts, with the intention of bringing about particular results.

That planning is a process is made conspicuous by some planners in their definitions of planning. Schaefer, for example, conceives of planning as an "orderly process of defining a problem through analysis, identifying unmet needs and demands that constitute a problem, establishing realistic and feasible goals, deciding on their priority, surveying the resources needed to achieve goals, and projecting administrative action based on the weighing of alternative intervention strategies for solving the problem."[3(p124)] Other planning theorists concur with this conception of planning, with some variation in the steps involved, and emphasize the importance of decision-making. Drucker, for example, views planning as a "continuous process of making entrepreneurial (risk-taking) decisions systematically and with the best possible knowledge of their futurity, organizing systematically the efforts needed to carry out these decisions and measuring the results of these decisions against the expectations through organized feedback."[8] Decision-making is viewed here as an important activity inherent in every step of the planning process regardless of the number of steps involved in the process. An important concept emphasized by Drucker, yet lacking in other planning definitions, is feedback.

A variety of planning models exist, with as many variations in steps. The following outline of planning is derived from the four general purposes of planning previously discussed. However, this nine-step model is deceptive, for we find that, in actuality, none of the individual steps is a discrete entity. Although the nine steps may appear discrete on paper, in practice, the planning process is rarely consecutive. Steps may overlap or occur simultaneously, and concerns may be generated at any step that calls for reconsideration of previous steps. The nine-step planning model is outlined as follows:

1. formulation of overall goals and purposes
2. data collection and analysis
3. identification of problems and needs
4. examination of constraints, capabilities, resources, and interest groups
5. examination of alternative courses of action and probable consequences
6. definition of objectives and priorities
7. formulation of a plan of action
8. implementation of the plan
9. evaluation of outcomes according to predetermined criteria

Each step of the overall long-term-care planning system is viewed as a subsystem because of its characteristic nature of interrelatedness and interdependency. Any step within the planning system is subject to change resulting from the activities and feedback generated by the operation of any other step or steps. A number of the steps may involve a number of people, and it is essential that cooperative and interactional colleagial relationships be developed if the total system is to be effective in achieving desired improvements or results. The various steps, as viewed within a systems framework, are shown in Figure 2-3.

It should be emphasized that formal planning can start at any step or steps. However, the author prefers to begin the process with an overall definition or statement of goals, needs, and purposes—an activity that normally sets into motion the steps of the assessment system.

28 / Part I: The Conceptual Frame of Reference

```
Assessment            Planning                  8. Implementation         9. Evaluation

1. Formulation        4. Examination               Planning                  Impact
   of goals and          of constraints,
   purposes              capabilities,             Organizing                Acceptability
                         resources, and
                         interest groups           Staffing                  Effectiveness
2. Data
   collection                                      Direction                 Efficacy
   and analysis       5. Examination
                         of alternative            Control                   Efficiency
                         courses of
3. Identification        action and                                          Adequacy
   of problems           probable
   and needs             consequences


                      6. Definition of
                         objectives
                         and priorities


                      7. Formulation
                         of plan of
                         action
```

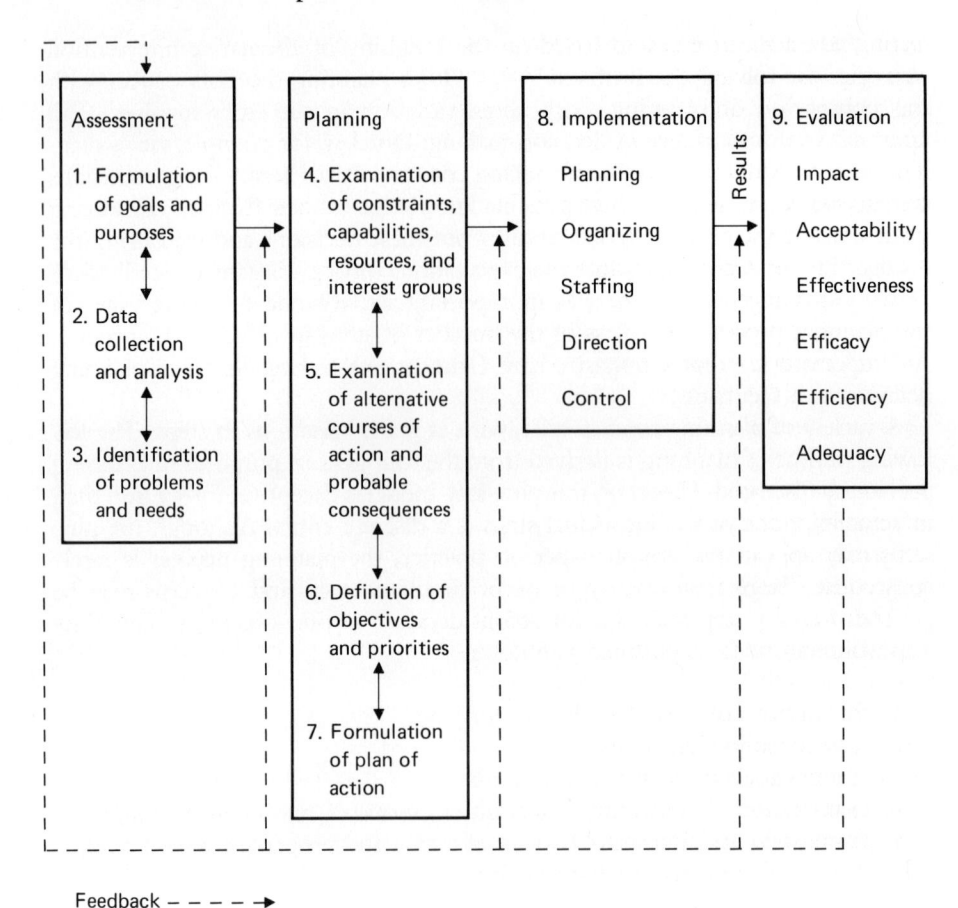

Feedback – – – – →

Figure 2-3. A Systems Approach to Long-Term-Care Planning

Step 1: Formulation of Overall
Goals and Purposes

Ideally, the first step in long-term-care planning is the formulation of stated goals and purposes; this step should be taken before a problem is encountered. The importance of defining overall goals cannot be overemphasized: it prevents the selection of solutions and the determination and specification of objectives before problems have been identified. This step is frequently omitted or superficially approached, resulting in programs without clearly stated goals.

Initiation of long-term-care planning is not necessarily an automatic response to a recognized need. Identification of the needs of the elderly may originate from a "hunch," "gut-feeling," or "belief" that all is not what the practitioner and others want it to be. Recognition of the need for particular long-term-care services may also originate from the concerns of long-term-care providers, personnel in health- or social-service-related organizations, or community members. This initial approach to planning may not be very systematic and can be relatively unfocused. The validity and reliability of these methods are dubious, and the accumulated information may not hold up under scientific scrutiny. Yet it is often the suspicions, hunches, and jumble of subjective data, together with the values and beliefs held by practitioners and community members, that are most relevant to establishing goals. Once goals are clearly defined, they can act as a springboard for further inquiry, with a particular focus on a target population group.

With the belief that a problem or need exists, the planner begins to formulate some idea of the problem, data needed, parties of interest who need to be interviewed to secure information, and a listing of related factors that might be associated with the problem. Issues that need to be given consideration at this time include the necessary expertise to implement various steps in the planning process, the necessity of conducting surveys of the target population of elderly, and the utilization of existing statistical information pertinent to the target population group (see Chapter 4).

The overall goals, once determined, provide direction and are related to the establishment of the problem. Overall goals and purposes can be based on need or some idea that a discrepancy or discrepancies exist. Since the author has indicated the importance of relationships as a systems concept, existing and nonexisting relationships that "should" or "could" exist need to be identified. *Discrepancies* are the qualitative or quantitative differences (or both) between what exists and what "could" or "should" exist. Problems and needs (the terms are used interchangeably) are defined as discrepancies. A discrepancy might be, for example, a lack of health-care and human services for a large elderly population when comprehensive services for this target population "should be an integral part of a community's long term care delivery system"; or "lack of transportation services" when transporting disabled elderly to health-care services should be provided. The various needs of the elderly population might also include further health supervision after hospitalization or assistance of family members in the care and health supervision of an elderly family member. The elderly individuals become, then, the basic referent for long-term-care planning and achievement.

Step 2: Data Collection and Analysis

In order to determine the nature of a problem or discrepancy, information about the various factors impacting on the health and social needs of a target population must be collected. This aspect of assessment is best described as "the attempt to measure the nature of the situation—the application of the measuring tool"[7(p160)] and includes information about past trends, present realities, and desired futures pertinent to the elderly population.

Information about past trends should include the number of elderly in the specific locality under consideration; predicted population increases, illnesses, and disease patterns; and health-care and social-service utilization. Such information provides valuable clues and ideas of the stages through which phenomena have passed to arrive at the present stage and allows the planner and practitioner to speculate on future direction. This process is referred to as *trend-extrapolating;* it requires that data be viewed from more than one point in time to determine the trends.[7(p187)] The time period chosen should be long enough to show any changes that may have occurred.

Information about present reality should include observations made by long-term-care providers, individual statements from key people in health-care and social-service organizations, statistical information from surveys of the target population, and needs. In collecting information about the present situation, the planner will need to obtain information from a variety of sources. Data collection can become an overwhelming project, and the planner must, therefore, be selective; it will be impossible to collect all relevant information.

Step 3: Identification of Problems and Needs

As data are generated, studied, and analyzed, needs should become apparent and the nature of the problem evident. Ultimately the data base that has been formulated should offer clues to needs, the care that should or could be made available, and some ideas about possible interventions. A data base relevant to a population group under study is crucial when the planner is seeking funding sources, scarce resources, and their allocation. Allocation of resources very well may depend upon a well-documented discrepancy and presented need for health-care and human services for a target population.

In analyzing the data, the long-term-care planner and practitioner must keep in mind the areas of input relevant to the optimal level of functioning of elderly population groups, such as their demographic characteristics, types of health-care and human services available, socioeconomic factors, political factors, and health status.

Present intervention strategies being applied to the system under study must also be considered, and their strengths and weaknesses examined in terms of impact on target groups of elderly. The planner should also seek the input of people with personal, professional, legal, or business responsibilities in the problem area, for their input can contribute significantly to the identification of problems.

During the process of examining the data, a number of needs may become evident; these needs must be sorted in terms of their relative importance. Some planners weigh needs in order to assign them priorities. Others use a sorting process based on the economic principle of opportunity costs—that is, resources spent for one kind of program or activity with some particular outcome cannot be spent for another program or activity with the same outcome. The author prefers to use the following guidelines suggested by Archer and Fleshman in assigning priorities:[5(pp47-48)]

1. Determine those needs in which change can be brought about.
2. Recognize those needs that, given time, will resolve themselves without assistance.
3. Recognize those needs requiring more resources—time, money, personnel (collaboration with other agencies)—than we can reasonably spend on them (without assistance).
4. Recognize those needs beyond the scope of the practitioners' expertise (and obtain required expertise).
5. Recognize those needs requiring actions by others or other agencies.
6. Recognize those needs that can be met by any nonprofessional.
7. Recognize those needs that can be met by health- and social-service professionals.

A sorting of needs can help define the parameters of the long-term-care needs of a target population group and the resources necessary to meet specific needs.

In summary, the assessment system is composed of a number of interrelated and interdependent subsystems, which include: the formulation of overall goals and purposes, appropriate data collection and analysis, and identification of the problems, needs, or discrepancies. Once the problems have been identified, they become the input for the planning system.

Step 4: Examination of Constraints, Capabilities, Resources, and Interest Groups

The next step in the nine-step model is based on the identification of problems or discrepancies—the output occurring from the assessment system. This output becomes the input for the planning system. Having identified discrepanices or long-term-care needs, the constraints, capabilities, and resources available must be examined in order to begin formulating an approach to solving needs and eliminating discrepancies.

Resources that must be examined include financial support—especially if it is deemed necessary for program implementation involving manpower, facilities, and necessary equipment.

Various constraints need to be examined since they could be barriers to the implementation of a specific program of solution or some desired plan for improvement. These constraints may include certificate-of-need procedures in some states or localities if a new long-term-care organization or structure is being proposed at considerable cost. Opposing community groups need to be considered, as well as any local legal mandates that may impede the implementation of the plan. Some states require letters from various professionals and agencies that validate the need for desired improvements in the delivery of long-term care to the elderly, such as an adult day-care program. These letters, which should be written on stationery with appropriate agency headings, would have to be obtained.

Identification of supportive interest groups can be beneficial to the long-term-care planner and practitioner since they may provide additional information and assistance in promoting implementation of a program. Large numbers of people can have an impact on facilitating change.

Step 5: Examination of Alternative Courses of Action and Probable Consequences

With knowledge about the problem generated from examining the constraints, capabilities, resources available, and interest groups, planners next must consider alternative courses of action to resolve the discrepancies or problems identified. In most cases there is more than one way to deal with a problem, as well as differing beliefs about the value of certain long-term-care services over other types of long-term-care services. Thus, some particular approach to a problem must be specified. The planner might opt to search for one particular solution—"a satisfying approach"—or search for a number of solutions and choose the most appropriate or best solution.

A number of adult day-care models exist. In some localities a health-care model may be more appropriate than a social model. Other planners may view a comprehensive model including social, medical, nursing, and other health-related services as the best solution. Although one particular approach to adult day care is described in Chapter 12, this approach is not the only alternative.

In choosing the most appropriate or best alternative to meet a target population's needs, the planner can use a number of familiar criteria. These criteria include an examination of the costs, benefits, feasibility, and acceptability of the proposed program, as well as a consideration of the scope of the problems that the program of long-term-care services is proposing to attack. Such criteria can help reduce the number of choices made solely on intuition. The criteria can be changed or additions made to reflect more critical criteria. Ultimately, however, some decision must be made. A plan must be formulated.

Step 6: Definition of Objectives and Priorities

Definition of objectives and priorities is part of the planning system and must occur before plans are put into action. The planner must specify program objectives and the specific criteria that will be used to determine whether these objectives have been achieved.

Objectives differ from goals in that objectives are quantifiable. Goals should indicate an outcome but are usually too general to be measured in a specific situation. Confusion still exists between the two terms, and they are frequently used interchangeably.

Objectives should be derived from the overall goals in step 1 and must be stated in measurable terms because they yield performance criteria. Performance criteria are used for analyzing alternatives for problem solution as well as individual behavior in determining whether and to what extent we did what we set out to do. Methods of evaluating elderly behavior based on predetermined performance criteria are discussed in Chapter 14.

Step 7: Formulation of a Plan of Action

Once a decision has been made concerning the most desirable alternative solution that will achieve particular outcomes identified, a specific plan must be laid out. This plan provides some direction and specifies what the planner is going to do, who in particular is going to do it, and when it is going to happen or be completed. Some planners develop a time chart describing various activities to be accomplished. Setting forth tasks or activities in this fashion can be an aid to program planning and can ensure that certain necessary steps will not be overlooked.

The final plan ideally should be reviewed by others involved before its implementation in order to identify missed items or issues. The plan then becomes the input for the implementation system.

Step 8: Implementation of the Plan

Planning that has been well performed should help clear the way for the adoption of its outputs—the plan. *Implementation,* simply stated, means that you are now going to utilize your materials, methods, and resources to do what you said you were going to do about a particular problem.

The actual process of implementation involves *planning, organizing, staffing, direction, and control.* The idea that "planning and implementation are two distinct and separate activities dies hard."[9] *Planning* that occurs during the process of implementing any program will be concerned with objectives, policies, procedures, and budgeting.

The *organizing* required during the process of implementation may involve such activities as teaching staff and personnel about the procedures necessary for implementing program activities, procedures for meeting with referral agencies, and procedures for client admission.

Staffing involves deciding on who does what for whom, in what order, when, and with what resources. Once staffing activities have been dealt with and understood, *direction* needs to be provided to ensure that program activities, goals, and objectives are carried out.

The last factor involved during the implementation of a plan is *control*. Control refers to the environmental manipulation carried out by the implementor so that decisions made can be carried out and tasks performed. The implementor essentially monitors the extent to which plans are being carried out. Thus, control is also cybernation enabling the implementor to receive *feedback*. Feedback is used as a means of guiding or correcting a system's course of action. Plans may be changed as feedback indicates. The actual process of implementing a selected model of adult day care is discussed in Chapter 12.

Step 9: Evaluation of Outcomes
According to Predetermined Criteria

Although evaluation should be built into every step of the long-term-care planning process, program evaluation is considered here as a separate entity. Evaluation is one of the most important elements in program management and is performed *after* the plans and programs are set in motion and during the operation phase.

The process of program evaluation includes all necessary steps to determine the extent to which predetermined objectives are met. Evaluation therefore requires measurement of results in terms of agreed-upon performance criteria. Criteria are indicators or characteristics by which one recognizes, ascertains, measures, or tests whether and to what degree a norm has been attained.

The selection of performance criteria is value-laden and is the major distinction between evaluative research and basic research concerned with hypothesis testing.[10] Values influence professionals in determining what is "good," "bad," "desirable," "understandable," "improved," and "not improved." The evaluation process is circular, stemming from and returning to the formation of values as illustrated in Figure 2-4. At the conclusion of the evaluation effort, a new value might arise, or an old value might be modified or reaffirmed.

The ultimate goal of program planning, implementation, and evaluation is the successful operation of the program. The evaluation provides a measure of the extent to which program activities attain the desired results.

Summary

As long-term-care professionals, planners, and practitioners face the problems inherent in the health-care and human-service delivery system and seek ways to change it, the systems approach embodied in this chapter may be one way to make significant improvements in the quality of life of many of our older citizens. The key to planning for change in the long-term-care delivery system lies in people, and any approach or sequence of steps as described here can only be as good as the people who use it. Neither the concept of a systems approach nor the phases of planning with their respective steps should be looked upon as a panacea; rather, the hope is that an exposition of these concepts and methods will fill a void and motivate those concerned with the inequities and gaps in the existing long-term-

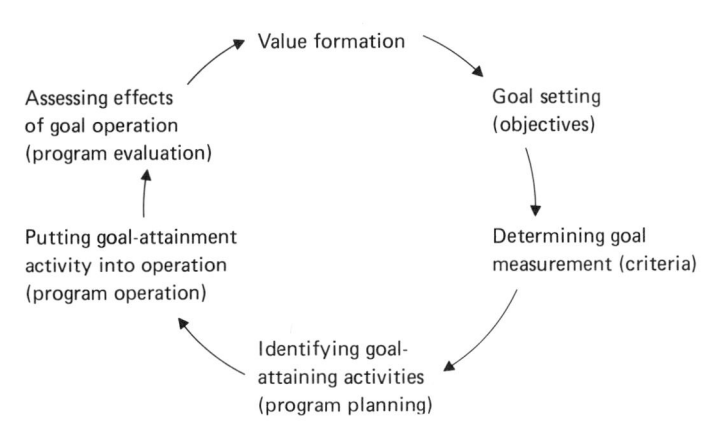

Figure 2-4. The Evaluation Process

care system to explore, develop, implement, and evaluate new and different organizational structures and processes for the care of the elderly who are disadvantaged or otherwise disabled.

References

1. VonBertalanffy L: General systems theory. *Main Currents in Modern Thought* 11: 75–83, 1955.

2. Hall AD, Fagan RE: Definition of a system, in Buckley W (ed): *Modern Systems Research for the Behavioral Scientist*. Chicago, Aldine Publishing Co, 1968, p 81.

3. Schaefer M: *Administration of Environmental Health Programs: A Systems View*. Geneva, World Health Organization, 1974.

4. Drof Y: The planning process: A facet design, in Lyden FJ, Miller EG (eds): *Planning, Programming, Budgeting: A Systems Approach to Management*. Chicago, Markham Publishing Co, 1975, pp 96–99.

5. Archer SE, Fleshman R: *Community Health Nursing: Patterns and Practice*. North Scituate, Mass, Duxbury Press, 1978.

6. Davidoff P, Reiner T: A choice theory of planning. *J Am Instit Planners* 27: 103–115.

7. Blum H: *Planning for Health: Development and Application of Social Change Theory*. New York, Harper & Row, 1959.

8. Drucker PF: Long-range planning: A challenge to management science. *Management Science*, Apr 1959, p 240.

9. Friedman J: Notes on societal action. *J Am Instit Planners* 35: 311–318.

10. Suchman E: *Evaluation Research*. New York, Russell Sage Foundation, 1967, p 32.

3

Planning for Adult Day Care Within a Continuum of Long-Term-Care Services

Ann Clark, RN, MS

Introduction

A plan sets forth a direction, values, and general strategies for achieving goals and/or solving problems.[1] Although the plan can be distinct and separate from the implementation phase of the planning process, the author suggests that the plan and the action associated with it are, in fact, parts to an integrated whole and should be carried out by the same planning person or service agency.

Planning at the agency level focuses on the development of goals and strategies to provide direction and support for program services. Planning tasks at this level include the identification and coordination of resources, materials, and personnel necessary to implement the plan. The outcomes of the planning process include the following:

1. Formulation of a policy statement declaring the agency's commitment to adult day-care services. This statement usually includes a philosophical basis for the policy.
2. Development of goals and strategies for participant services. Goals may deal with a reduction in disability and premature institutionalization and an

increase in socialization with peers. Strategies include the development of planned programs, integration of these programs with other community services, staff development, and research.
3. Development of an organizational structure to administer the program services. This structure must include administration physicians, therapists, nurses, social workers, nutritionists, and other support personnel. It then becomes necessary to clarify the responsibilities of each of these persons, the relationship between them and the community, and the funding sources needed to pay for them.
4. Identification and establishment of the linkage system, both internally and with other community resources.
5. Establishment of data-collection methods, both for internal and external use.

Two widely recognized principles of planning merit attention. The first is that the participants should be included in planning services that affect them. The second is that, in highly structured agencies, the planning effort should be sanctioned by the board, the director, and staff. If the needs for a proposed program are not recognized and supported by these persons, the resultant programs are likely to fail.

One successful approach to dealing with planning is the use of a task force. This body can work collaboratively with the individual planner or agency. The task force should be interdisciplinary, with its membership reflecting the composition of the larger community.

The following presentation of a model for a comprehensive continuum of health-care and social services for the elderly is based on the concept of a system of options and parallels of service. The implementation of a coordinated program of services in more communities is long overdue.

Our current system of long-term care for the elderly is afflicted with confusion and fragmentation. The number of programs available to the elderly in some communities often seems never-ending, whereas, in a neighboring town, services may be scarce, or even totally lacking. Even when services are available, it is often difficult for professionals, and even more so for consumers, to sort through the bewildering maze of programs and regulations in an attempt to determine the function of each program and, more importantly, which one service or combination of services might be most appropriate for whom. To complicate matters further, programs within the same community many times offer duplicate services, thus decreasing the effectiveness that a more coordinated program could offer.

It is important to note that eradication of all duplicative services is not recommended in a community. Crawford and Leadly state that the "complete elimination of a duplication through consolidation carries the threat of over-bureaucratization," whereas "complete independence of multiple providers is associated with a loss of clients 'through the slats' and a wasteful use of resources."[2] The challenge for long-term-care planners is to arrive at that fine balance between total independence of all providers and a complete integration of all programs and services—in other words, to devise a system of working interdependence. Such a system will ideally provide an optimum mix of cost-effectiveness and complete client service.

An integrated system of options services and the resultant coordination in between the service and care modalities are a major means of enhancing ease of transfer between these services and agencies. Flexibility in the levels of care and services provided to the elderly is critical because of the occurrence of changes in health status, of either a temporary or permanent nature, that may derive from the process of aging or may be unpredictable.

Planning for any new community program necessitates a study of present resources available in order to identify any gaps in services, thereby determining needs and providing a focus for planners (see Chapter 4). The following section presents a model of a continuum of community resources for elders that will assist in the planning process. Described are various health-care- and social-service components that are available in communities and that need to be considered in the planning for an adult day-care center if it is to be truly a part of a comprehensive system of services for the elderly. Along with a brief description of each service component included in the model, the need for planning and coordination among the various community programs is addressed. Some special projects that outline different approaches to planning for elderly services are also described.

Model of Continuum of Community Services for the Elderly

The model of the continuum of services (see Figure 3-1) ranges from those services that provide the lowest level of support or care to those health-care and social resources that have the potential for providing total care and support to the elderly and their families. Thus, the most independent elderly person might require only the socialization support available at the local senior-citizen center or perhaps might enjoy and benefit from attending a congregate meal site during the week, both options of assistance found at the lower left end of the continuum.

Advancing along the model, the protective environment of a housing-for-the-elderly project might provide just the right level of assistance for this elderly person in later years. Other older persons, however, might require the added services component of a congregate housing development, while the even more frail elderly person might benefit from the intensive services and care available in a nursing home, rehabilitative center, or, when acutely ill, might require the specialized care provided in an acute-care hospital, depicted at the far right end of the continuum. Hospice care, a specialized care and services modality for the terminally ill, is also included at the right of the continuum since it also provides a range of intensive and specialized care.

Chapter 3: Planning for Adult Day Care / 39

```
←———————————[ ADULT DAY-CARE PROGRAMS ]———————————→
[Psychosocial Model] ←→ [Psychosocial/Medical-Rehab Model] ←→ [Medical-Rehab Model]
```

                                    Independent
                                     Housing

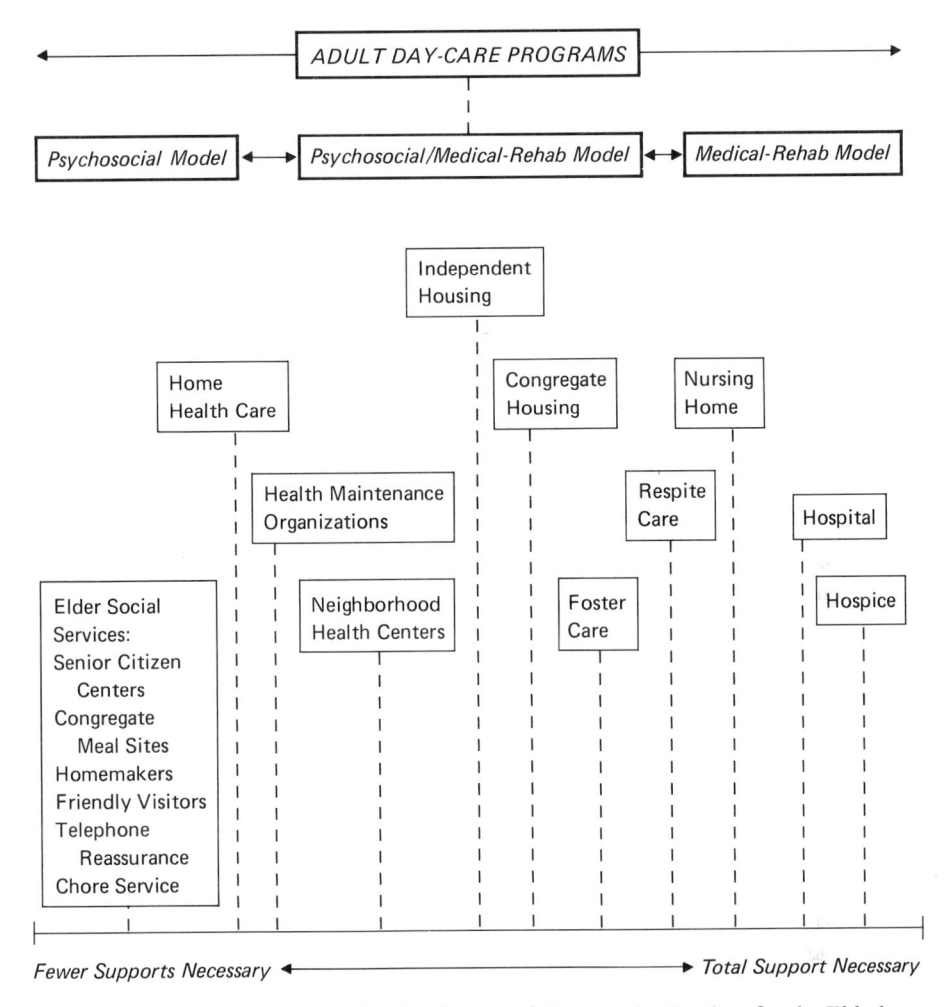

        Home   Congregate   Nursing
     Health Care   Housing   Home

              Health Maintenance   Respite
               Organizations   Care   Hospital

  Elder Social   Neighborhood   Foster   Hospice
  Services: Health Centers   Care
   Senior Citizen
     Centers
   Congregate
     Meal Sites
   Homemakers
   Friendly Visitors
   Telephone
     Reassurance
   Chore Service

Fewer Supports Necessary ←————————————————→ Total Support Necessary

Figure 3-1. Proposed Model of a Continuum of Community Services for the Elderly

At several points along the continuum, resources overlap. This overlapping of health-care and social service resources is intentional for two reasons. At any one point in time, it might be appropriate for the services of different resources to be utilized by the elderly in order to meet their needs most completely. Yet perhaps the most important reason for the system of overlapping services is that it gives the option of choice, since the same level of care and services may be available within more than one of the service components. The key factor is to provide a system that offers options to the elderly and their families.

Different individuals, depending on condition and ability, will require different service arrangements. Thus, the long-term care system will maintain maximum independence and quality of life for its clients if it provides for each a service package tailored to the individual's needs.[3]

For example, it might be very appropriate for an elderly person to attend an adult day-care program while learning to safely control newly diagnosed diabetes. Yet, for many reasons, such a person may not wish to, nor be ready to, attend the center. Perhaps he or she is not yet ready for the busy interaction with others at the center because of the recent death of his or her spouse. Instead, the person may choose to manage and learn about his or her diabetes with the assistance of the area community-health nursing agency, in conjunction with a homemaker provided through the local elder-services agency. Whatever the choice, a range of services and care are readily available.

Adult day-care-center programs, depending on the type of model chosen (refer to Chapter 10 for a discussion of types of models), may be present at different points along the continuum. A more socially oriented model of adult day care would fit into the lower left section of the continuum, whereas a more intensive center with a strong rehabilitative-therapies program would be more accurately located at the right side of the continuum.

The continuum of community services is an attempt to visually represent the range of care and services that might be considered by area health-care and social-service planners. Adult day-care-center planners should be familiar with the range of services available in their community, identify gaps in present services, and mobilize program planning and implementation to lessen those gaps and provide a more comprehensive system of choices for the elderly.

Model Components

Planners need to be aware of the various components of the model depicted in Figure 3-1 in order to utilize the appropriate resources already available within their community and to develop a well-planned, efficient, cost-effective, and quality adult day-care program. The components of the model will be discussed as they are presented from left to right along the continuum. Not all components are now represented in all communities, but they do reflect the stated needs of our elder population.

Elderly Social Services

Elderly social services comprise those service and care resources, categorized primarily as social supportive services, that enable the elderly to remain self-sufficient for as long as possible within their own home environments. These services are available to the elderly through a variety of funding sources and may include homemaker services (an individual is available to enter the client's home and assist with light housekeeping chores, shopping, and preparation of meals); transportation services; meal sites for the elderly; legal assistance and advocacy programs; counseling services; friendly-visitor programs; telephone-reassurance programs; and senior-citizen drop-in centers. The provision of a well-balanced meal to a homebound older person through a Meals-on-Wheels program and assistance with heavier household tasks and repairs (often called *chore service*) are other important resources that might provide just the appropriate level of assistance required by some elderly people in the community. Education and training programs (available under the Older Americans Act) are also welcome resources for many of the elderly.

Two other vital components of a network of social services to the elderly concern the coordination of services: (1) information and referral and (2) case management. *Information and referral* is the process of responding to requests from the community, usually from a starting point on the telephone, distributing accurate information about available community resources, and making referrals to appropriate resources when the elderly or their families telephone. The additional *case management* service refers to the processes of needs assessment, counseling and direct assistance in coordinating services from community agencies, and resources that are vital follow-through mechanisms for many of the elderly who are unable to perform this coordination themselves.

Many of these community services to the elderly are made available through the funding and organization of the elder-services network, primarily through the respective titles of the Older Americans Act, which are discussed later in this chapter.

Volunteer programs developed in direct conjunction with the elder-services network through the Older Americans Act are the *Foster Grandparent Program* and the *Retired Senior Volunteer Program*. The Foster Grandparent Program provides volunteer opportunities to the elderly age 60 and over, who may enroll in a program to provide time and services to children with special needs. A Foster Grandparent Program is a welcome asset to a comprehensive community program since it concurrently benefits and meets the needs of two special population groups, the very young and the very old.

The Retired Senior Volunteer Program (RSVP) provides volunteer opportunities to the retired elderly in a variety of settings, for example, hospitals, nursing homes, schools, and day centers. Transportation is arranged for the volunteer, when necessary, and a meal may also be included. In many areas of the country, local civic and community organizations (such as councils on aging and church clubs) provide such services as meals assistance, transportation, and visitor support to the elderly within their community. These local resources are a vital part of the total picture of social-service supports to the elderly.

The social-services component of the model thus itself encompasses a wide range of supportive services that might well provide just enough assistance to maintain the independence of the more stable elderly within their own communities.

These social supportive services are often augmented by home health-care services, which are described in the following section. This blending of services is often developed to offer a comprehensive plan of care to the elderly in need of social and health-care assistance at home.

Home Health Care

There is no one universal definition of home health care. The range of services available to persons in their homes (and the elderly comprise the highest users of home health care) varies from agency to agency and from state to state, mainly because of differences in organization and funding sources of home health care. Generally speaking, home health care is the provision of a wide range of services in the home, from frequent, highly skilled services, which may be medical, nursing, or therapies provided to persons in unstable condition, to the level of maintenance care required by a person with a relatively controlled chronic illness, but who may require periodic health monitoring and treatment on a less frequent basis. A home health-care agency certified to participate in the federal Medicare program must provide at least the following services to persons in their homes: skilled nursing and therapies along with home health-aide (unskilled personal-care assistance) services. Many home health-care agencies, also called community health agencies, also provide social work and counseling assistance along with close liaisons to area social-supportive services for the elderly.

The ministering to the sick at home is nothing new; one need only look through town and home-health agency histories to obtain an awareness of the totality of care that was provided for many years, including the delivery of babies before the town doctor arrived, if, in fact, there was even a doctor in the area.

Providing for care in the home is a type of service that is still much valued in today's health-care system.

> Home health care is responsive to ... diverse needs of the individual patient. It maximizes an individual's ability to function ... while minimizing dependency and loss of human dignity that frequently accompany illness. With appropriate home health care, many persons can achieve and be maintained at an optimum level of functioning with greater control over decisions affecting their well-being.[4]

Specific examples of care that might be delivered under the sponsorship of a home-health agency include such skilled nursing services as dressing changes and monitoring the status of wound healing following surgery; diabetic teaching; cardiac monitoring and teaching regarding status and care regime; the physical assessment of the patient with chronic lung disease; and many more nursing-care areas, including the all-important aspects of preventative health-care teaching to both the client and the entire household.

Skilled therapy services, including physical, speech, occupational, and dietary therapies, are also part of the home health-care component, and all or some of the specialized therapies may be necessary to a person's improvement or maintenance at home. Physical therapy for the client with a recent stroke might include skilled range-of-motion and strengthening exercises and training the client and care-support persons in techniques of easier transfers (bed to chair, chair to toilet) and progressive ambulation and stair climbing directed toward a rehabilitated state of independence and optimal level of functioning. If a loss of speech function has occurred, a speech therapist may be enlisted to assist in the essential relearning of speech patterns. An occupational therapist is another important member of the health-care team who facilitates independence in activities of daily living that enable a person to continue as an important family participant. Simple homemaking tasks become major obstacles to many clients who have impaired motor function and coordination skills following a stroke, and who must learn new techniques for such functions as peeling potatoes, cooking at the stove, and many more routine yet life-sustaining tasks. Adequate nutrition is essential to life, and the skills of a dietitian may be crucial to a person's management at home.

As in institutions, the key to successful provision of health care at home is the interdependence of the health-care team members. Admittedly, home health care may not be the choice for all elderly people, but it is an option that is gaining increasing momentum with the spiraling costs of institutionalized health care and the current expansion of the range and depth of home health-care services.

Health Maintenance Organizations

Health Maintenance Organizations (HMOs), or systems of financing and delivery of health care that provide comprehensive health-care benefits to voluntarily enrolled members at a prepaid fee,[5(p1)] are one option of health-care services that is gaining increasing popularity in the United States and one that adult day-care-center planners must be aware of along the continuum of health-care services. The complex organizational and financial aspects of the health-maintenance organizations at the present time do not include a component for an adult day-care program. However, it does not appear incongruous to conclude that it may very well be a component included in the future with the increasing emphasis within the United States on community-based options of preventative health care.

Although the term *health maintenance organization* was not coined until the early 1970s, comprehensive prepaid health-care plans have existed in the United States for many years. One of the early examples of this form of health-care delivery and financing is the Kaiser Foundation, an industry-based, prepaid plan founded in 1947 that is still one of the largest in the country.[5(p2)]

It was not until the 1970s, with our government's increased emphasis on exploring cost-efficient alternatives to health-care delivery as a result of spiraling health-care costs, that the concept of HMOs gained government sanction and support. The 1971 White House Paper entitled "Towards a Comprehensive

Health Policy for the 1970's" provided the rationale for government support of HMOs and paved the way for the adoption of Public Law 93-222—the Health Maintenance Act of 1973—which first provided government grants for the development of HMOs. (This initial act was very stringent; amendments to this act in 1976 have loosened the requirements somewhat for HMO certification.)[5(p2)]

The comprehensive-care benefits available to HMO members include a full range of medical, nursing, dental, pharmaceutical, laboratory, and radiological services. The broad spectrum of health-care services, both preventative and acute, focuses on a preventative-wellness rather than a disease-oriented approach to health care.

The HMO concept, with its emphasis on delivery of comprehensive health-care services in a group-practice setting, may very well be a major organizational system of health-care delivery for the future, especially with our country's move toward a national health policy.

Although legislation for HMOs does not now address the need to include an adult day-center component, many HMOs incorporate a program of home health care, and it seems logical to speculate that as adult day-center models become a more viable option of health care in more communities, that the adult day care may very well become a recognized component of the HMO system.

Neighborhood Health Centers

Neighborhood health centers began to arrive on the health-care scene in the 1960s in response to the decreased availability of health care in inner-city and rural areas, as an attempt to provide comprehensive health care within these underserved communities. A neighborhood health center may offer a wide range of services for common health problems and is usually staffed by nurses, doctors, social workers, dentists, nurse-practitioners, optometrists, nutritionists, and other health-team members, with back-up services available through a nearby hospital. Health-care personnel from the community are often enlisted to work in the facility, a situation that produces a "health center" in the neighborhood, of the neighborhood, for the neighborhood, and by the neighborhood.[6] A planning committee for an adult day-care center would be well advised to incorporate valuable personnel and resources found in a neighborhood health center and should begin vital outreach and public relations efforts toward this purpose from the early stages of program planning and implementation.

Independent Housing for the Elderly

The term *independent housing* refers to conventional housing-for-the-elderly projects: that is, state- or federal-aided housing projects for the elderly, in which no special arrangements are made for the provision of supportive health-care or social services, as is the case with congregate housing, discussed below. In actuality, projects of merely protective housing for the elderly are becoming a phenomenon of the past as increasing numbers of projects incorporate plans for health-care and social services as a component of the housing development. At present, there are programs of state- and federally-supported independent housing for the elderly, along with privately owned, subsidized housing programs that work in conjunction with local housing authorities.

Many adult day-center participants may come from housing projects. This fact becomes increasingly important as the need arises for greater levels of support and services than are presently available in a particular project. The adult day-center director may very well be the appropriate person to mobilize and coordinate the services needed or to intiate the referral to the primary assessment and screening agency, which will assume responsibility for the required followup.

In many communities, the needs of the aging population of elderly people in such housing projects for increased health-care and social-services support are being addressed through arrangements with community agencies that may, on a regular basis, come into the center to provide such services as health-care screening, provision of congregate meals, social activities, educational and resource meetings, and many other services and programs. Restrictions for residence in a particular housing project vary from location to location, based on a range of income- and age-related ordinances from local housing authorities to limitations imposed by state and local funding programs.

Congregate Housing

Congregate housing is not a new concept; yet it is a housing alternative experiencing new growth as a significant lifestyle option for the aged. One way of viewing congregate housing might be to consider the concept of federally-supported housing for the elderly and take that concept one step further.

Congregate housing was first officially defined in the 1970 Housing and Urban Development Act, and later in the 1974 Housing and Community Development Act, as "low cost housing in which some or all dwelling units have no kitchens and in which there is a general dining facility."[7] Hence, early definitions and development of congregate housing focused on the aspect of providing congregate meals within an area of planned housing. Leaders in congregate housing are now, however, voicing dissatisfaction with this limited definition and are addressing the concept that "the essential 'congregating' is that of services rather than either living units or old people...." Concentration of services within a residential setting is one way of focusing relevant services and making them available to residents.

It is this type of thinking that pervaded at the First National Conference on Congregate Housing for Older People, held in Washington D.C., November 11–12, 1975, under the auspices of the International Center for Social Gerontology (ICSG) and planned in response to requests from representatives of both the housing industry and planners of services for the elderly.

The following definition of congregate housing was proposed at the conference:

> Congregate housing is an assisted independent group living environment that offers the elderly who are functionally impaired or socially deprived, but otherwise in good health, the residential accommodations and supporting services they need to maintain or return to a semi-independent life-style and prevent premature or unnecessary institutionalization as they grow older.[7(p7)]

This type of congregate housing provides for many different models with various options of service assistance, hopefully in response to what the needs of the elderly would be in a particular geographic area. "The heart of congregate housing . . . is the special services that are made available to the residents of the congregate housing facility. These services make it possible for an older man or woman to live independently and make his or her own decisions regarding daily activities."[8]

A model of congregate housing might include the sharing of many daily activities within a single housing project. Private facilities would be available for a bedroom, sitting room, and bathroom, while meals and their preparation might be shared among several occupants. Services might also include housekeeping aid, personal-care assistance, transportation, and many other supportive services.

These services might all be housed within the housing project, but they might very well be provided by relationships with other community resources. For example, the personal-care assistance required by some members of the housing complex may be contracted for through an area home-health-care agency; while the social services such as transportation and homemaking assistance might be available through a liaison with a local direct elder-services agency.

Two major barriers to the development of congregate housing that require further explanation and development are financing and the present lack of coordination between housing and other services for the elderly. However, these barriers may be easier to overcome, and congregate housing may be a more firmly entrenched option for the elderly because of a recent enactment (the Congregate Housing Services Act of 1978), which calls for furthering the concept of congregate services for the elderly and nonelderly who are permanently or temporarily disabled in low-rent housing provided through a public housing agency or a nonprofit corporation, in order to prevent unnecessary institutionalization.

Foster Care

Foster Care for Elders is a program designed for the "frail elder" person who needs 24-hour supervision and assistance with personal care and who may be intermittently confused, but for whom nursing-home placement is not the solution.

The Long-Term Care Division of Medical Assistance under the Massachusetts Department of Public Welfare has worked in conjunction with the Massachusetts Department of Elder Affairs on a program of Foster Care for Elders based on a New York model. In February of 1979, there were five sponsors of Foster Care for Elders programs in Massachusetts, chosen by the Department of Public Welfare, each of which carried approximately 20 participating households. The department has developed guidelines for the operation of the program along with criteria for matching families with the specific needs of the elderly. Each participating family is reimbursed a set amount per month to care for an elder person who requires a continuous level of supervision and care.

One sponsor in the Massachusetts program is the Foster Care for Elders program at Massachusetts General Hospital. If a person referred to their Transfer Office is believed to be an appropriate candidate for a foster-care program, a team consisting of a nurse and a social worker makes an evaluation visit to a household that has applied to participate. The household is evaluated for such aspects as safety, the general housekeeping, capabilities of providers, and the assessment of whether services available will meet the client's needs. If appropriate, the placement is made, including the mobilization of any community resources that are essential for the total care of the client: for example, a visiting nurse, home health aide, or skilled therapies assistance.

The team visits the site within three days after placement, every week for the first month, and then on a monthly basis to reevaluate the placement and the client's progress. Household participants are reimbursed at a basic rate, which includes an amount for client spending money. The basic reimbursement rate to the household was $300 per month in 1979. Two years later, the rate had increased to $15 per day, or $465 for a 31-day month. This basic rate may be supplemented if it is determined on an individual basis that a more intense level of services and care is required.

In the first year of the program, the Massachusetts General Foster Care Program for Elders placed 20 clients. As of the fall of 1981, 61 clients had been placed in foster-care settings. Foster-care programs might very well provide the answer for a significant segment of the elderly population and should be seriously considered as a possible option of care by community health-care planners.

Respite Care

Respite care is another crucial component of the services model for the impaired elderly. The term *respite* is defined as "a hiatus, an interval, a rest, or a recess."[9] Essentially, the concept of respite care refers to many different forms of providing a rest or relief to the primary care givers of an elderly person who gradually requires a great deal of care and support at home from the family and often from other community resources. The concept of respite care is intentionally not presented here as any one formally established program for the elderly, but rather as a concept of respite from the heavy burden of care responsibilities for the primary care givers, which can be provided through various means.

These means might include in-house placement by a community mechanism that allows for short-term-respite use of a small number of nursing-home or chronic-care facility beds. Respite care may also refer to relief assistance provided directly within the family home. This type of assistance has existed informally for several years, in the form of good neighbors and good friends or through private-care arrangements. The concept of respite care is merely formalizing this assistance mechanism and drawing it into a system of long-term-care options for the elderly. Certified home health-care agency personnel (nonproprietary) are available in many areas for 24-hour care, especially for short-term or emergency arrangements. Noncertified proprietary home-health agencies and, in many states, proprietary agencies who may be certified to participate in 24-hour care are another personnel resource for respite-care assistance.

The relief from care that is available through these various arrangements enables families to regroup and replenish their own resources and energies, which often will make the difference between being able to continue to care for the elderly within their own family settings and having to place them in a nursing home when that is not yet the desired option.

Funding mechanisms for a comprehensive and formalized program of respite care remain limited, thus preventing the further development of this care option for the elderly. Yet, as government agencies continue to act on legislation that provides broader-based community health-care services, it is hoped that respite care will become a more viable concept in increasing numbers of communities.

Nursing Homes

Nursing homes provide in-house care for the elderly and disabled and are generally classified according to the level(s) of care available. The designation of different levels of care is linked to the source of reimbursement that is accepted by the home.

In addition to room and board, Level I and Level II nursing homes provide around-the-clock nursing care, various therapies, and other skilled services. Level I and Level II encompass a more intensive level of health care and are referred to as Skilled Nursing Facilities. Level III facilities, or Intermediate Care Facilities, provide for a less intensified level of assistance with routine nursing care available. The person in a Level III nursing home is usually physically stable, requiring only a maintenance level of health-care assistance. Level IV facilities are termed Residential Care Facilities and merely provide protective supervision for residents who do not routinely require nursing or medical assistance. Currently, Medicare only reimburses for Level I nursing-home placement because Medicare only covers services for persons who are progressing, and therefore rehabilitable, or whose health condition is deteriorating. In other words, Medicare does not reimburse for the maintenance level of long-term care that the more stable elderly person requires.

Many facilities offer a range of levels of care in one setting, thus providing an increased flexibility for the client within the facility who may require varying levels of health-care support and supervision because of changes in health status.

The institutionalized setting of a nursing home is the appropriate choice for many elderly people, and it is a choice that adult day-care-center providers must be cognizant of, even from the early planning stages of the program. An area nursing home might be a perfect site for a proposed adult day-care center, depending on the type of program needed and purpose. A definite advantage to this arrangement (which is described in Chapter 12) is the potential for utilizing many of the same resources—that is, specialized-therapies equipment, dietary services, and activity programs, especially major activities or excursions planned around whole-day times. The availability of emergency back-up staffing is another advantage to planning an adult day-care center in a nursing home. Many nursing homes have rehabilitative therapies departments, whose services would be a necessity in a rehabilitation-oriented adult day-care program. Another advantage of a nursing-home setting that is often overlooked by planners early in the search for a site, but which gains increasing importance as the search progresses for accessible and appropriate space, is that nursing homes are usually already barrier-free, with accessible bathroom facilities.

Disadvantages to the use of nursing-home space for an adult day-care center (at least in Massachusetts) are the complicated and time-consuming certificate-of-need process that must be followed, and many proponents dislike linking the day-care center with an institutional-care center, which may evoke an image of "sick elderly" rather than the less frail elderly who might attend the center. The key to overcoming this kind of community prejudice if a nursing-home site is chosen for the site of an adult day-care center is the provision of extensive and ongoing public relations and outreach efforts that will help project the positive image of the adult day-care program.

Regardless of whether a nursing home is actually designated as a viable space for a planned adult day-care center, it is essential that public relations and research attempts for documentation of need for the facility include the nursing-home administrators and social-work departments. These actions are important not only from the standpoint of providing valuable data necessary for the proposal-writing process, but they may also help decrease a sense of competition between the programs that would block collaborative planning for services to the elderly in the community.

Nursing homes can be a vital resource for an adult day-care center in a community, offering assistance in the direct provision of services, as well as in-kind services (for example, lights and heat), emergency back-up facilities and personnel. Nursing homes can also be a resource when respite care is needed by family members on a temporary basis or when a longer-term placement is required because of the declining health status of an adult day-care-center participant. Adult day-care-center planners and providers are encouraged to learn the nursing-home resources available in their community in order to most effectively plan the type of adult day-care center that is needed within the area and to incorporate the most efficient use of available resources.

Area hospitals are another valuable resource for an adult day-care center. The obvious liaisons are for the provision of emergency treatment and as a vital referral source, yet it may also be profitable for the center to contract with the hospital for certain specialized services (for example, therapies, dietary consultation, education).

The areas of interdependence between community resource components are many, and only a few possible liaisons that would benefit an adult day-care center have been addressed here. The challenge is one of striking the right balance between total bureaucratization and "losing people through the slats." Adult day-care-center planners and administrators must be especially aware of the available community resources with these key agencies to provide a system of supports that will enable more elderly people to remain safely within their homes for as long as they choose and for as long as is feasible.

Hospitals

Hospitals are generally classified as either acute- or long-term-care facilities, and the types of care provided, along with the reimbursement for the two types of facilities, may also vary.

Acute-care hospitals supply full emergency-treatment services and a comprehensive range of medical and surgical services to the community. Nursing services are a key component of hospital care, as is the expertise provided by rehabilitative therapy, dietary, radiology, pharmacy, laboratory, and social service personnel.

Hospitals may voluntarily choose to become accredited through the Joint Commission on Accreditation of Hospitals (JCAH), which is jointly sponsored by the American College of Physicians, the American College of Surgeons, The American Hospital Association, and the American Medical Association. Periodic accreditations of enrolled hospitals include a survey against established standards and criteria for hospitals, thereby ensuring an accepted level of health-care practice and quality patient care.

Long-term- or chronic-care hospitals are those hospitals whose emphasis is on restorative and long-term care rather than on the primary treatment of a disease or illness. Rehabilitative chronic-care hospitals also provide a highly skilled level of care and may include all the services available through an acute-care hospital—that is, medical, nursing, pharmaceutical, dietary, therapy, social-work, home-health-aide, and laboratory services, but care is directed at long-term management and adjustment rather than initial curative treatment.

The area hospitals, whether acute or long-term care, are a major health-care and social-services resource in a community and provide crucial assistance to our aging population; they are thus a vital component within the comprehensive services continuum.

Hospice

Hospice is not a place but a philosophy. Hospice encompasses both at-home and inpatient care for persons who have a terminal illness with a limited prognosis. Curative and restorative treatments are determined to be no longer reasonable, and prolonging life is no longer the focus of medical care.

A primary goal of hospice care is to enable clients to live as completely and as free of pain as possible during the terminal phases of their illness. The family of the client is an integral part of the unit of care, as is the client. The aim is to keep the family involved in the dying client's care and to provide the supports necessary to the family to help them cope with the death and adjustment to life without the client.

The care is coordinated and provided by an interdisciplinary team composed of nurses, doctors, social workers, clergy, pharmacists, and any other care givers. An assessment of needs (physical, emotional, spiritual, and financial) is made by the total hospice team with input from the client and the family. It is then determined whether hospice care is appropriate and consented to by all involved. An individual plan of care is developed and continuously updated through regular conferences including the entire hospice team. In addition to medical services, team members provide personal care to the client (feeding, bathing, toileting, and grooming assistance), homemaker services (household tasks, grocery shopping, and food preparation), along with specific nursing treatments and the teaching and counseling of both client and family. Medications to relieve pain are given frequently and usually on a regular schedule, since most hospices believe that helping the client to meet death is impossible unless pain is controlled.

The term *hospice* in medieval times referred to a way station for travelers, a place of sanctuary for weary travelers.[10] Hence, hospice is viewed as a place to provide care for the terminally ill and their families, who are indeed weary travelers in the journey of life and who need special support.

The beginning of the hospice movement, focusing on care for families as well as clients, is marked by the founding of Saint Christopher's in London in 1967. The first hospice program in the United States was Hospice, Incorporated, begun in New Haven, Connecticut in 1971 and was expanded in 1974 to include home-based care. There are now more hospice programs in existence, with many in various stages of development. A key issue preventing rapid expansion of the hospice movement is the barriers to reimbursement imposed by many third-party insurance mechanisms that preclude reimbursement for the level of care provided by much of the hospice program.

In 1980, Blue Cross of Massachusetts initiated an experimental program of third-party reimbursement for hospice care. Hopefully, this program will prove successful and lead to an expansion of this and other funding sources. Greater numbers of clients and their families would then be able to utilize hospice.

Outreach

All systems have interfaces that must be bridged. In the long-term-care system, these interfaces are between systems and between a care giver and the community in which it exists. Outreach is the organized human intervention that bridges the caps. It is a process that disseminates information, reaches out to actively engage in interaction the people who are at an interface, and encourages the development of trust and acceptance of the long-term-care facility, the people in it, and the concepts governing it.

Adult day care is young and not well known, which makes outreach not only desirable but essential to its development. The impact of outreach will be visible in its outcomes. Five of these outcomes—cooperation, coordination, use, support, and integration—and examples of community members toward whom outreach can be extended are described below.

Cooperation

The community within which an adult day-care center wishes to operate has an established decision-making and power-sharing system. Alliances must be formed with key people to gain access to this system and share in it. Some of the key people within this system are the mayor, selectmen, local physicians, the city or town council on aging, administrators of the local hospitals and nursing homes, the health department, the city or town planning board, and the police and fire departments. Some of the desired outcomes of cooperation with these members of the existing power structure could be an interpreting and writing of local ordinances in favor of adult day care, referrals, access to local information, mutual respect, support in meeting local health ordinances, ease in obtaining zoning changes and handling transportation access problems, and having police and fire plans in the event of trouble.

Coordination

The long-term-care options addressed previously are used simultaneously and sequentially by many of the elderly. Planned interaction among these systems can maximize the use of scarce resources, prevent the duplication of services, and facilitate the transfer of information for optimum participant care. For instance, if the Visiting Nurse Association (VNA) is visiting a participant several times a week and one of those visits is for a blood-pressure reading only, coordination can permit the transfer of that function to the adult day-care center and the transfer of the blood pressure reading to the VNA. A sense of unity between an adult day-care program and other long-term-care options can result in new support sources being brought to the attention of the adult day-care center by the other facilities. The greater lobbying power of all long-term-care options combined can be used to strengthen the position of adult day care.

Use

Disabled adults and the elderly are the participant population of adult day care. Any form of outreach that does not reach them both directly and indirectly through others can fail for want of enough participants. Outreach workers, case managers, and homemaker/home-health aides can all be used to make the primary contact. Word-of-mouth of participants and their families can be the single most effective means of reaching other prospective participants. Open-house days, health fairs on site, programs before community organizations, information booths at local activities and gatherings, and publication of information in local newspapers, especially those addressed to the elderly or disabled adults, are all means of reaching and informing the public.

Support

The community can be a wealth of support if only adult day care wishes to tap it. The adult day-care advisory board is usually composed of members of the community as well as members of the adult day-care center. These people can become the core of a cadre of volunteers, employees, consultants, and good-will supporters drawn from the community. This cadre in turn can be the basis of a combined private and business financial-support network. With this phalanx of involved people, the adult day-care center can become trusted and accepted. Without it, the center can exist in a sea of isolation, distrust, ignorance, indifference, or vague antagonism.

Integration

Outreach efforts that seek to have the outreach workers become well known to the entry personnel of other agencies and to the transporters, and then to have the same outreach workers be the key people for transfers, can facilitate the easy and smooth movement of participants from one facility to another. Personal involvement of the key personnel with each other can make the difference between the system being a continuum and its being fragmented.

Planning Organization

The presentation of the various components of the service model is complex; yet, in many areas, the discussion is far from complete, since services may vary widely from agency to agency and from state to state. The need for awareness of these different services and active planning and coordination with them is essential for the adult day-care-center planner and provider. In fact, the very reason that a discussion of the available services is included in the context of this book is that adult day-care-center planners have the responsibility to be as fully informed as possible regarding the available resources in the community if the center is to truly serve a need and be an appropriately and efficiently utilized component of the health-care and social-services system without unnecessary and costly duplication of services.

Some strong concerns need to be voiced regarding the speed with which many adult day-care-centers are emerging. Massachusetts alone had 6 programs under Medicaid sponsorship in 1976; in the spring of 1978, 18 programs were listed. In the fall of 1981, there were 46 adult day-care centers operating in Massachusetts; an additional 7 centers were certified for operation but had not yet opened. Although there is a definite need for adult day-care centers, their proponents may very well be performing an injustice to the public, especially in this time of spiraling health-care costs and fragmentation of services, if the growth of these centers is allowed to go unchecked. The resulting situation might well parallel the errant and unchallenged growth of some substandard nursing homes that occurred in the mid- to late '60s, rather than the desired development of quality that would ensure a comprehensive continuum of long-term-care services. Despite guidelines and criteria promulgated by some state programs, the evaluation requirements of proposals for adult day-care centers remain weak, thus posing a barrier to the development of better-planned programs.

A move toward increased coordination and integration of health and social services is originating from a multitude of directions; this trend has major implications for the adult day-care center. Spurred on by testimony presented at a series of public hearings on home health care held throughout the United States in 1976,[4] home health-care advocates are now working toward the development of a broader definition of home health care, which will impact on the total community long-term-care services system. Much testimony was presented against the current structuring of federal reimbursement programs, which promote a narrowly circumscribed, medically oriented, and age- and income-specific approach to home health care. The public and the health-care providers were clamoring for a broader definition and a system of home health care that would include aspects of disease prevention and health-promotion services, which are important components of the care and services to the elderly in the home.

The recommendations voiced at the public hearings have not gone unheeded. The hearings served as a major impetus for the current trend toward expansion of home health services. Both the American Nurses Association, in their statement *Health Care at Home: An Essential Component of a National Health Policy,*[11] and the National League for Nursing have developed broader definitions that encompass an expanded view of care at home. The definition proposed by the American Nurses Association now stresses the importance of health promotion and maintenance activities, whereas the National League for Nursing expands the definition even further by advocating that home health care be defined in terms of a blending of health-care and social services.[12] This concept of blending the direct health-care services (for example, nursing; physical, speech, and occupational therapies; home-health aide; and social worker) with types of social supports that are needed by many persons in the home setting, especially the elderly (for example, homemaker, chore service, transportation, and hot meals) is a logical combination that was the subject of much debate at the public hearings and has been a topic of increased interest and study since those hearings.

Persons involved in the planning for adult day-care development need to be aware of the type and number of home-health agencies present in their area and what services they provide. Depending on the focus of the specific adult day-care center and the level of care that is to be provided, it may be very possible and cost-effective to make arrangements for home-health providers to be included in the program of the adult day-care center.

At the present time, many adult day-care centers cooperate with home-health agencies to provide certain skilled services (for example, nursing and therapies) right at the day center, as needed by the individual participants. In addition, many participants in an adult day-care center may not be able to attend the program every day of the week and may need the services of a home-health agency on the days that they cannot, or prefer not to, attend the adult day-care program. The need for excellent coordination and communication between the adult day-care center and an area home-health agency is obvious and lends support to the current push toward coordination of all services available in the community from the very onset of program planning.

Current trends in the network of elderly services indicate an even stronger move toward community services integration. In Massachusetts, the home care corporations are viewed mainly as a social-service component. However, as their ties to other community services are strengthened (for example, with hospital discharge planners and social-service personnel, neighborhood health centers, deinstitutionalization programs, and community health-maintenance programs) the home-care corporation becomes a prime force in the movement of integration of various social- and health-service systems—the very integration of services that has been called for by the proponents of home health.

Many adult day-care centers are developed with start-up funding assistance from an area elder-services organization, such as a home-care corporation. Close relationships between the day-care center and the area elder-services organization are already occurring in many localities, especially in regard to the provision of transportation and nutrition services. As elder-services agencies grow and expand their range and depth of services, it seems only logical that even stronger ties should be established to decrease unnecessary duplication of services and to better utilize the social-services and health-care dollar for the elderly.

Local councils or agencies on aging are a key "grass-roots" resource for anyone planning an adult day-care center, because of their strong link to the elderly of the community. It is possible that the local council on aging could assist the center in certain areas—for instance, with transportation to and from the center. Awareness of local programs for the elderly and an awareness of programs and services of state and regional elder-services agencies is essential for effective and appropriate use of available resources.

Liaisons with elder-housing-project personnel in the community are also crucial. Many state- and federally-supported housing projects for the elderly constructed in recent years have made great strides, through links with other elder-concerned agencies within their community, in providing a range of services to the elderly, such as blood-pressure and health-counseling clinics and regular meals at sites within the housing complex.

Elder-Services Network

The 1961 White House Conference on Aging provided the impetus for the formation of a special federal agency to serve the elderly. At the conclusion of the conference, the Special Staff on Aging in the Office of the Secretary of Health, Education and Welfare (HEW) began to work on legislation for a special program for the elderly that became a reality with the passage of the Older Americans Act of 1965. This act established the Administration on Aging, the federal department that would be responsible for the development of special programs for the elderly, while at the same time serving as the administering organization for any program. According to President Lyndon Johnson, the Older Americans Act

> clearly affirms our nation's high sense of responsibility toward the well-being of older citizens. . . . Under this program every state and every community can move toward a coordinated program of both service and opportunities for older citizens.[13]

The Older Americans Act has been amended eight times since its passage. The most recent amendment was in 1978, when the act was reorganized into six titles instead of the previous nine. This amendment resulted in reorganization, expansion, and strengthening of services to the elderly. Despite the changes, the primary purpose of the act remains to establish program objectives and funding to plan, administer, and provide services to meet the needs of citizens 60 years of age and older.

The Administration on Aging, a division of HEW, is in essence, the federal parent organization to regional, state, area, and local agencies for aging. Title III

(1973 amendments) of the Older Americans Act mandated that each state develop one agency whose responsibility would be to plan and provide services to the elderly. States were to designate Area Agencies on Aging (AAAs) for the purpose of planning and coordinating a comprehensive system of services for the elderly.

Figure 3-2 shows the hierarchy of the elder-services network, from the federal level down through local agencies. Titles and organizations of the agencies vary from state to state—for example, Department of Elder Affairs (Massachusetts), Council on Aging (New Hampshire, Vermont), Office for the Aging (New York).

Due to demographic and geographic characteristics, some state agencies on aging also serve as the federally mandated AAA. Both the state agency and the AAA must develop priority plans for the organization and delivery of services to the elderly within their area. The AAA plan must correlate with the state plan, and, in turn, the state plan must identify with federal objectives of the elder-services program. The AAA develops its priority plan for the area, and, once accepted, this agency has the power to channel funding into the direct elder-services agencies.

In Massachusetts, an additional component was developed within the elder-services network just prior to the federal mandate for the establishment of state and area agencies on aging. Massachusetts sanctioned the establishment of home-care corporations, and, at the time of this writing, this state is divided into 27 home-care corporations—nonprofit elder agencies with boards of directors and advisory councils comprised mainly of the elderly. The Massachusetts home-care

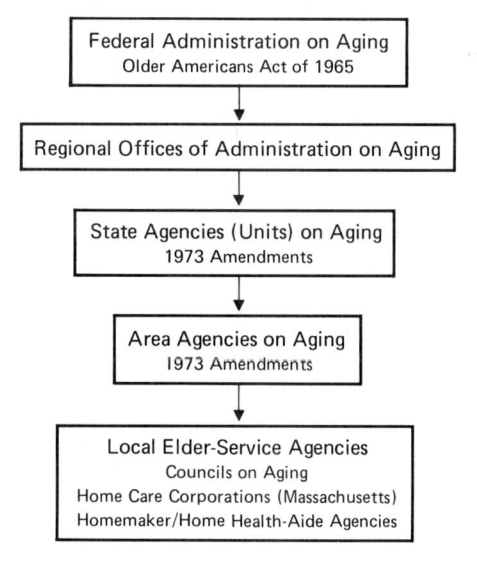

```
┌─────────────────────────────────────────┐
│   Federal Administration on Aging       │
│      Older Americans Act of 1965        │
└─────────────────────────────────────────┘
                    │
                    ▼
┌─────────────────────────────────────────┐
│  Regional Offices of Administration on Aging │
└─────────────────────────────────────────┘
                    │
                    ▼
┌─────────────────────────────────────────┐
│    State Agencies (Units) on Aging      │
│           1973 Amendments               │
└─────────────────────────────────────────┘
                    │
                    ▼
┌─────────────────────────────────────────┐
│        Area Agencies on Aging           │
│           1973 Amendments               │
└─────────────────────────────────────────┘
                    │
                    ▼
┌─────────────────────────────────────────┐
│      Local Elder-Service Agencies       │
│           Councils on Aging             │
│   Home Care Corporations (Massachusetts)│
│   Homemaker/Home Health-Aide Agencies   │
└─────────────────────────────────────────┘
```

Figure 3-2. Elder-Services Network

corporations center around five major functions: case management, chore services, homemaker services, information and referral, and transportation services. Other services may include housing, nutrition, and legal and advocacy assistance and vary from area to area throughout the state. For the most part, the home-care corporation system is part of the planning and coordination mechanism of elder services since the direct services are then contracted for through local service agencies.

Local service agencies may refer strictly to elder-concerned agencies—that is, a council on aging, or they may be home-health-care or social-services programs that provide a range of services to the elderly in a community. Representatives of local service agencies are usually included on boards of directors and advisory councils of the next higher level on the elder-services model.

Due to the duplicative nature of Massachusetts' organization of home-care corporations and the mandated AAAs, the trend is currently toward consolidation of these two units. Increasing numbers of home-care corporations are applying for status as federally recognized AAAs.

The organization of the elder-services network, though far from complete, has facilitated major advancements in the development of increased services to the elderly throughout the country. Adult day-care-center planners are urged to familiarize themselves with the elder-services structure within their own community and to work with the appropriate agencies to strengthen the network as true advocates of planned system change.

Health-Systems Agencies

An important legislative development in health planning was the signing into law of the National Health Planning and Resources Development Act of 1974 (Public Law 93-641). This legislation required the Secretary of Health, Education and Welfare (now titled Department of Health and Human Services) to establish National Health Planning Guidelines and mandated the organization of a comprehensive health-planning network (see Figure 3-3). The law established over 200 regional planning agencies, called Health Systems Agencies (HSAs), throughout the country, whose main function is to determine health-systems changes that will lead to improved health status while restraining increasing costs of the system. Each HSA is responsible for preparing its statement of goals and recommendations in the form of a Health Systems Plan (HSP). As Figure 3-3 indicates, some HSAs are further broken down into regional subcouncils, depending on the population of the area. These subcouncils must then provide information for the HSP to the HSA. Sixty percent of the board of directors for each HSA must be comprised of consumers; the other 40% of the seats are allocated to health-care providers.

The various HSPs within the state are then reviewed by both the Statewide

Health Coordinating Council (SHCC) and the State Health Planning and Development Agency (SHPDA). The SHCC is a governor-appointed body consisting of representatives from each HSA and other key health-planning members within the state. The SHPDA generally falls within the structure of the state government and is responsible for the planning of state health and human services. Following these reviews, and keeping in mind the National Guidelines, a State Health Plan (SHP) is then drafted.

The law also established that the Secretary of Health, Education and Welfare must consult with and receive recommendations and comments from HSAs, SHPDAs, SHCCs, and the National Council on Health Planning and Development, which is the advisory council to the secretary, in the development (and revision) of the National Health Planning Guidelines.

The two components in the lower left corner of Figure 3-3—the Area Agency on Aging and the Local Government Planning Councils—are not actually part of the health planning network but are linked with this main network to demonstrate the fact that these are two major groups that need to be involved in planning health care in communities, especially in planning health care for the elderly.

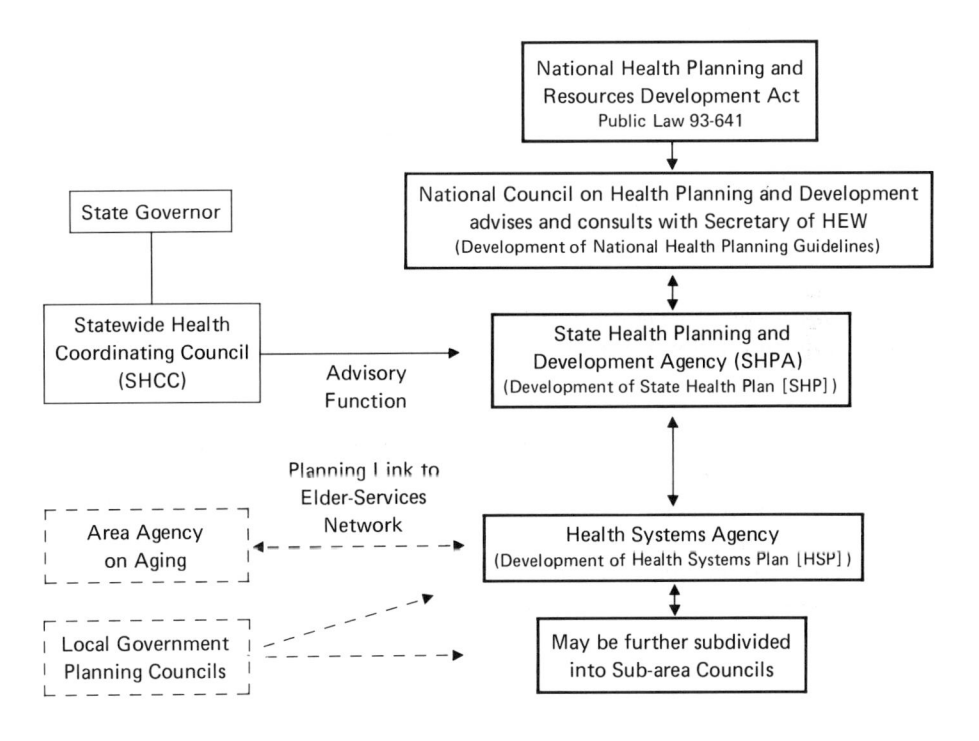

Figure 3-3. Health-Planning Organization

The organization, development, and impact of the various health planning agencies differs from area to area and from state to state. The Health Planning and Resources Development Act provides an organized means of enabling local communities to play a major role in the planning for health care for their area, and potentially, in making an impact on both the state and federal level.

Major strides are being taken in the integration of the different divisions of state health-care systems and health-planning agencies in the formulation and implementation of state health-care plans.

Links between the elder-services network and the health-planning system exist informally in many areas through representation on boards of both the AAA and the HSA. Methods of integrating and linking the HSA and the AAA on a formal basis are now being tested by the Administration on Aging.[14]

Role of Physicians, Adult Practitioners, and Social Workers

Any presentation of supports required by an aging person would be incomplete if it did not address the importance of key groups of independent health-care providers, the physician, the adult or geriatric nurse-practitioner, and the social worker, all of whom may be important contact people within an individual participant's plan of care, including a plan within an adult day-care center. Their roles in the total health-care system are myriad; they are mentioned here briefly only in relation to their possible links with an adult day-care program.

Area physicians need to be alerted early in the adult day-care center plans in order to gain their input in the program development. This input should be encouraged in some form as an ongoing process, perhaps by enlisting a physician representative on the center's board of directors, since physicians are often the sole health-care provider in direct contact with an older person. Physicians are obviously important referral sources for an adult day-care program. Adult day-care programs do not always provide on-site physician services, but nursing care is provided under the orders of the participant's doctor.

The growth of the nurse-practitioner movement in the United States has brought about the rise of the geriatric nursing specialist, who may be functioning within a community in conjunction with a health facility or who may have an established independent practice in the area. The nurse-practitioner with expertise in the field of geriatrics is a key resource person who could be well utilized in an adult day-care-center program. The services of a geriatric nurse-practitioner might be enlisted through an arrangement with an area agency that employs the practitioner (many community nursing agencies employ geriatric specialists) or through direct employment by the adult day-care center.

Social workers in the area, either through institutions or through community-based agencies, are also key contact people who, by the nature of their work and contacts with the elderly and their families, are important resource people to involve in the planning, implementation, and ongoing operation of an adult day-care-center program.

Adult day-care-center planners are encouraged to work within this systems approach to health planning and along with any area or local planning boards if they are to provide a comprehensive range of services that will allow more choice and help ensure quality of life for many elderly.

Model Coordination Projects

Increasing numbers of communities are engaging in projects to decrease costs of services to the elderly and enhance coordination and delivery of a comprehensive range of services. Means to do this range from the establishment of information-sharing committees and task forces, composed of representatives from various elder-concerned service agencies, to full-scale government-supported construction projects, in which complexes of services are linked together.

The following four projects each presents a unique contribution toward the coordination of services for the elderly:

1. Project Triage, Connecticut
2. Holyoke Geriatric Authority, Massachusetts
3. Project Find, New York City
4. Friendship Center, New York City

Project Triage, Connecticut

The trend toward exploration of expansion of community-based services rather than institutionalization for the elderly encouraged the state of Connecticut to undertake a study in 1972 to determine what elder services were available in the state to enable a person to remain at home rather than be institutionalized. The results of the study indicated that not much was available for the elderly and that what services were available were fragmented and difficult to utilize because of third-party insurance constraints.[15]

As a result of the study, federal funding was awarded for a research and demonstration project that would provide a coordinated system of care for the elderly in a seven-town region in central Connecticut. The objectives of the program were:

1. To develop a single entry point for evaluation of all needs of the elderly. An assessment team, composed of a nurse-clinician and a social worker, was formed. Upon receiving a referral, the team would conduct an in-depth, multifaceted assessment of the participant in his or her home. A plan of care would then be developed by the team, in conjunction with the client and

the family. This plan would be initiated, referrals made, and services coordinated with the appropriate health-care and social-service agencies.
2. To create new services when gaps existed. (This objective included the development of a meals program.)
3. To develop an integrated service-delivery system at the local level. Initial plans called for the coordination to occur solely between existing agencies in the area, without any superimposed coordinating agency. However, experience soon showed that the providers did not want to be coordinated and that the plan would not work. The triage system was then devised as the primary screening and referral mechanism, which might also be thought of as "the interface between the consumer and the system."
4. To develop financial support for the full spectrum of care. Due to the problems with traditional third-party insurance-reimbursement mechanisms, the project was granted special waivers of many of the Medicare restrictions. In essence, these waivers enabled Project Triage to proceed unhindered by many of the funding constraints usually present in home health care. The project also became the primary clearinghouse for all expenses accrued by an individual, including all medical and social-services expenses for both inpatient and at-home care and support.
5. To explore the value of preventive and supportive services.
6. To demonstrate the cost-effectiveness of coordinated care. Cost-effectiveness was explored from the aspects of both the outcomes and benefits to the individual and the results on total costs to the federal government. In order to test the triage model, a control group was formed, consisting of elderly citizens in neighboring communities who were going through the traditional long-term-care system. Periodic evaluation of both groups is ongoing.

The study results reveal that Project Triage, a system of coordinating services, has made a difference, and that the objectives named above were met. Preliminary findings had indicated that, compared with the federal government Medicare expenditures of 1976 for those greater than 65 years of age, Project Triage resulted in a decreased percentage of expenditures for the areas of inpatient hospitalization and physician services. As expected, the percentage of Triage monies spent on home care for the year 1976 was above the government percentage of Medicare monies spent on home services. The final study results have demonstrated that a comprehensive array of medical and social services can be provided for the elderly at a cost that is not significantly higher than the cost of delivering fewer, more fragmented, services to a comparable group served within the traditional system.

The Project Triage experience has also provided recommendations for change in our traditional health-care delivery system for the elderly. In 1981, several of the recommendations have been implemented through changes in the traditional payment mechanisms for home health care.

Geriatric Authority, Holyoke, Massachusetts

Another project addressing the issue of coordination of services for the elderly, but on a smaller scale than the coordination evident in Project Triage, is one undertaken by a municipal group in Holyoke, Massachusetts. The Geriatric Authority of Holyoke was formed as an autonomous public organization to provide direction to the project and a means of acquiring and channeling the funds for the development of a geriatric campus or village.

In 1973, the Geriatric Authority of Holyoke received monies from the Administration on Aging to assist the planning process, which included a community-wide survey and assessment of existing services, and which identified needs of the elderly of Holyoke. Efforts were then directed toward obtaining funding to construct the type of geriatric center that was needed by the community. The center now houses both a skilled and an intermediate nursing-care facility, a supportive-services center, administrative offices, rehabilitation services, food services, dining and recreational areas, and health-care facilities. Transportation is provided within the complex and is extended to the surrounding community. A geriatric outpatient clinic is also available, and funding was recently pursued for low-income housing that would include both congregate housing and independent housing for the elderly. An adult day-care center opened in Holyoke in December of 1977, and a second adult day-center opened at the geriatric center in 1979.

The Geriatric Village in Holyoke is designed to offer a wide variety of residential and supportive services in one location to elders in order to assist them in maintaining their optimal independence.

Project Find, New York City

Project Find is a community-based senior-citizen program that encompasses a network of service sites, two multipurpose senior citizen centers, two coffee houses, two nutrition programs, and an information and referral booth in the waiting room of the New York Port Authority bus terminal. Project Find also sponsors low-rent housing units, a hotel for senior citizens in Times Square, and participates in the CETA (Comprehensive Education and Training Act) Adult Work Experience Program.

This comprehensive program of senior services on Manhattan's West Side began in 1967 as one of the demonstration projects funded through the National Council on Aging with federal Office of Economic Opportunity funds. The entire project began with an extensive survey and documentation of community needs.

As the project developed, programs and services were added according to an established priority plan. Currently over 4000 senior citizens are served by the range of these programs.

Friendship Center, New York City

Another program for the elderly in New York City is called Friendship Center. This service project started in 1973 and is sponsored by the Community Service Society of New York City and the New York City Department for the Aging, with assistance from grants received from the National Institute of Mental Health, the Federal Administration on Aging, and Bellevue Hospital. The store-front center is based on a busy inner-city street in a highly populated neighborhood of elderly people. It is geared towards providing services to the more disoriented and frail elderly rather than the more healthy elderly, who are more socially active.

This service model offers a drop-in center that provides group socialization, information and referral, advocacy, consultation, escort services, shopping assistance, case-management, health screening at weekly mini-clinics, and visits to homebound elderly. In 1977, nutrition services were added through congregate meal sites and Meals-on-Wheels. The program's aims are to serve the less able and more isolated elderly and make referrals to other appropriate community resources.

The success of the Friendship Center paved the way for the 19th establishment of the Frail Elderly Team Program in another section of New York City. Here the same types of services are available. The New York programs of comprehensive services provide necessary supports at easily accessible, community-based centers that emphasize prevention of isolation and early detection of illness.

Theoretical Model

The integrated community-services model presented in Figure 3-4 is based on the concept of providing a single entry point into an integrated system of health-care and social services—a single entry point that is readily accessible to those in need of assistance. This single-entry point would consist of an intake and assessment process conducted by a multidisciplinary assessment team, whose members would be drawn from community representatives in the fields of health care, social services, mental health, and housing. The core of the team might consist of a nurse and a social worker.

This team of professionals would be responsible for conducting an assessment of the person's need for services and care. The team, in conjunction with the participant and family, would determine what level and type of assistance are needed and then develop a plan to mobilize and implement the appropriate resources. The primary responsibility for mobilizing these resources would be delegated to the assessment team, but it might be possible, and very appropriate,

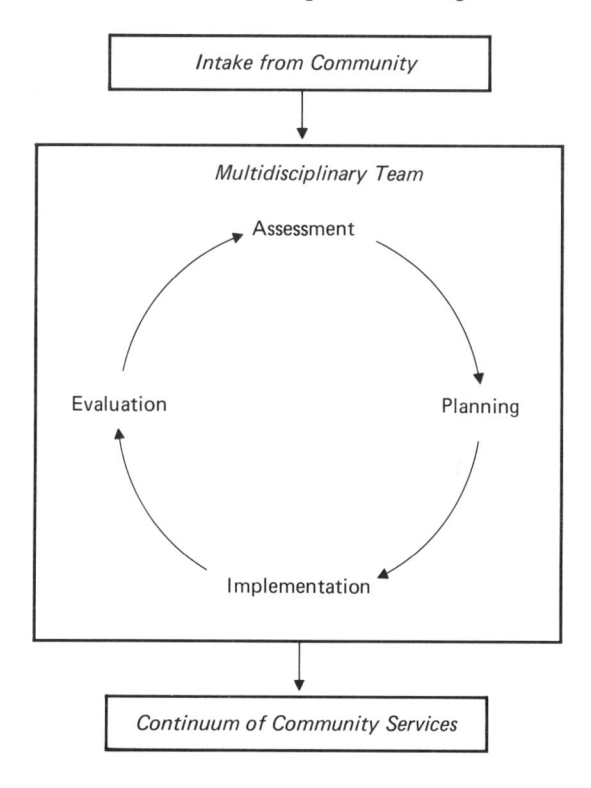

```
                    Intake from Community
                              │
                              ▼
        ┌─────────────────────────────────────────┐
        │         Multidisciplinary Team          │
        │                                         │
        │              Assessment                 │
        │           ╱           ╲                 │
        │     Evaluation         Planning         │
        │           ╲           ╱                 │
        │            Implementation               │
        │                                         │
        └─────────────────────────────────────────┘
                              │
                              ▼
                Continuum of Community Services
```

Figure 3-4. Integrated Community-Services Network

to incorporate the participant and family in this process. As an example of the process, the initial assessment might establish a need for assistance with shopping and light housekeeping; the area home-care corporation would then be contacted by the social worker on the assessment team, and the services would be readily put into motion. Too often, in our present services "nonsystem," this process is unnecessarily delayed as the elderly person attempts to telephone inappropriate resources in the community, resulting in undue frustration on both the part of the person needing assistance and the agency personnel, who have spent costly time and energy fielding an inappropriate request. Obviously there would need to be a substantial amount of public relations and consumer education to ensure that the persons in the community were knowledgeable about the initial intake process.

If it is determined at any given time (by the service or care providers or by the participant) that a change in the level or type of service is needed, the situation would be referred back to the primary assessment team for reevaluation and development of another component of the plan.

Joan Quinn, the project director of the triage program in Connecticut, a single-entry-services project, terms this type of an assessment system the "interfacing component" between the consumer and the various community agencies. The responsibility for and task of "wading through" the requirements and restrictions of the respective programs are lifted from the consumers and delegated to the assessment team.

A separate bureaucracy for coordination is established to conduct the processes of intake assessment, referral, case management, and overall evaluation of services. In essence, one is describing the planning process—the need for careful assessment and development of objectives and a plan of care for an elderly person—and then the implementation of the plan through services mobilization and ongoing evaluation of those services. The "planning" functions of this multidisciplinary team become superimposed over the continuum of health-care and social services (see Figure 3-4).

The rationale for this kind of system—that is, for the development of a separate bureaucracy to assume the responsibility of coordination, rather than simply stating that the coordination will occur between existing agencies—is based on the following assumptions:

1. The availability of services in a community does not necessarily ensure accessibility and coordination of service delivery. If mere availability did ensure accessibility and coordination, our present "system" of health-care and social services for the elderly would not be as confusing and fragmented as it is.
2. Developing an integrated service-delivery system at the local level that depends upon the incorporation of the appropriate personnel in all present agencies and service organizations is unrealistic. This kind of planning would be very costly to agencies, and the burden of this cost could not readily be assumed by agencies whose resources are already stretched to the limit in order to meet their primary functions.

The kind of system described has potential for, and would be well suited to, a series of computer-based programs that could assist the transition stages with any change in the individual's health status or needs. Obviously there are restrictions to this kind of proposal. Funding for such a wide-scale project is a key issue; yet, as described in the triage project discussed earlier, it is a problem with possible solutions.

Another major concern is that of providing the appropriate personnel for the multidisciplinary assessment team. This team serves as the key link for ongoing case management and information and referral. Since these are two major functions presently performed by many elder social-service agencies and AAAs, it does not seem illogical that these existing agencies could assume the assessment responsibility, especially with some expansion of current services and funding to include long-term-care team members attuned to assessment skills and resources available within the community.

Summary

The long-term-care resources discussed in this chapter admittedly do not include all possible resources available within every community; the resources chosen were those familiar to, and deemed most appropriate by, the author. Yet, whatever the community, the primary issue is that adult day-care-center planners be aware of the various resources currently within the specific community and incorporate key community people and agency representatives in the initial planning, implementation, and ongoing update of the services of the adult day-care center. It is also important that this new awareness not be limited by local boundaries, but be expanded to consideration and incorporation of current research and trends in regional, state, and national long-term-care-services planning and delivery.

Recent trends within society and the health-care system have provided the incentive for a major exploration of community-based options of long-term care for the elderly and chronically disabled. A well-planned adult day-care center with close ties to the appropriate health and social services within the community is a long-term-care option that more communities need to consider. All comprehensive long-term-care planners should address adult day-care centers as a viable option within a coordinated range-of-services continuum if we are truly to profess that "health care is a right and not a privilege [with] options available and accessible for all."[16]

References

1. Hyman HH: *Health Planning A Systematic Approach*. Germantown, Md, Aspen Systems Corporation, 1975, p 77.

2. Crawford CO, Leadley SM: Interagency collaboration for planning and delivery of health care. *FCH Community Assessment,* Nov 20, 1978, pp 43–44.

3. *Statement Encouraging Parallel Services*. Burlington, Mass, Association of Massachusetts Homes for the Aging, Inc, 1979, p 1.

4. *Home Health Care Report on the Regional Public Hearings, Sept 20–October 11, 1976*. DHEW Publication No. 76-135. Dept of Health, Education and Welfare, 1976, p 3.

5. Zelten RA, Bray S (eds): *Health Maintenance Organizations*. Presentations to the 1976 Training Program in Health Maintenance Organization Management, Leonard Davis Institute of Health Economics, the Wharton School, University of Pennsylvania, May, 1977. Philadelphia, University of Pennsylvania, 1977.

6. *A Directory of Neighborhood Health Centers in Massachusetts*. Roxbury, Mass, Massachusetts League of Neighborhood Health Centers, 1976, p 6.

7. Carp, FM: The concept and role of congregate housing for older people, in *Congregate Housing for Older People: An Urgent Need, A Growing Demand*. Selected papers from the First National Conference on Congregate Housing for Older People conducted by The International Center for Social Gerontology, DHEW Publication No. (OHD) 77-20284, United States Dept of HEW, 1977, p 3.

8. Williams C: *Congregate Housing for Older People in Massachusetts. A Staff Report*. Boston, Citizens Housing and Planning Association, Inc, 1978, p 1.

9. *Random House Dictionary of the English Language,* college ed, sv "respite."

10. Rezendes D, Abbott J: Hospice movement: Way stations for the terminally ill. *Perspectives on Aging* **8:** 6, 1979.

11. *Health Care at Home: An Essential Component of a National Health Policy*. Kansas City, Mo, American Nurses Association, Publication No. CH-9 3M, 1978.

12. *A Prospectus for a National Home Care Policy*. Prepared by the Assembly of Ambulatory and Home Care Services, American Hospital Association; Council of Home Health Agencies and Community Health Services, National League for Nursing; National Association of Home Health Agencies; National Council of Homemaker-Home Health Aide Service, Inc., 1978. DHEW Grant # HSA 77-88(p) 4/26/77.

13. Summary of the Older Americans Act, (P.L. 95-478) in *Aging Program Factsheets*. National Association of Counties Research Foundation, Wash DC, November 1978, pp 1–6.

14. Benedict RC: Making the health care system responsive to the needs of the elderly. *Aging,* May-June, 1979, p 25.

15. Quinn J: Triage: Coordinated home care for the elderly. *Nursing Outlook* **23:** 570, 1975.

16. Mitchell M: Long term care. *Hospitals,* Apr 1, 1972, p 23, cited in *Nursing and Long Term Care: Towards Quality Care for the Aging*. Kansas City, Mo, American Nurses' Association, 1974, p 64.

4

Needs Assessment: Methods and Data Sources

Elizabeth Ballas Daly, RN, MSN, DNSc

Introduction

Before long-term-care planners can begin planning for long-term-care services for the elderly, needs and discrepancies between what is and what is desired must be identified and defined. Thus, at the very core of planning is an assessment of needs. The first step in this process is the collection of pertinent information about the community or geographic area of concern.

What kinds of information are important for assessment of the elderly population's needs? While this may appear to be a very simple question, the answer is far from simple. There is no apparent agreement about the depth or breadth of knowledge that is specific for determining the health problems of an elderly population group residing in some particular area. However, experience has shown that baseline data can provide the kind of information necessary for planning adult day-care programs. Certain kinds of factual information can provide an overall picture and serve as a framework for the identification of chronic problems of the elderly, from which long-term-care needs can be determined—of which nursing and social needs are an inherent part. This chapter presents the kind of data considered baseline, as a guide to long-term-care planners, so that the multitude of factors relating to the health and social needs of elderly population groups can be viewed in their proper perspective and relationship. The kind of information collected falls into two broad categories: (1) data about the community and (2) information about an elderly population group.

Much of the information relative to a community and specific age group, such as the elderly age 65 and over, can be found in summary form from census reports, annual reports, records, and survey studies that already have been done. Thus, long-term-care planners in studying the needs of an elderly population group and a community should first find out whether pertinent and related studies have already been done, what kinds of information can be obtained from key professionals, organizations, and agencies in the community of concern before launching into additional surveys. This chapter presents some of the major sources of information. Existing survey summaries, statistics, and annual reports can save precious time and money.

Although much of the data required to identify needs is available at the national, state, and regional levels, often such data are neither reported, assembled, nor documented at the local level; thus, the planner may be faced with an inadequate data base. In such cases, planners can collect pertinent data about an elderly population group through other various data-collection methods that have been used or developed to determine health-care needs of population groups. This data collection does, however, require some basic understanding of the research process and the scientific method. Although somewhat complex, the research process is a logical and systematic progression through a number of steps in an orderly fashion and should conform to scientific principles so that the information produced is explicit, objective, and reliable.

This chapter presents data-collection methods that have been used or developed to determine the needs of population groups within the framework of scientific research in order to encourage the formulation of a data base that is objective and reliable. No attempts are made to determine the best method of collecting data for a particular situation since it is not possible to know all the circumstances under which particular methods will be used. Furthermore, the various methods of data collection noted in this chapter may vary considerably in complexity, cost, usefulness to the planner, and length of time needed to obtain the information. Planners will therefore be faced with making decisions concerning which method to use and the appropriate technique for the method. However, the amount of time/cost expended may be minimal in terms of the data's usefulness in presenting a picture of the needs of the elderly in their proper perspective.

The chapter first introduces some important concepts and ideas used throughout this book and then proceeds to a description of a defined data base, existing sources from which data may be obtained, and data-collection methods.

Basic Concepts

Needs Assessment

A needs assessment is generally undertaken by individuals, groups, or agencies that have a service component, such as long-term-care facilities, hospitals, and community-service organizations. In each case there is some desire to learn about the needs of elderly persons. A nursing home, for example, may wish to assess the needs of the elderly in the community or communities they serve. Thus, a needs assessment may be designed to

1. describe an existing situation
2. explain circumstances
3. extend existing knowledge
4. verify past trends and currently existing knowledge

We have previously indicated that a needs assessment is an important component of research. As such, we have defined this concept in the following way, based on several characteristics of scientific research:[1(p11), 2(pp20-21)]

> A needs assessment is a systematic, empirical and critical investigatory process aimed at obtaining and discovering relevant facts and information that may ultimately lead to revisions or confirmation of accepted beliefs (theories or laws) in light of new information and facts.

Several points made in the above definition need to be emphasized and clarified. First, a needs assessment that is systematic means, in effect, that the approach used to acquire information and facts is so ordered and disciplined that long-term-care planners, community people, and health-care and social-service professionals, organizations, and agencies can have confidence in the assessment outcomes.

Second, a needs assessment that is empirical is one in which the investigation is grounded in reality and experience, as opposed to an assessment based on personal beliefs. The planner who conducts an empirical assessment is essentially subjecting certain held beliefs about the needs of an elderly population group to a test in the real world. Objectivity is imposed on the assessment situation, including the data-collection situation.

Lastly, a needs assessment that is a critical investigation is one that involves careful judgment throughout the process. Judgments must be made concerning the appropriate assessment approach, reliable data sources, and reliable and objective methods of collecting data. Judgments must also be made about what types of information to collect and what constitutes enough information. It would be presumptuous to claim that a planner must have *all* the facts about an elderly population group in order to gain some understanding of its health-care needs. However, that which is believed significant and relevant must be sorted out from that which is irrelevant.

Data

Data are all the pieces of information that the health-care planner systematically collects in the process of implementing the first step in a needs assessment. Data can be, for example, the number of elderly persons residing in a particular area, obtained from a census report; the number of disabled elderly, obtained from surveys or statistical reports; or the number of potential referrals to an adult day-care program, obtained from various community groups and agencies.

Data can also be numbers obtained through questionnaires; for example, a long-term-care planner might wish to know the degree of interest disabled elderly persons might have in adult day-care services if they were made available. Subjects might be asked to rate themselves on a four-point scale, ranging from very interested to no interest. In this example, two pieces of information would be generated: the number of disabled elderly persons and the degree of their interest in adult day-care services. Data can also be in the form of opinions, attitudes, and descriptions of the elderly in need of services. This information can be obtained through interviews with key health professionals or through a literature search. It is from data carefully collected and summarized that the health-care planner seeks to describe, understand, explain, and verify a situation and then to make suggestions, recommendations, or predictions.

Baseline Data

Baseline data are all the information or facts that provide a foundation for making an evaluation based on preestablished criteria. Planners, for example, who desire to become adult day-care providers are frequently required to submit an application or proposal to some particular authoritative body. Such proposals include supporting documentation of need for a day-care program. The supporting documentation or baseline data are frequently evaluated on criteria such as degree of need in the community or geographic area for an adult day-care program; the poverty or income levels of persons age 65 and over; functional status and health statistics of persons age 65 and over; and the degree of support and cooperation of health professionals, organizations, and agencies in the area to be served. Baseline data must be of the utmost concern since any type of evaluation made will be affected by both the quality and completeness of the data base.

The feasibility of acquiring a complete data base or all possible information and facts will vary for a variety of reasons, such as the availability of specific information, the cost and time in collecting necessary information, and differences between data-collection methods. Time is an important factor. Collecting data for a needs assessment may require days, weeks, or even months. However, health care planners are encouraged to make a concerted and conscientious effort to obtain at least baseline data that reflects in an objective manner the need for new and different organizational structures and processes for care of the elderly.

If information to be collected is determined in advance, both the quality and completeness of the data base can be enhanced. Time can be devoted to collecting necessary information and facts rather than to figuring out which data should be collected. The following outline defines baseline data as an overall guide for the health-care planner interested in determining the needs of some particular elderly population group. Long-term-care planners interested in applying to become adult day-care providers or interested in submitting a grant proposal may also find the baseline-data guide useful. It should be noted that the ordering of the items presented may vary with the organizational format of some application forms. However, the basic elements within each section should be included at some point in the proposal.*

Baseline-Data Guide

Baseline data as defined here include data concerning two major areas: the community and the elderly population group. These data are further broken down into categories of indicators: demographic, socioeconomic, environmental, health-status, and long-term-care system. These indicators are generally associated with the long-term needs of the elderly, and thus data are collected relative to these items.

Long-term-care indicators deal with information relative to the potential demand for adult day-care services. Factors such as accessibility, availability, and acceptability can determine the degree to which population groups who have long-term-care needs will translate those needs into a demand for long-term-care services. Thus, the planner should obtain data relative to the number of potential elderly who might benefit from adult day-care services and who are willing to attend such a program in the area of concern.

The planner may begin with any category of items. Ultimately information should be obtained regarding all the categories of indicators, as well as a brief description of the community of concern. The following guide outlines the information that should be collected.

 I. Data Concerning the Community
  A. Describe the community, town, or geographic area of concern. Record the community, town, or geographic area of concern by name. If a

---

*The planner is referred to "Writing Project Applications for Funding"[3] for further tips and discussion relative to the writing of a proposal.

number of towns are being assessed as a collective, record the name of the collective.
   B. Record the total number of people residing in the area of concern.
   C. Obtain a map of the area of concern. At some point in time, all long-term-care facilities can be recorded on the map, as well as barriers and road patterns.
II. Data Concerning the Elderly Population
   A. *Demographic Indicators*
      1. Obtain and record the total number of persons age 65 or over in the area of concern. When a number of towns are involved, the sum total of persons age 65 and over is recorded, as well as the number of elderly in *each* town.
      2. Obtain and record the percent of the total population age 65 and over. Compare this data with data from adjoining communities, the state, or the nation as a whole. Describe statistics that are higher at the local level.
      3. Obtain and record projected population estimates of persons age 65 and over for *each* town or community. Note whether projections have already been reached.
      4. Obtain and record population trends. In particular, note and describe increases occurring in the past five years.
      5. Describe the mobility patterns of the elderly population group in each town or community.
   B. *Socioeconomic Indicators*
      1. Obtain and record the number or percent of the total population with income levels below the poverty line ($5,000 or below).
      2. Obtain and record the number or percent of elderly population with income levels below the poverty line ($5,000 or below).
      3. Obtain and record the number or percent of elderly receiving welfare assistance. Compare this data with data from adjoining communities, the state, or the nation as a whole. Describe statistics that are higher in the area of concern than those of another community, the state, or the nation as a whole.
   C. *Environmental Indicators*
      1. Describe transportation patterns and routes to existing long-term-care facilities.
      2. Identify and describe densely populated areas. Note those areas in which large numbers of elderly reside.
      3. Describe housing conditions in the area of concern. In addition, note:
         a. percent of the total population lacking some or all plumbing facilities
         b. percent of the total population lacking complete kitchen facilities

c. percent of the elderly population living in low-income housing.
4. Data on items a, b, and c can be compared with data from another community, the state, or the nation as a whole. Describe statistics that are higher in the area of concern.
D. *Health-Status Indicators*
 1. Obtain and record age-specific death rates by cause for the elderly in the area of concern. Compare data with similar data from adjoining communities, the state, or the nation as a whole. Describe statistics that are higher in the area of concern.
 2. Obtain and record specific disease rates of the elderly population in the area of concern. Compare data with data from adjoining communities, the state, or the nation as a whole. Note statistics that are higher in the area of concern.
 3. Obtain and record functional disability statistics, including the following:
    a. number or percent of elderly limited in ability to work
    b. number or percent of elderly who need assistance in living chores, such as food shopping and preparation and housekeeping
    c. number or percent of elderly who need assistance with personal care
    d. number or percent of elderly with limitation in traveling
    e. number or percent of elderly with limitations in social activities
    f. number or percent of elderly needing medical or social-service assistance on a continuing basis—for example, regular injections, prescription medicines, speech therapy, rehabilitation therapy, professional counseling, nursing services or social services in the home, or special care.
E. *Long-Term-Care-System Indicators*
 1. Identify and state the number of long-term-care facilities serving the elderly in the area of concern (specifically document the lack of). In addition, note:
    a. current bed-occupancy rates in all these facilities
    b. the presence or absence of waiting lists
    c. future plans for building additional facilities
    d. the number of elderly currently residing in long-term-care facilities who might potentially benefit from adult day-care services.
 2. State the presence or absence of all types of adult day-care services in the area of concern, including adult mental-health day care. Some programs service only those with specific conditions, such as mental-health problems.

In summary, we have presented the kind of data relative to community and elderly population group that we believe should be included in a needs assessment.

The next step in a needs assessment process is obtaining this information. The following section presents some of the major data sources available to health-care planners and practitioners.

Data Sources

Once the long-term-care planner has some idea about the kind of information to be included in a needs assessment, the next step is to determine whether studies pertinent to the elderly have already been done; what kinds of information and health-care and social-services data these studies provide; what kind of information can be obtained from the various published sources; and what kind of information can be provided by key health and social-service professionals and key community people and resources.

A large number of data sources are available to the planner. It is most helpful to know these sources, for existing survey summaries, statistical reports, and health-care and social-services data summaries can save both time and money. The major sources for different types of information are listed in Table 4-1.

The *population at risk* indicated in Table 4-1 deals with the number and characteristics of the population under study—the elderly—residing in some geographic area. Germane to the concept of population at risk is the recognition that risks are not evenly distributed throughout the population.[4] Some population groups are more susceptible to illness, disease, disfunctioning, dissatisfaction, and disabilities than are others because of a variety of factors, including age, income level, sex, area of residence, and available health-care services. A population at risk should be specified in order to obtain a descriptive statistic that is relevant for the risk or risks studied.

Table 4-1
Selected health-related data sources

Category of Information	Data Sources
Population at Risk	
Census profile	U.S. Bureau of the Census
Population estimates	U.S. Bureau of the Census Federal-State Cooperative Program for Local Population Estimates
Distribution of the elderly, age groups	Local agencies: summary reports State health departments Universities Local planning agencies City planning department

Table 4-1 (*continued*)

Category of Information	Data Sources
Health Status	
Vital statistics Mortality data	Death certificates U.S. Bureau of Vital Statistics City or town reports
Morbidity data	National Center for Health Statistics Disease registries Local surveys Public health department, health agencies State health-data annual reports
Disability data	Industry records Mental-retardation registries Disability claims Welfare programs for the blind or partially disabled School records Home health-agency records Visiting Nurse Association records Uniform Hospital Abstracts Local surveys State and local mental-health authorities Employment commissions State and local family-service authorities Human-service councils Public-welfare department Health-systems agencies State administrators of vocational rehabilitation American Board of Physical Medicine and Rehabilitation National Center for Health Statistics
Inpatient Facilities and Services	
Characteristics of facilities	Hospitals Administrators Nursing homes Extended-care facilities National Center for Health Statistics American Hospital Association Joint Commission on Accreditation of Hospitals Licensure boards Professional organizations Chambers of commerce Department of Public Health: health-data annual reports (nursing homes and extended-care facilities included)
Capacity of facilities	Hospital reports State Hospital Association Hill-Burton Agency

Table 4-1 (*continued*)

Category of Information	Data Sources
Capacity of facilities (*continued*)	American Hospital Association National Center for Health Statistics Cost-review commissions

Services and utilization	Boards of health
	Hospital associations
	   American Hospital Association Guide
	   Hospital Statistics
	   Area Resource File
	Hospital records
	Nursing-home records
	Department of Public Health (nursing homes and extended-care facilities included)
	State health-data annual reports
	State and local health-planning agencies
	Extended-care facilities' records/reports
	Special studies
	Directories of nursing-home facilities

Mental health	Psychiatric hospitals Mental-health agencies Department of Health, Education and Welfare National Institute of Mental Health Police reports
Road patterns to health care	Local planning commissions, road maps, chambers of commerce
Status and disposition of elderly clients	Individual hospitals that utilize the hospital-abstract system or aggregated data from reports or commissions Hospital continuing-care departments Hospital home-health-care coordinators Visiting-nurse associations Survey data Health professionals: physicians, social workers, directors of nursing Meals-on-Wheels organizations Nursing homes Extended-care facilities Councils on aging Elderly self-reports Family reports
Payment for services	Social Security Administration Social and rehabilitation services Blue Cross–Blue Shield, *Source Book of Health Insurance Data* State and local governments Hospitals Social-service agencies Government finance agencies State welfare departments

Table 4-1 (*continued*)

Category of Information	Data Sources
Quality of care	National Center for Health Statistics: length-of-stay statistics
	Professional Activity Study, Medical Audit Program
	Hospitals, nursing homes, extended-care facilities, community health agencies
	Commission on Professional and Hospital Activities
	Professional Standards Review Organization
	Discharge abstract systems (ambulatory and hospital)
	Individual facilities
	Hospital commissions
	Surveys, research reports
Home Care	
Admission or intake data	Home-health agencies
	Health departments
Ongoing-service data	Homemaker-service organizations
Discharge data	Visiting Nurse Association
	Social-services agencies
	Meals-on-Wheels organizations

From *Guide to Data for Health System Planning and Resources: Health Planning Information Series.* U.S. Department of Health, Education and Welfare, 1976.

Once the population-at-risk descriptive statistic is determined—providing a population count of the *total number of elderly* residing in a defined area of concern—it can serve as a *denominator* for purposes of constructing rates, ratios, and percentages. The *numerator* would be the *actual* or *estimated* number of persons having long-term-care needs, including those with temporary or long-term reduction in activities who are potentially in need of health-care and human services, such as adult day-care services.

The *numerator* (estimated number of elderly in need) and the *denominator* (the total number of elderly residing in an area of concern) provide an index relevant to the particular elderly population at risk. The objective of producing such a statistic is to describe the elderly population as clearly and accurately as possible. For example, 25 disabled elderly in an area comprising 1500 persons 65 years and over might constitute a need for adult day-care services, whereas in another area comprising 10,000 persons 65 years of age and over, the need for adult day-care services for 25 disabled elderly might be given low priority.

Selected Health-related Data Sources

Planners needing a more specific total population count can often obtain such data from agencies or universities involved with the U.S. Bureau of the Census in the Federal-State Cooperative Program for Local Population Estimates—a program in which the federal government works with states to produce "official" population estimates for state and federal programs requiring such figures. A selected list of agencies currently involved in this program is given in Appendix B.

Population estimates can also be obtained from many state, regional, and local areas that conduct their own surveys. Long-term-care planners and practitioners conducting needs assessments should not overlook findings from previous surveys conducted by health agencies, social organizations, small towns, city health-related departments, and local university graduate students. Before launching time-consuming and costly investigations, planners should investigate whether previous work already exists and whether previous findings are related to present needs-assessment investigations.

Data Sources by Health-Need Indicators

The major indicators generally associated with the health status and health needs of the elderly are listed in Table 4-2. These indicators can be used in various combinations to determine health needs. The various sources from which information can be secured regarding the indicators are also listed.

Table 4-2
Data sources by health-need indicators

Health-Need Indicators	Data Sources
Demographic	

Elderly population
  Age distribution
  Sex distribution
  Mobility patterns
  Population trends
	Town census reports
	State census reports
	U.S. Census Bureau reports: summaries by state
	Obtained from: local town halls, health departments, planning councils, and libraries

Socioeconomic	
Number of persons receiving public assistance (specifically elderly)	Local or state department of social welfare or social service
Number of elderly receiving medicaid	
Number of elderly receiving Medicare	Social Security Administration: local offices
Income levels of area by age	Local or state department of social welfare or social service

Table 4-2   (*continued*)

Health-Need Indicators	Data Sources
Environmental	
Location of health and other related facilities	Local planning councils, maps, chambers of commerce
Traffic patterns and routes to health-care facilities	
Natural barriers	
Housing conditions	Local planning councils, government, state or local-survey summary reports found in local health departments, councils on aging
Transportation services for elderly and disabled	

Health-Need Indicators	Data Sources
Health-Status	
Age-specific death rates by cause and residence	State profiles of mortality data by area of residence: reports found in university, local libraries; state or local health departments; area-wide planning councils; local office of vital statistics; local surveys
Incidence of specific diseases	State profiles of morbidity: the same as above; also local surveys done by some health-related agencies
Functional disability annually per 1000 population	
Incidence or prevalence of impairment	

Long-Term-Care System	

Long-term-care facilities
  Number and type
  Location
  Admission policies
  Number of beds
  Referral mechanisms
  Occupancy rates
  Number of elderly who might benefit from adult day care
	Agency administrators
	Published reports found at state or local health departments, area-wide planning councils

Health-Need Indicators	Data Sources
All Other Health-related Agencies	
Number of elderly served Types of conditions Admission policies Occupancy rates Location Services provided Referral mechanism Elderly who might benefit from adult day care	Directors, hospital administrators, Department of Mental Health administrator or director Department of Health and hospital administrators or directors State or local health departments

State Units on Aging

State units on aging have been listed frequently in the preceding data sources. The National Association of State Units on Aging should facilitate the collection of data from more than one state.

Gerontology Centers

Many colleges and universities have developed centers for study of the elderly. These centers frequently do original research; hold workshops, courses, conferences, and summer institutes; accumulate all available data pertinent to the elderly; disseminate this information both to professionals and to the lay public; and act as a general resource center.

Professional Organizations

Professional organizations should not be overlooked as they also may be able to provide the long-term-care planner and practitioner with valuable information. Many organizations regularly publish information useful to planners, and many have state, regional, or local chapters. The organizations listed in Figure 4-1 can provide information pertinent to the elderly.

Although much of the data deemed necessary for a needs assessment of population groups is available at the national, state, and regional levels, data are often absent at the local community level. The planner should thus determine what kind of information existing survey statistics and studies provide. Any other information considered essential for a minimum data set can be identified and obtained through various data collection methods that have been used or developed by the health-care system to determine health-care needs of population groups. Several methods are briefly discussed in the following section, with particular emphasis being given to the questioning method. A more in-depth study and discussion of observation and measurement methods can be obtained from almost any introductory book on research.[1,2]

Data-Collection Methods and Techniques

Data can be collected by a number of techniques. All of these techniques are, however, variations of three methods: observation, measurement, and questioning. In general, most long-term-care practitioners and planners are already familiar with the observation method, whereby data are collected by observing phenomenon. Measurement is a research method in which data are obtained through the application of measuring instruments, such as those concerned with physical measurement, chemical measurement, or microbiological measurement.[2(p275)] Questioning is a research method whereby information is collected through the use of a formal instrument, such as an interview schedule or questionnaire. It is

```
                    DATA SOURCES

American Association of Homes for the Aging
    347 National Press Bldg., Washington, D.C. 20004
American Association for Hospital Planning
    2284 Main St., Concord, Mass. 01742
American Board of Preventive Medicine
    615 North Wolfe St., Baltimore, Md. 21205
American Cancer Society
    219 E. 42nd St., New York, N.Y. 10017
American Geriatrics Society
    10 Columbus Circle, New York, N.Y. 10019
American Medical Association
    535 N. Dearborn St., Chicago, Ill. 60610
American Nurses Association
    2420 Pershing Rd., Kansas City, Mo. 64108
American Nursing Home Association
    1200 15th St., N.W., Washington, D.C. 20005
American Public Health Association
    1015 18th St., N.W., Washington, D.C. 20037
Blue Cross Association
    840 N. Lake Shore Dr., Chicago, Ill. 60611
Community Health Association
    13936 Woodward Ave., Highland Park, Mich. 48203
Joint Commission on Accreditation of Hospitals
    875 N. Michigan Ave., Chicago, Ill. 60611
National Association of Blue Shield Plans
    211 E. Chicago Ave., Chicago, Ill. 60611
National Council on the Aging
    1828 L St., N.W., #504, Washington, D.C. 20036
National Geriatrics Society
    212 W. Wisconsin Ave., Milwaukee, Wisc. 53203
National League for Nursing
    10 Columbus Circle, New York, N.Y. 10019
```

Figure 4.1. Professional Organizations as Data Sources (From *Guide to Data for Health System Planning and Resources: Health Planning Information Series.* U.S. Department of Health, Education and Welfare, 1976.)

this last method and the two techniques within this method—interviews and questionnaires—that will be described in this section.

Due to the formidable nature of dealing with all aspects of questioning, such as the development of appropriate questions, we cannot do more than introduce the planner to the several options available within the questioning method for purposes of collecting reliable and valid data.[10] No attempts are made to determine the best technique for a particular situation since it is not possible to know all the circumstances under which particular methods and/or techniques will be used.

Long-term-care planners frequently use both techniques—interviews and questionnaires—profitably to supplement one another in a single needs-assessment study of elderly population groups. The techniques described in this section are not mutually exclusive. They can be used in combination as parts of an integrated, sequential assessment project or they can be used independently of one another.

The long-term-care planner who has a clear understanding of the advantages of the two techniques, however, will be in a position to make a decision on the appropriate instrument for collecting data in a particular situation. Thus, the advantages of the two techniques are also described in this section.

Questioning Methods and Techniques

Survey research studies large or small populations.[1(p410)] Its principal method of gathering information is through questioning subjects. Questioning subjects is generally accomplished through use of formal instruments, such as the interview schedule or the questionnaire.

The interview. The interview is probably the oldest and most often-used technique for obtaining information from people—a technique not unfamiliar to most health-care and social-service professionals. An interview, when used with a well-developed and designed schedule, can obtain a wealth of information. Such a technique is most frequently used in face-to-face situations or over the telephone. Using the interview schedule as a guide, the interviewer poses questions for the respondents and records the responses.

There are two types of interview schedules: structured and unstructured.[5,6] In the structured interview, the planner determines in advance both the questions and the content of the responses in terms of the choices offered the respondents. This type of question is commonly referred to as "closed-ended." The respondents must choose from a number of alternatives the one that best approximates the "right" answer. Alternatives can range from a simple yes/no to complex expressions of behavior. An example of a closed-ended type of question, with a set of rather complex response options, is presented in Figure 4-2. Since a structured interview format should also be designed for easy analysis, Figure 4-2 also illustrates the checklist format.

The unstructured interview, on the other hand, poses questions to the respondent without offering possible answers. The respondent must decide on both the content and form of the response. This type of question is commonly referred to as "open-ended" or "free-response." In this style of questioning, questions are generally asked of each respondent in the same way and in the same order. The interviewer records the responses verbatim, or as close to it as possible.

The questionnaire. The questionnaire technique is not unlike the interview technique in that the nature of the questions posed may include mul-

---
CLOSED-ENDED QUESTION

Which of these three statements best describes your present transportation pattern?

☐ 1. I am completely free to go and return as I want.
☐ 2. I go out for most things I need.
☐ 3. I only go out for special occasions and/or basic necessities.

Figure 4-2. Example of a Closed-ended Question

tiple-choice, checklist, open-ended or free responses, or any combination of these. The major difference is that the questionnaire is self-administered by respondents. In most cases, the planner is not present when respondents complete the questionnaire. Many questionnaires are mailed to respondents.

Regardless of the type of questions posed, the respondent should have absolutely no doubt about what is expected. Thus, everything asked should be clear and defined if necessary. Directions for answering questions should be given, with examples of responses if the questions are complex. Directions should be given on how the questionnaire is to be returned, and self-addressed envelopes should be included to facilitate returns of the questionnaire. Some assurance that the information will be handled in a confidential manner and with anonymity should also be given. Last, but not least, some expression of appreciation for the respondent's cooperation should be stated.

Advantages and Disadvantages of Interviews

The interview technique has several advantages. First, the planner using this technique can know whether the respondent understands the question(s). When misunderstanding occurs, a planner can, within certain limits, restate or rephrase the question. Second, in face-to-face situations, the response rate tends to be very high. Respondents are frequently more reluctant to refuse to answer questions when the interviewer is present. Third, many people cannot fill out questionnaires because of blindness, illiteracy, or some disabling condition. The elderly, for example, may have difficulty with questionnaires because of small print, the texture of the paper, or the length of the questionnaire. The interview technique has the advantage of being potentially feasible with most kinds of people and age groups. Fourth, the level of questioning can be more in-depth than in a questionnaire. In-depth information can be obtained through probing questions. Lastly, the interview technique is relatively inexpensive.

A major shortcoming of this technique, regardless of the type of questions used, is that it takes time. Interviewing elderly subjects can take even longer than expected. Obtaining information from one person can take as long as one or two hours, depending upon the length of the interview schedule. The cost in time can be high.

Advantages and Disadvantages of Questionnaires

A major advantage of using the questionnaire technique is the enumeration of the most valid and reliable information. Because of the impersonal nature of the questionnaire, the planner can generally assume that respondents will be frank, especially if anonymity can be guaranteed. Second, the planner can obtain relatively large samples representative of the total population through mailed questionnaires. In some cases in which the total population is relatively small, such as the total number of elderly residing in some small community, it might be possible to survey most of the total population. Such a survey can enhance both the amount and the quality of the information obtained.

Along with the advantages, there are also some disadvantages to this technique. First, if questionnaires are mailed, there is a tendency for low returns. If returns are low, generalizations cannot be made, and results can be open to question. The second limitation of this technique is the cost involved, especially when large numbers are sampled. The costs of mailing and questionnaire reproduction can be high when sample numbers run high. However, the cost expended may be minimal in terms of the potential usefulness of the data acquired.

Criteria for Data-Collection Techniques

For data-collection instruments, such as a questionnaire or interview schedule, to produce the best results, they must meet the following criteria: (1) reliability, (2) validity, (3) objectivity, and (4) appropriateness.[1(pp442–476), 2(pp421–445)]

Reliability. Reliability is the most important criterion. Reliability is a multidimensional concept, frequently equated with such terms as stability, dependability, consistency, and accuracy. Thus, in one important sense, reliability is the degree of consistency with which an instrument measures some attribute it is supposed to measure. Does the instrument consistently yield the same or similar data results today as it did yesterday? If, for example, the same questions put to elderly persons concerning their ability to carry out activities of daily living were asked over and over again, would the same or similar responses be obtained? Obviously the answers would vary in specific details, but they should be related in nature to the question asked. Another important aspect of reliability is accuracy. An instrument considered reliable is one in which the measures obtained are the "true" measures.

Validity. Validity is the second most important criterion an instrument should meet to ensure quality data. Validity refers to the extent to which an instrument actually measures what it is supposed to measure or what the planner intends it to measure.

Validity is dependent upon reliability—that is, reliability is a precondition for validity. A measurement device or instrument cannot be valid unless it is reliable. However, although perfect reliability may indicate a high possibility for instrument validity, reliability does not indicate the extent to which validity has been achieved. It is possible to have a highly reliable instrument that is not valid; for example, a long-term-care planner might wish to measure the functional-disability status of elderly persons by measuring the number of elderly who have chronic diseases. While accurate information may be obtained about the numbers of elderly with chronic diseases, such measures would not be valid indicators of functional-disability status (see Chapter 5). What, in fact, was measured might be measured quite well, but it did not measure what the long-term-care planner intended.

Objectivity. Objectivity is also a criterion that should be considered in developing or selecting an instrument or measuring device. Objectivity refers to the extent to which information obtained is a function of what is being measured. This ideal can be influenced by a variety of factors. For example, interpersonal relationships in the data-gathering situation can affect objectivity. The face-to-face situation of questioning is particularly sensitive to the loss of objectivity. Ample evidence indicates that a respondent's role behavior can be elicited by the *demand characteristics* of the situation.[7] Respondents may care about the outcome of the data-collection process or investigation and may change their behavior and response content because they wish to help the interviewer. Factors such as age, sex, race, manner of dress, and profession of the interviewer may also affect the data obtained. Thus, in this sense, objectivity of data from the face-to-face interview situation can be suspect.

Another but more subtle factor that can influence objectivity adversely is the nature of the instructions printed on questionnaires. We have previously indicated that directions for answering questions should be included, with examples of responses given if questions are complex, for purposes of facilitating completion of the instrument. However, the response examples should not in any way suggest the content of the responses. Responses may disproportionately reflect the model response. Examples given in the directions should be given from a content area other than the one in which the respondent is expected to answer. In this way objectivity can be maintained.

Objectivity cannot be formally estimated. It is a judgment that the planner must make in the process of developing or selecting a data-collection instrument.

Appropriateness. Appropriateness is a characteristic that must be seen in terms of the relationship of instrument to respondents. This criterion refers to the extent to which respondents can meet the demands imposed upon them by a measurement instrument. Interview and questionnaire instruments place demands upon respondents, ranging from understanding English, reading, writing, and following directions to revealing delicate, sensitive, and personal information. Thus, consideration must be given to the most appropriate means of obtaining information and the types of questions that will best elicit desirable information in the least objectionable way for the particular group of respondents.

Writing Questions

The most difficult aspect of constructing an interview schedule or questionnaire is the writing of the questions. This section introduces a number of considerations that should be taken into account by the long-term-care planner in developing and selecting questions. When confronted with the actual wording of open-ended and closed-ended questions, the planner should consult more extended treatments, since the ensuing discussion is intended only as an introduction.[2(p326),8,9]

It is first necessary to consider the nature of a question. Basically, a question has two elements: the stem itself, which poses the question, and the response or answer. Responses or answers, as we have previously indicated, can vary in their form. Questions can be closed-ended, in which respondents are offered a number of options, or they can be open-ended, in which respondents are not offered any options. If responses or answers are offered, the long-term-care planner is faced with making decisions about the content of the question (the stem) and the form the responses will take if questions are closed-ended. If particular information and facts are desired, the content of the questions will be guided by the planner's particular purposes. Kerlinger offers some useful criteria that can provide a guide in the development and selection of questions.[1(pp485-486)] These criteria are as follows:

1. *Are the questions related to the investigation's objectives?* Each question of an interview or questionnaire should have some particular function—that is, the content of each question should elicit information for certain purposes. For example, a planner might want to know how many elderly people in a small community have limited mobility. The content of the question should be structured in such a way as to elicit information indicating the respondent's mobility limitations. Responses might be offered in the form of a closed-ended question.
2. *Are the questions appropriate?* The planner must decide which question form, closed-ended or open-ended, will best obtain the desired information or material. Closed-ended questions are best for obtaining some information—

such as age (a range of options can be offered), sex (male or female can be checked), income levels (a range of options can be offered)—particularly when all that is required of respondents is their preferred choice.
3. *Are questions clear and unambiguous?* Questions that can be interpreted differently by different people are unlikely to produce meaningful information or reliable information. Statements or response options that are ambiguous invite differing responses. Thus, questions or responses containing two different, distinct ideas should be avoided. The statement "I go out for most things I need or like," might generate responses of both agreement and disagreement by the same respondent.
4. *Do questions suggest an answer?* Leading questions that suggest answers can result in disproportionately large numbers of "yes" or "agree" responses. They should be avoided, otherwise distorted or biased results can occur.
5. *Do the questions consider the ability of respondents to respond?* The planner should not assume that respondents know or understand complex terminology, concepts, or issues familiar to the health-care or social-service professional. Words in each question should be made as simple as possible. Questions should be avoided that might offend respondents or make them feel uncomfortable if they do not know the answer. One way to avoid invalid responses due to lack of information is the use of what is frequently referred to as a filter question. Such questions are posed for the purpose of determining the respondent's level of information before he or she proceeds to questions that might ask for opinions, feelings, or attitudes relevant to a particular subject or topic. For example, before asking a key person in the community about his opinion on adult day-care services in the area, first find out if he knows what adult day-care services are.
6. *Do questions demand personal, sensitive, and delicate information the respondents may not wish to provide?* Questions that deal with sensitive material represent an intrusion on the respondent's privacy. Some respondents may be very willing to participate and answer questions; others may not be so willing. Some useful techniques in dealing more effectively with material of a delicate and personal nature are as follows:

   a. Pose questions of an impersonal nature at the beginning of an interview. Later in the interview, questions of a personal or controversial nature can be asked after a rapport has been established.
   b. Develop unobjectionable questions and response options whenever possible.
   c. Use closed-ended questions in an interview or questionnaire when dealing with sensitive or controversial material. Closed-ended questions are less intrusive than open-ended questions. It is generally easier for a respondent to check off an item that might be socially-disapproved of or sensitive than to verbalize it in response to an open-ended question.

d. Provide a nonjudgmental atmosphere. Indicate that some people behave or believe one way, and others behave and believe another way.
e. Always be courteous, conscientious, and sensitive to the needs of respondents.

In summary, the decision to use open-ended and closed-ended questions must be made by the planner. Decisions can be based on important considerations, such as the amount of time available, the nature of the investigation's objectives, the nature of the population group being investigated, and the cost involved. Planners might use a combination of both types of questions in order to offset the strengths and weaknesses of each.

Application of the Questioning Method

An important approach to research and obtaining data is the research-survey approach. Survey approaches assume that while the data necessary to answer questions raised do not exist or have not existed, the setting or source needed to generate information does exist. For example, information can be obtained from key health-care or social-service professionals, the elderly themselves, consumers of health care or social services, and health-care and social-service providers from various organizations and agencies.

Several survey approaches to doing a needs assessment have been categorized into three broad major areas by Siegel and his associates:[10]

1. the community-nonsurvey approach
2. the social- and health-indicators approach
3. the community-survey approach

A similar, but more useful, set of categories is offered by Warheit, Bell, and Schwab:[11]

1. the social-indicators approach
2. the key-informant approach
3. the rates-under-treatment approach
4. the field-survey approach
5. the community-forum approach
6. the service-population approach

These six approaches to a needs assessment can be used profitably in combination to supplement one another in a single needs-assessment investigation. Although it is difficult to suggest any one approach that is clearly superior to all others, decisions can be made based on: (1) the kinds of information the planner desires, (2) the most appropriate and reliable source, and (3) the cost in time and money to obtain appropriate and valid information.

The Social-Indicators Approach

The social-indicators approach deals with obtaining demographic data, health statistics, and data on population trends and shifts. These data are the first information planners must collect in order to obtain some idea about the nature and the potential size of the population under study. Such descriptive data can be found in public records and reports and have been discussed earlier. However, it is important to note that all the information necessary for minimum data in a needs assessment of elderly groups will not necessarily be found in public records. Additional information can be generated from a number of other sources, all of which involve using questioning techniques. Thus, the key-informant, rates-under-treatment, field-survey, community-forum, and service-population approaches are research approaches that the planner might also find useful in obtaining necessary information for a needs assessment.

The Key-Informant Approach

The key-informant approach involves securing data about the needs of a particular group of people from key people within some defined area who are in a good position to know what the group under study needs and what their health-care patterns are like.

The criteria for selecting key informants should be based on the individual's knowledge of and experience with the population group under study. Informants can include public officials and health-care providers in various positions within the long-term-care-delivery system, as well as others engaged in the delivery of services to the elderly, such as administrators and long-term-care-program personnel. The steps in using the key-informant approach would include

1. developing a list of key informants who would be most familiar with the needs of a particular elderly group and existing discrepancies in long-term-care services for the elderly
2. identifying specific investigatory objectives
3. constructing questions relevant to the specified objectives
4. developing an interview schedule or questionnaire
5. administering the questionnaire or interview schedule. Information can be obtained by
    a. person-to-person interview—most frequently done as it allows for free exchange of ideas

b. mailed questionnaire
   c. telephone interview
6. tabulating questionnaire data summarizing interviews' data
7. writing a report, including a description of group's consensus on various questions asked, such as the needs of the population group under study and their priority

The key-informant approach has several advantages. It is relatively easy to conduct and can elicit a broad range of information from knowledgeable individuals about the needs of the elderly. In the process of obtaining information, key informants can become important contacts for later involvement in planning adult day-care services, such as writing letters of validation of need or becoming involved in implementing an adult day-care program. Providing for increased participation by key informants increases the likelihood of an integrated community-services approach to the needs of the elderly. Specific information on health practices, utilization of health-care and social services, and lack of services for the elderly can be obtained. An additional and important advantage in questioning key informants is the low cost involved in carrying out interviews.

Obtaining information from key informants can, however, have certain limitations. Some informants may have personal biases that could inadvertently leave out disadvantaged elderly who have not come to their attention. Second, the information obtained is difficult to evaluate objectively, particularly if the data obtained reflect a set of opinions. Third, if questionnaires are used rather than interviews, valuable information can be lost if the response rate is low. Contacts for future planning may also be lost.

The Rates-Under-Treatment Approach

The planner desiring information concerning the utilization of services in the community can use the rates-under-treatment approach. This approach has been widely used in research dealing with the prevalence and treatment patterns of general population groups. Thus, it is appropriate in studying the needs of the elderly. The rates-under-treatment approach (RUT) is based on the assumption that one can estimate the needs of a population group from a sample of persons who have received care or treatment. That is, those using a service are assumed to be representative of those elderly in the community needing the service, but not necessarily using it. Thus, the long-term-care planner using this approach must be aware of the underlying assumption of this approach. The steps usually involved in this approach would include

1. developing specific investigatory objectives.
2. identifying agencies and persons in the community who provide health-care

services to the elderly and obtaining permission to secure information pertinent to the population group under study.
3. developing questions for an interview schedule or questionnaire related to the specified objectives. Such questions might be directed towards eliciting information concerning the age, sex, and place of residence of persons utilizing the services, the health and social problems treated, the health and social problems and number of persons needing continuing long-term-care supervision, and the number of persons who could potentially benefit from adult day-care services. Data might also include outcomes of services provided.
4. implementing the questionnaires or interview schedules. Individuals being asked for information should know in advance why it is needed and how it will be used.
5. summarizing the information in a written report. Simple tables can be used where appropriate.

The rates-under-treatment approach is a relatively low-cost approach to collecting a large amount of data pertinent to the types of elderly individuals being seen in the health-care system, the types of services available for continuing care, and how they are being utilized. This kind of data, plus data about the community's population trends, can help the long-term-care planner estimate the needs of elderly population groups. Surveys of use are advantageous since they can demonstrate some basic principles of utilizations.[12,13]

There are also some disadvantages and limitations in the RUT approach. First, those using the services do not always reflect the true prevalence of those in need of health care and human services. Factors such as cost of care, acceptability of services, and accessibility of health-care and social services can determine the degree to which elderly people translate their needs into demands. Many more elderly needing long-term-care services exist than actually receive them. Second, information from the private sector can be more difficult to obtain than data from public records in the public domain. Last, data may not be aggregated by area of residence to the service area of concern or to the elderly population group therein. Many people receive and obtain services outside their service area. Thus, available data may be difficult to interpret.

The Field-Survey Approach

The field-survey approach is based on drawing representative samples of the population and analyzing data obtained from the sample. If conducted properly, with appropriate sampling techniques and valid, reliable, and appropriate questioning techniques, the survey can yield the most valid and reliable findings on the long-term-care needs of elderly population groups. Surveys of elderly population groups can elicit in a direct way the long-term-care needs of those elderly residing in some area of concern. The steps of this approach would include

1. developing specific investigatory objectives.
2. enlisting the cooperation of interested and relevant agencies to ensure their cooperation or involvement in implementing the survey and a wide range of pertinent questions.
3. determining a technique for collecting data—questionnaire or interview schedule—and constructing questions and format.
4. determining an appropriate sampling procedure. Procedures for collecting samples are discussed in most introductory research texts.
5. implementing the questioning technique.
6. coding collected data according to predefined criteria or format
7. writing reports on the findings. Simple descriptive tables, charts, or graphs can be used to convey material. Agency administrators and community people can better understand material described in simple terms. If the audience of the written document is more sophisticated, an explanation of statistical methods might be in order. More often than not, community members agency personnel and long-term-care providers are more interested in the substance of the report and its relevance to professional practice and long-term-care programming than the scientific community, who may be more interested in the processes used to obtain information.

A major advantage of the field-survey approach is the enumeration of a wealth of information that can be generated and obtained. It is also a direct method of studying the elderly's needs, as opposed to other approaches of an indirect nature.

Several limitations to the field-survey approach are noted. First, mailing costs and questionnaire reproduction can be high when sample numbers are high. Second, the limitations of the approach are those associated with the questioning method used. As previously indicated, mailed questionnaires have a high nonresponse rate. Planners might wish to determine ahead of time an acceptable nonresponse rate. Despite the limitations noted, this approach to collecting information is the most widely used means for obtaining information from large segments of the elderly population.

The Community-Forum Approach

The community-forum approach to a needs assessment involves an open public meeting in a community. This approach is useful for eliciting information relative to the needs of an elderly population group residing in some area and the needs that are perceived as being of high priority. A second purpose of this approach is to attract as many community members as possible and the greatest numbers of viewpoints. Such information can provide the planner with some idea of the priority ratings the community group is giving to problems being uncovered. The steps of this approach would include

1. establishing a committee, who would define its goals and objectives (a committee might include health-care planners, social-service providers, and consumers)
2. constructing some agreed-upon questions to elicit information
3. securing a meeting place, designating a time, and posting a public notice of the meeting and its purposes
4. securing a moderator, who elicits responses from the group using the agreed-upon structured interview schedule
5. tabulating responses from the respondents
6. summarizing in a written report the needs identified and their priority

The community-forum approach has several advantages. It is relatively easy to arrange a community forum and a broad range of community expression can be uncovered. It is also relatively low in cost compared with other approaches we have discussed. An important advantage is that, in a large community of elderly individuals, interested persons who wish to become involved in adult day-care services might be uncovered who otherwise would go unidentified. Individuals who might suffer from or be related to the problem in one way or another might also be uncovered. Community participation may not only cut through value biases that otherwise might allow certain problems or needs to be forgotten, but also call attention to the peculiarities and discrepancies currently existing in our long-term-care delivery system as they relate specifically to the elderly. The community-forum approach can also provide a medium through which an awareness of what is possible in the way of adult day-care delivery can be presented.

The community-forum approach has certain limitations, as do most of the other approaches discussed. First, it can be difficult to ensure that a wide cross section of community members will attend. Those with the greatest interest frequently are not those whose needs should be receiving attention. The data collected may also therefore be more value-laden or impressionistic and thus also difficult to quantify and evaluate objectively. Despite these limitations, the data may be useful in terms of needs assessments by providing another aspect of information relevant to the elderly residing in the community.

The Service-Population Approach

The service-population approach is based on inference of need drawn from information obtained from various sources, such as visiting-nurse associations and nursing homes. The purpose of this approach is to elicit information regarding how people using a service feel about it; what changes they perceive as being desirable with respect to it; what services they need but are not being provided with by the agency; the nature of the problems and needs elderly individuals perceive they have; and the problems and needs that prompted their seeking health-care and human-service assistance. The long-term-care planner in using this approach might wish to focus on only several purposes with regard to a needs assessment. The steps generally used in this approach would include

1. developing a list of agencies or health-care and social-service organizations providing long-term-care services to the elderly population in a defined area, such as nursing homes, extended-care facilities, and homemaker agencies
2. developing specific objectives relevant to the investigation and overall needs assessment
3. constructing a questionnaire or interview schedule with appropriate, valid, and reliable questions
4. implementing the chosen questioning technique
5. tabulating questionnaire data and/or summarizing interview data
6. writing a report of findings, using simple charts and tables where appropriate

The service-population approach is advantageous in that questions posed to elderly respondents in various institutions can elicit their needs in a direct way. This approach may appear to be similar to that of the key-informant approach because the settings may be the same. However, the approaches differ in regard to the type of sample generating the information. The key-informant approach is an *indirect* method of obtaining information about the needs of the elderly. Thus, the population surveyed is the provider of services. The service-population approach on the other hand, is a *direct* method of obtaining information about the needs of elderly since it is the elderly individuals themselves who generate the information based on questions posed. The planner might find it useful and profitable to use both approaches, resulting in two points of view about the needs of the elderly—that of the providers of service and that of the elderly. The two points of view might even be compared to determine similarities and differences.

Several limitations are cited for the service-population approach to a needs assessment. First, those using the service might have different needs, problems, and/or characteristics than those in the general population. Findings, therefore, cannot be generalized to the elderly population of the area. Those using services of a particular agency or institution are a select population group. Despite these limitations, the planner might discover that some institutionalized elderly are in that setting because there is no other choice.

The Delphi Technique

In addition to the six approaches we have discussed above, several other approaches are also used to determine the health and social needs of population groups. One such approach worthy of mention is the Delphi technique.

The Delphi technique is an approach developed by a research and development organization (Rand Corporation) for forecasting short-term social and organizational futures. Until recently, the Delphi technique was used predominantly in the field of technological forecasting.[14] More recently, however, it has been used in the long-term-care field for determining the needs for health and social services, problem-solving, and planning.[15,16]

Simply described, the Delphi technique is a procedure for obtaining consensus from a panel of experts who are asked to complete a series of questionnaires. It differs from other survey approaches in several respects. First, the technique consists of three to four rounds of questionnaires administered to a selected panel of experts. Panelists generally do not know each other's identity, nor do they interact with each other except through an intermediary. As with the key-informant approach, the selection of panel members is generally based on their expertise and knowledge about a certain area, such as gerontology, health-care services generally required by the elderly, and health-care needs of the elderly.

The multiple-enumeration approach required by the Delphi technique permits knowledgeable panel members to present their estimates without being biased by dominant personalities overpowering others, as might occur if the members were gathered at a meeting or in a face-to-face situation. It is a means employed for effecting group consensus of opinion, predictions, or judgments concerning a particular identified topic.

A second characteristic of the Delphi technique is the use of feedback to various members of the panel. Responses to each round of questionnaires are analyzed, summarized, and returned to the panel members before each succeeding round. The net effect is to slowly eliminate extreme positions by forcing their holders to the median. With the knowledge of the panel's viewpoints, members have the opportunity to reformulate their opinions, judgments, and forecasts. Over time, through refinement and clarification of each member's position, a consensus is reached.

In using the Delphi approach, a planner would have a predetermined acceptable consensus percentage. For example, a planner might wish to conduct a study using the Delphi technique to ascertain priorities in long-term-care services for an elderly population group or the need for a long-term-care agency to have a range of options for future use of its facilities by disabled elderly. Consensus might be defined as 75% of the panel members coming to an agreement on the need for adult day-care services. The steps in using the Delphi technique would include

1. defining the objectives.
2. identifying individuals who are knowledgeable about the health-care needs of elderly and familiar with the concept of adult day care services.
3. enlisting the cooperation of interested and relevant experts.
4. constructing an initial questionnaire and determining an acceptable consensus percentage.
5. implementing the initial questionnaire.

6. analyzing and summarizing the initial questionnaire. The data can be presented in terms of average responses or range of responses. Data from the first questionnaire becomes the basis for the second questionnaire.
7. presenting questionnaire two together with findings from questionnaire one to panel members.
8. analyzing and summarizing questionnaire two. Data from questionnaire two becomes the basis for questionnaire three.
9. presenting questionnaire three together with findings from questionnaire two are presented to panel members.
10. analyzing and summarizing questionnaire three. Determining whether there is consensus and the percentage of consensus.
11. writing a report, including the priorities identified or probabilities of need for a range of health-care options in some particular agency or institution.

The Delphi technique has a number of advantages. It can provide a broad range of information from knowledgeable people. It is an efficient and efficacious method of obtaining information from a relatively large group. In addition, the cost in time and money for participating panel members is relatively minimal. Panel members are spared the necessity of time-consuming group meetings. Face-to-face confrontation is avoided; thus the possibility of dominant personalities or a vocal few overpowering others is nonexistent. Perhaps the greatest advantage of the Delphi technique is the anonymity that it ensures. Because panel members do not interact with one another, a greater frankness of opinion and judgment can be generated than might occur in a face-to-face situation.

As with other approaches to a needs assessment, the Delphi technique does have several limitations. First and foremost, the technique can be costly and time-consuming for the planner implementing it. A number of time-consuming steps are involved, such as soliciting knowledgeable people and constructing a series of questionnaires, analyses, and data summaries. Second, a poor selection of panel members and/or poor questionnaire response rates can lead to the occurrence of biases. Panel members might become fatigued during the latter questionnaire-mailing phases and/or might drop out, leading to premature closure or agreement when, in fact, panel members have not reached a consensus. A final limitation of the approach is that the assessment data is subjective in nature. A different group of panel members might very well come up with a different set of results. The validity and reliability of the data can, therefore, be questioned. Since results are based on judgments and opinions, it should not be assumed that the data are representative of available information.

In summary, the seven approaches to a needs assessment presented are similar because questioning techniques are used to both generate and obtain information. However, the approaches differ in the data plans they require. Difficulties of collecting data will vary. Decisions to use an approach or combination of approaches for a needs assessment and minimum data base are based on important considerations, such as the type of necessary and/or additional data needed, the most appropriate source or sources from which information might be generated, and the time and cost involved. Long-term-care planners are encouraged to add, delete, modify, or change the approaches to suit their own purposes and particular situations. Various approaches might be combined profitably in a single needs assessment in order to obtain enough information that can serve as "indicators of need." In this way, the limitations of one approach can be offset by the strengths of other approaches.

It would be presumptuous to claim that a planner must have all possible facts about an elderly population group in order to gain some understanding of its needs. Obviously complete information is impossible. However, the planner must collect information that is significant and relevant to the elderly system under study. Mobilizing long-term-care resources is an expensive proposition. Allocations of resources to one particular group often means that another group is denied something. As a result, knowledge of elderly population groups in need and discrepancies and gaps in existing health-care and human services geared towards disadvantaged and disabled elderly must be documented in a scientific manner in order to justify the mobilization of scarce resources. Those in decision-making positions controlling the allocation of resources are more likely to attend to those problems that are well documented and presented in a scientific manner than those voiced solely on intuition.

Application of Assessment Data

The application of assessment data is in many ways analogous to evaluation in the concepts used and in the purposes served—primarily guidance and direction of decision makers. Data relevant to health statistics, disability statistics, long-term-care resources and their utilization by the elderly, and the health and social needs of disabled elderly all must be assembled. Data must be ordered and synthesized into some meaningful whole in order to be able to draw inferences that become the basis for program planning. Thus, it becomes important to examine the various pieces of information from both time and value perspectives.

Examining Data in a Time Perspective

Current information about numbers of elderly and the health, social conditions, and numbers of elderly with limited ability to function in activities of daily living represents just one point in a lengthy process. Planners must also examine their assessment data in the perspective of time—that is, trends must be recognized. For example, age, sex, and income-distribution characteristics of a particular elderly group residing in a particular geographic area can reveal predictable concerns. Shifts in age distributions must be examined since they can be both revealing and disconcerting when considered in relation to services and resources. The fact that a particular community has a population of 10,000 elderly is important. Further knowledge, however, that the elderly population has increased over the last five-year period by 10% adds another dimension. Have the numbers of elderly disabled and/or limited in their capacity to carry out activities and function also increased within the same time period? If data are seen in the perspective of time, their meaning can be amplified.

Statistics must also be viewed in the perspective of larger environmental forces that might have significance. For example, the greater likelihood of institutionalizing elderly individuals might be related to changing family patterns, unavailable adult day-care services, inaccessible long-term-care resources in particular geographic areas, and/or past and present reimbursement policies and referral mechanisms. Are nursing homes in the area filled to capacity with waiting lists and no plans to build future facilities? The planner looks for those things in the environment that indicate the needs of an elderly group under study.

Examining Data in a Value Perspective

Data about health-care and human services in an area can also be viewed in a value perspective. The National Commission on Community Services has, for example, suggested several criteria that can be used as a frame of reference when examining health-care resources of an area.[17] These criteria include:

1. *The comprehensiveness of long-term-care services.* To be comprehensive, services should be provided for all people in a community who need them, wherever they need them. This criterion applies not only to the more familiar institutional models of care but also to noninstitutional day-care services. Some areas might have large numbers of elderly with chronic diseases, functional disabilities, and psychosocial problems. Existing data on the types of long-term-care services in the area might not include adequate community services or adult day-care services. The bulk of services provided might, in fact, be geared to mothers and children. Thus, it might become evident that the needs of the elderly population are not being adequately met if they are, in fact, being met at all.
2. *The adequacy of facilities, personnel, and financial resources.* Unless adequate long-term-care services are provided, comprehensive care cannot be provided by any community in which elderly reside. Further analysis of an area might indicate that the financial situations of organizations, together with the availability of income from federal sources, have been influential in directing the types of long-term-care services and programs that currently exist in many communities—all too frequently categorical and away from adult day-care services for the elderly. What, in fact, might exist are hospitals and nursing homes. However, if hospital or nursing home beds are available but admission or referral policies are so rigid as to cause undue delays and

long waiting lists, then the end results are inadequate in relation to the needs of the elderly in the area. If the only types of adult day-care services being provided to a community with large numbers of elderly are geared toward mental-health problems, then the end results are inadequate in relation to the total needs of an elderly community.
3. *The availability, accessibility, and acceptability of long-term-care services.* Long-term-care services must be available, accessible, and acceptable. In some communities, data might indicate that health-care and human services are available but not easily accessible especially for those with limited functioning abilities. In addition, many elderly who are institutionalized do not require 24-hour institutional medical care, nor do they wish to be in nursing homes. Most communities provide few options. Data should be examined in terms of the acceptability of a new and different model of long-term-care services—adult day-care services by the elderly group themselves as well as by the professionals and providers in the area.

Summary

The simplicity or complexity of conducting a needs assessment of an elderly population group will vary from one community to another and from one geographic area to another. While useful data might be available at the state and national levels, information considered essential for inclusion in a minimum data base may in fact be nonexistent at the local level or level of concern. The long-term-care planner is obligated to conduct sufficient investigatory studies that generate relevant data so that the combination of these findings and existing statistical data at the local level forms a sensible, relevant, and sufficient foundation for the needs assessment. It is at this point that the questioning method of obtaining information is considered since it is the principal means by which data are generated and obtained in survey research that studies large and small populations. Long-term-care planners do have several techniques from which to choose—questionnaires or interview schedules—in order to generate relevant information about the needs of elderly population groups. The planner must realize that both have advantages and disadvantages. Thus, the task is to discover and use the most appropriate technique for a particular population group and for a particular purpose. Frequently the best course of action will be to use both techniques. In this way, the weaknesses of one technique can be offset by the strengths of the other.

Consideration must be given to the sources from which relevant information can be generated and collected. A number of approaches, therefore, have been discussed, from which essential information can be obtained through the use of questioning techniques. Each approach must be examined in light of the population generating the information. In some cases, the health-care planner might need information from key long-term-care providers in a specific service area pertaining to numbers of elderly referrals—elderly who might benefit from adult day-care services—and/or information from the elderly themselves who reside in some particular community. Thus, in a single needs assessment project, consideration might be given to combining survey-research approaches in order to obtain basic and essential information.

Data that has been collected and assembled must be seen in some perspective in order to be worthwhile as a basis for planning health-care and human services. Some criteria have been discussed that can provide the planner with a frame of reference. These criteria can also be valuable guidelines for organizing and assembling all the pieces of information obtained by the planner. Once relevant data are assembled and examined in some perspective, inferences or conclusions can be drawn, and a specific plan of action can be developed.

References

1. Kerlinger F: *Foundations of Behavioral Research,* ed 2. New York, Holt, Rinehart & Winston, 1973.

2. Polit D, Hungler B: *Nursing Research: Principles and Methods.* New York: J B Lippincott Co, 1978.

3. Hall C: Writing project applications for fundiing. *American Librarian* **1:** 779–780, 1970.

4. U.S. Department of Health, Education and Welfare. *Guide to Data for Health System Planning and Resources: Health Planning Information Series.* Wash DC, US Government Printing Office, 1976, HEW Document No. HRA 76-14502, p 25.

5. Cannell C, Kahn R: The collection of data by interviewing, in Festinger L, Katz D (eds): *Research Methods in the Behavioral Sciences.* New York, Holt, Rinehart & Winston, 1953.

6. Cannell C, Kahn R: *Interviewer's Manual Survey Research Center,* rev ed. Ann Arbor, Institute for Social Research, University of Michigan, 1970.

7. Orne MT: On the social psychology of the psychological experiment: with particular reference to demand characteristics and their implications. *Am Psychologist* **17:** 776–783, 1962.

8. Noelle-Neuman E: Wanted: Rules for wording structured questionnaires. *Public Opinion Quarterly* **24:** 191–201, 1970.

9. Kornhauser A, Sheatsley PB: Questionnaire construction and interview procedures, in Selltiz C, Wrightsman LS, Cook SW: *Research Methods in Social Relations,* ed 3. New York, Holt, Rinehart & Winston, 1976, Appendix B.

10. Siegel L, Atkinson C, Cohen A: *Mental Health Needs Assessment: Strategies and Techniques.* Wash DC, National Institute of Mental Health Report, 1974, p 10.

11. Warheit G, Bell R, Schwab J: *Planning for Change: Needs Assessment Approaches.* Wash DC, National Institute of Mental Health, 1975, p 47.

12. Berger DG, Gardner EA: Use of community surveys in mental health planning. *Am J Pub Health* **61:** 110–118, 1971.

13. Anderson RM: Health service use: National trends and variation 1953–1971. Wash DC, US Department of Health, Education and Welfare, National Center for Health Services, Research and Development, HSM Publication No. 73-30004, 1972, pp 1–5.

14. Helmer O: On the future state of the union, in Jantsch E: *Technological Forecasting*. Institute for the Future, Report R-27, Menlo Park, Calif., May, 1972:116–32.

15. Starkweather DB, Gelwicks L, Newcomer R: Delphi forecasting of health care organization. *Inquiry,* **12:** 37, 1975.

16. Lindeman CA: Delphi survey of priorities in clinical research. *Nursing Research* **24:** 434–441, 1975.

17. National Commission on Community Health Services. *Health Is a Community Affair*. Cambridge, Mass, Harvard University Press, 1966, pp 196–223.

5

Assessing and Meeting the Needs of the Long-Term-Care Person

John N. Morris, PhD
Carl U. Granger, MD

Population at Risk

Growth Trends of the Aged

In order to understand the present concern with the condition of the elderly in this country, one need only look at the growth trends for the 65-and-over age group. In the period between 1900 and 1970, there was a *six and one-half* times increase in the over-65 age group, as compared with an only *two and one-half* times increase for the under-65 age group.[1] With respect to the future, the *Annual Report to the President* from the Council on Aging (1976) points out that

> projections for 1980 indicate an overall 65 years and over population of some 24.5 million with some 38 percent, or 9.1 million, 75 years and over.... By 2000 the U.S. may have an estimated 30.6 million 65 years and over, of which an estimated 44 percent, or 13.5 million, are expected to be 75 plus.[2]

Given the magnitude of this growth, it is important to generate a reasonable estimate of the proportion of elderly persons who will require support services. Precise estimation is always difficult, and, as is often the case, we must both draw upon fragmented epidemiological data and cope with the lack of congruence in the intent of the projected service interventions themselves. Are our chief concerns cost containment, maximizing personal independence, functional improvement, and/or the improvement in the quality of life of the elderly population? For our part, we would say that all of these are important and what is needed is an integrated cost-conscious system for maintaining and improving the life situation of the elderly long-term-care clients.

Who does, therefore, fit within the definition of the long-term-care client? To begin, there is a general consensus that the elderly as a group differ in their health status from other segments of the population. Episodes of acute problems, for example, are much more likely to be characterized both by restricted activity days (a mean of 11.0 days for those 65+ as opposed to 5.0 days for persons aged 17–64) and bed-disability days (a mean of 4.5 days for persons 65+ as opposed to 2.1 days for persons aged 17–64).[3] In addition, the elderly are more likely to suffer from multiple health conditions of a permanent nature. Cures like those we have come to expect from the acute-care sector are lacking for chronic diseases. As pointed out by Ryder,

> progress in preventive measures against infectious diseases has sparked what might be termed a revolution in disease, and has resulted in a significant shift to chronic ailments in the health profile of the American population. Those prevented from dying of typhoid fever, smallpox, pneumonia, and other diseases with high mortality rates a generation ago are now living on to die of cardiovascular disease, cancer, diabetes, or another chronic disease with high prevalence among older people.[4]

Prevalence of Chronic Diseases

From the perspective of chronic disease, it may seem reasonable to assume that the long-term-care client could be designated simply on the basis of the presence or absence of specific medical problems. Unfortunately, according to a Department of Health, Education and Welfare (DHEW) estimate, 86% of the noninstitutionalized population of persons 65 years of age and older report that they have one or more chronic diseases.[5] Thus, almost 19 million of the roughly 21.9 million elderly persons estimated to be living in the community in 1976 have such a problem. This figure is obviously a gross overestimate of the number of elderly who should be considered candidates for long-term care. With respect to the specific conditions reported by elderly persons living in the community, survey data gathered between 1969 and 1973 indicated the prevalence rates shown in Table 5-1.

Number of Vulnerable Aged Persons

Once again, there may be those who would assume that long-term client vulnerability could be defined simply by reference to *one* of the chronic conditions shown in Table 5-1. For example, all elderly diabetics could conceivably be considered

Table 5-1
Prevalance rates of chronic diseases in noninstitutionalized elderly

Disease	Noninstitutionalized Elderly %	Millions
Arthritis and rheumatism	38.0%	8.3
Heart condition	19.9%	4.4
Hypertension	19.9%	4.4
Diabetes	7.9%	1.7
Impairments of back or spine	6.7%	1.5

From *Health United States 1976–1977*. DHEW Publication No. (HRA) 77-1232. U.S. Government Printing Office, 1977.

candidates for active long-term-service supports. Unfortunately, this type of definition would also result in an overestimation of the number of long-term-care clients in need of support. For example, estimates derived from 1978 DHEW data show that, even in the presence of these chronic conditions, many elderly persons are able to live quite adequately in the community (see Table 5-2). Concentrating on those elderly persons in the community who were found to be either limited or unable to carry out a major activity, DHEW data indicate that there was no single medical condition for which 50% or more of the persons with the condition were also found to be restricted in an activity (although 49% of those with a heart condition were, in fact, restricted).

It should be clear from the foregoing that it is only when a medical condition leads to a loss of previous independence, or is found in conjunction with func-

Table 5-2
Percent of elderly persons with chronic diseases who were and were not limited or unable to carry out a major activity

Disease	% Restricted	% Not Restricted
Arthritis and rheumatism	26	74
Heart condition	49	51
Hypertension	19	81
Diabetes	33	67
Impairments of back or spine	20	80

From *Health United States 1978*. DHEW Publication No. (PHS) 78-1232. U.S. Government Printing Office, 1978.

tional dependence, that it becomes of prime concern. Sherwood has defined the situation as follows:

> Someone is a long-term care person who has reached, either suddenly or gradually, a state of collapse or deterioration in human behavioral functioning which requires—for survival, slowing down the rate of deterioration, maintenance, or rehabilitation—the services of at least one other human being.[6(pp3-79)]

According to the most recent estimates, 22% of the elderly population report some type of limitation in a major activity, and 17% indicate that they are unable to carry out one or more major activities.[7] Nagi, going beyond these findings, has reported on a particularly useful national data set, in which finer functional distinctions were made. The Nagi data concentrate on adults 18 years of age and older and are based on interviews with 6493 persons in the community. In this study, 11.6% of the total sample, both aged and nonaged, had some form of disabling condition.[8] Table 5-3 shows the extension of this percentage to an estimated community population of 148,097,000 persons 18 years of age and older.

From this data base, the number of elderly with functional impairments can be estimated at some 7.7 million persons, or 35% of the elderly age group, which is comparable to the 39% DHEW estimate. If one limits the definition to the latter two categories in Table 5-3, in which the persons included are those who require help at home, there are some 4.4 million elderly persons with such needs, or 20.1% of the elderly population. At the same time, it should be emphasized that some 68% of this high-need group do not require help with personal care and are thus capable of grooming, feeding, and dressing themselves.

A further refinement of the 20.1% estimate of needy elderly can be drawn from data reported as part of the U.S. Government Accounting Office (GAO) Cleveland Study, in which 14% of the total community population were found to be

Table 5-3
Adults 18 years and older with disabling conditions in a population of 148,097,000

Degree of Disability	Adults 18 Years and Older %	Millions
Not limited in work or independent living	88.4	131
Limited in work but judged to be functionally independent	6.3	9.3
Needed assistance with living chores (including outdoor mobility, shopping and housework)	3.5	5.2
Needed assistance with personal care and mobility	1.8	2.7

From *Health United States 1978*. DHEW Publication No. (PSH) 78-1232. U.S. Government Printing Office, 1978.

extremely impaired.[9] This estimate of 14% can be seen as part of the 20.1% group estimated by Nagi, or about 70% of this more generally needy group. In an independent study of Massachusetts elderly, data were presented that further substantiate the 14% estimate.[10] In this latter study, based upon a random-probability sample of Massachusetts elderly, 13.5% of the community elderly were estimated to have extreme needs, needs that if not met would result in the individual being institutionalized.

On the basis of these two comparable findings, the minimal estimate of the number of vulnerable elderly persons in need of long-term supports is 14% or about 3.1 million people. This estimate is smaller than the 4.4 million arising from the Nagi data, but is quite similar to the one provided by LaVor of some 3,400,000 aged who require care at home.[11] Finally, with respect to the future, there is every reason to expect an increase over time both in the number and proportion of vulnerable elderly. Most importantly, the distribution of vulnerable elderly is not constant with age, and it is only with the most advanced segment of the population, those who are 85 years of age or older, that general disability becomes the rule.[10] In this regard, it is interesting to note the predicted disproportionate growth in the 85+ age group, from 1 in every 16 elderly today to 1 in 10 in the year 2035.[12]

Service Support Systems

Distribution of Vulnerable Aged in the Community and Institutions

Given the earlier estimates of long-term-care vulnerability, the question of how best to serve the needs of these persons must be addressed. Institutional placement has become an increasingly used option, and questions can be raised concerning whether most or even a large segment of the vulnerable long-term-care elderly are making use of such environments at any given point in time.[13,14,6(pp3–80), 7(pp91–126)]

In the GAO Cleveland study, 14% of the community elderly were found to meet this definition. Similarly, 1976 DHEW data found 83% of institutionalized elderly to need regular assistance or to be totally dependent.[7(p239)] Extrapolating from these data, and assuming that about 5% of the elderly population are in institutions at any one point in time, one can estimate that only about 25% of the extremely vulnerable long-term-care elderly are in institutions and that the other 75% are in the community.[7(p. 235)] The vast majority of aged in need of long-term care continue to remain outside of institutions; from this perspective, the community, and not the institutions, is the normative setting for the vulnerable elderly. There has, however, been extensive reliance on institutions as a dominant

Chapter 5: Assessing and Meeting the Needs of the Long-Term-Care Person / 109

alternative for care in the family setting. Thus, if institutions are to be seen in a true perspective today, they are a minority alternative.

For a minority service, there is no question that institutional placements are of major concern. The cost of institutions, the confinement of the elderly, and the quality of care have led to a serious national debate on how best to meet legitimate needs of the long-term-care elderly client. Therefore, who is it that is being institutionalized?

With respect to institutional placements, there are few who would take exception with the statement that the decisions concerning the most appropriate service-support setting for the long-term-care person should involve consideration of the likely consequence of the action taken, hopefully based on knowledge rather than on beliefs. Unquestionably there are persons for whom institutions are appropriate and, in fact, the only possible alternative, given the long-term-care client's needs for high intensity, 24-hour care. In a longitudinal 20-year study of 207 aged persons in the community carried out by Palmore, 26% had been institutionalized one or more times, suggesting that a high proportion of elderly eventually experience an institutional placement.[15] Studies also suggest that, for many elderly persons, institutional placement is not capricious. Family members of institutionalized elderly have expended considerable efforts to keep these people in the community prior to their placement. When institutionalization is necessary, many families continue to maintain high levels of contact with and helping behaviors for their elderly institutionalized relatives.[16,17] It should also be noted, however, that persons without close relatives are more likely to enter long-term-care facilities with lower levels of disability than those who have relatives.[18] Thus, there is a genuine concern that many persons are placed in institutions who, with proper supports, might have been able to remain in the community.

As pointed out by Hammerman, Friedsam, and Shore, "the 'consumers' of services of long-term care facilities are increasingly older, female, widowed, economically dependent, and affected by multiple physical and psychological disorders."[19] It has been estimated that persons 75 years of age or older are three times more likely to be found in nursing homes than the 65–75-year-old group.[20] The male-female differential in long-term-care facilities widens with advancing age; the percentage of women is 62% for the 64–74-year-olds as compared with 75% for those 85 and over.[21] Gottesman and Brody cite evidence indicating "that childless old people and those with only one surviving adult child are over-represented in institutions."[22] Although 82% of the total elderly population have at least one adult child, Townsend and Gottesman both estimate that only about half of the institutionalized have an adult child.[23,24] Townsend found "that the most common events precipitating admission were the deaths or sudden illnesses of close relatives." The institutionalized, then, are likely to have fewer informal resources than their counterparts in the community and depend in large measure on the institutional resources for their quality of life.

*Variables That Tip the
Balance Toward Institutions*

In a Canadian study comparing community and institutionalized elderly, those who were institutionalized were seen, among other things, to have much more trouble in the control of bladder and bowel and much greater recent loss of independence in activities of daily living (ADL).[25]

In a study carried out by the Hebrew Rehabilitation Center for Aged (HRCA) in conjunction with the Vermont Peer Standards Review Organization (PSRO), an evaluation was made of the potential of placing individuals who were clinically deemed appropriate for intermediate-care facilities, but who had the potential for placement in a community-care home or domiciliary-care facility.[26] In a discriminant-function analysis, in which an attempt was made to understand the basis on which the clinical group selected the roughly 180 dischargeable clients from among 2000 total clients, it was found that functional health accounted for about 29% of the variance.[27] When a multiple-regression equation was attempted, in which social, psychological, and health variables were also entered, it was found that functional health was the single most important predictor, with the other variables making smaller, but important contributions. In this instance, it was found that individuals who were seen as dischargeable had minimal needs for services in such areas as bathing, dressing, and other personal care areas, but higher levels of need for services in more instrumental areas, such as cooking, cleaning, and shopping. The large residual population judged not to be dischargeable were much more likely to have personal-care needs.

In this same PSRO study, when combined mathematical and clinical validation procedures were used to identify newly admitted patients with the potential to return to the community, a full 25.6% were so identified. Interestingly, in a PSRO study of a sample of nursing-home residents in Denver, 28% were identified "could probably function at home with home help supportive services."[28] In an earlier investigation carried out as part of a larger study of applicants to the HRCA in Boston, clinical judgments concerning a sample of 344 applicants revealed that over half were capable of functioning in the community with appropriate community supports and living arrangements. Evidence from this study indicates that many of these persons accepted admission to the center presumably because of the lack of such resources.[29] It should also be noted with respect to this HRCA estimate that the average applicant had to wait for some two years to be offered residence, and many applicants to this facility at the time of the study were applying, to some extent at least, on a contingency basis as a hedge against projected escalating needs in the future. In point of fact, many persons who enter long-term-care facilities do not necessarily spend the rest of their lives in these facilities. In 1972, 1.1 million persons entered nursing homes, and approximately 750,000 persons were discharged alive.[30] In the state of Massachusetts, similar discharge ratios were reported for 1975, and, in this instance, data were also presented showing about 31% of the persons who were discharged alive returned to live in the community, the vast majority of the remaining persons discharged alive were transferred to acute-care hospitals, and a small number were transferred to another long-term-care facility.[31]

Functional Assessment of Disability

Nagi's Conceptual Model of Disability

Appropriately serving long-term-care clients by maximizing their quality of life and preventing needless institutionalization requires the application of a conceptual model. The model should help us understand the complex relationships between physical, mental, or emotional conditions, social supports, and demands of the environment. Use of the model requires a comprehensive functional assessment that relates to the full range of possible services that might meet patterns of need uncovered by the assessment. The plan of services that might be derived should include specification of appropriate levels of care and optimal sites for treatment, as well as specification of outcomes of care (in terms of quality of life) as a result of the service program. The conceptual model of disability developed by Nagi is a useful starting point:

pathology ◊ impairment ◊ functional limitations ◊ disability[8]

Diagnoses of pathology and impairment are usually considered to be the linchpins of medical characterization and classification; however, diagnosis may not necessarily be the most important variable to describe various states of disability for the long-term-care client. As noted by Greer, Sherwood, and Morris, diagnostic classification for those with chronic illness is not simple.[32] Diagnoses tend to wax and wane in importance with the passage of time. Diagnostic designations often are not permanent, identical diagnoses may have variable impacts on different clients, and diagnostic terminology may not be relevant to the cluster of problems to be resolved from the perspective of long-term care.

Functional Limitations on Independent Living as Measured Through Activities of Daily Living and Levels of Social Support

While the International Classification of Diseases is widely used to describe pathology and impairment, methods for describing functional limitations and disability are much less well developed, understood, or accepted and are infrequently used in practice.[33] Functional limitations are those activities in which the client's performances are deficient to the extent that the individual is unable to meet the demands of the environment or the expectations of society. The environmental demands and social-role expectations that are most relevant to long-term care are within the domain of independent living. The strengths and weaknesses of an individual for living independently are measured through assessment of ability to perform personal and instrumental activities of daily living (PADL and IADL) and through assessment of the level of social and psychological supports available to the individual. In order to avoid endless listings of multiple variables, it is necessary to utilize only those bits of descriptive data most appropriate to the purposes and analyses being sought.

The Department of Gerontological Research of the Hebrew Rehabilitation Center for Aged (HRCA) for a number of years has employed a multidisciplinary team of research-oriented clinicians, who have screened populations applying to alternative long-term-care programs, from institutions to sheltered housing to home care. In each instance, a primary predictor variable that emerged in statistical analyses developed for replicating these judgments is functional status.[34] The variables included personal and instrumental activities of daily living. While these were important primary items in the equations, they were not the sole items and in order to successfully replicate the clinical decision-making process, it was necessary to go into other areas, such as anxiety, emotional status, cognitive status, housing conditions, social isolation, and general social participation. The point is that the decision about appropriate placement is complex and that physical-functioning status plays an essential role.

Purposes and Analyses Served Through Functional Assessment

Key-Characteristics Profile

A major purpose of functional assessment is to profile the key characteristics of persons in need of long-term care, whether through acute-care hospitals, outpatient care, rehabilitation programs, vocational programs, educational programs, home care, day care, or long-term-institutional care. Whereas assessment of absolute health status is important (though difficult to do consistently), it is more important in long-term care to know how a client uses whatever health status he or she possesses. Ability or inability to maintain independent living is the principal determinant of need for long-term-care services, whether in a community setting or within an institution. Assessment of the activities of daily living and the level of social supports is the method of measuring these abilities.

Comprehensive Plan of Services

Following characterization by functional assessment, a plan of services can, to a large extent, be developed that is specific to the needs of each client or a whole group of similar clients. Because the assessment is comprehensive, the plan of care

Chapter 5: Assessing and Meeting the Needs of the Long-Term-Care Person / 113

can integrate all necessary services while avoiding gaps due to failure to take note of pertinent problem areas. Serial assessments at different points in time allow tracking of changes that occur through the course of the individual treatment program. Assessments of groups of clients at any point in time allows the service program to estimate the aggregated level of need for those individuals being served, and thus an appropriate plan for staffing and manpower can be developed. Comprehensive functional assessments allow for an orderly review of the status of individuals in fulfilling the requirements of the activities of daily living. The effects of the treatment program for correction and management of disability are more readily monitored and measured. Communication among interdisciplinary members of the treatment team is enhanced through the use of a common language. Quality assurance can be developed around collection of standardized data for audits and program evaluation in order to detect, document, and correct any deficiencies in care. A basis is established for answering research questions regarding benefits of treatment, uses of alternative treatments, interventions, and for studying cost-effectiveness. The area of long-term care is a mixture of medical, physical, psychological, social, economic, and other issues. To meet the challenge of integrating all of these issues, functional assessment must be a dynamic appraisal of activities, skills, performances, environmental conditions and needs.

The data base developed on each person served needs to address several key questions:

1. What are the medical, physical, and psychosocial characteristics of persons served?
2. How are these characteristics translated into personal needs?
3. How are services provided that are appropriate to maintain a level of functional performance with as much improvement as possible on the one hand, or else the least degree of deterioration on the other hand?
4. How are the service specialists integrated into a comprehensive and continuous plan of care?
5. How are individual persons tracked over time in order to measure the stability or change in condition that occurs in order to derive outcomes of care?
6. How do the outcomes of care become translated into benefits achieved and cost-effectiveness measures?

Methods of Functional Assessment

With respect to assessment, a number of useful measures already exist, and others are in various stages of development. At the same time, there is no single system for optimizing assessment and planning goals, and major efforts are needed toward further developing such instruments. Within the gerontological and rehabilitation fields many interview schedules and functional-health batteries of scale items now exist that begin to address issues.[35–51] They represent a beginning.

In assessing the status of the individual, it will be necessary to look at performance at many levels and in a wide variety of situations. The placement of the long-term-care person in a community-living situation and the matching of an individual with a service program require a consideration of all those activities that a person must be able to accomplish in order to live in the community. We are not, however, suggesting an all-encompassing set of highly specific measures; rather, we are suggesting that key-indicator (proxy) measures be taken—measures that are relevant both to task dysfunctions and to the decision-making process that would be relative to intake and tracking within an adult day-care program that is working under a comprehensive system of client-care planning. That is, these measurement scales should be related both to the human conditions, as evidenced by dysfunction (for example, particular motor-coordination problems of the arms and hands), and to relevant personal activities—from the most obvious, such as dressing and transferring to and from a chair, to less obvious instrumental activities, such as using a utensil or dialing the telephone. While it cannot be expected that every human activity should be measured, at the very least it is necessary that major-task dysfunctional categories in relation to the major personal, instrumental, and affective areas be measured in a structured manner. The measurements taken should be capable of producing reliable information in a wide variety of situations on the basis of a requisite list of questions or tests that are as nonobtrusive as possible.

What, then, are the areas to be measured? The answer to this question will, of course, depend upon the nature of the placement decision being contemplated and the availability and extent of control over local resources. According to Weiler and Rathbone-McCuan, evaluation results should be relevant to the appropriateness of adult day care in the long-term-care continuum.[52] A wide range of factors must be considered in the formulation of policies about adult day-care service delivery. Two of the most important are definition of the role that adult day-care services will play in publicly financed long-term-care programs and the means for integrating adult day-care centers into existing human-service systems.

What follows are some of the areas of inquiry and potential task dysfunction in which test procedures have been and/or need to be developed and measurements have been taken. These areas have been selected because of their relevance to community functioning. The basic approach suggested emerged from the model of the problem-oriented medical record described by Weed.[53,54] Functional assessment represents the extension of the defined data base beyond the traditional components of the medical history, the physical examination, and laboratory data. Functional assessment provides a framework for a systematic review of those domains important to fulfillment of social roles and for a satisfactory quality of life.

Older Americans Resources and Services (OARS)

The Duke University Older Americans Resources and Services (OARS) instrument has been used in a number of long-term-care studies in recent years. Of particular interest has been the longitudinal GAO study of Cleveland's community elderly and the services they used. Five domains of functional health were identified by the Duke group as being basic and important:[55]

1. physical health
2. activities of daily living
3. mental health
4. social resources
5. economic resources

Each of these domains was defined within rather broad six-point scales, and they have been further reported as dichotomous variables. Of particular interest has been the reporting of the point-prevalence percentages of persons with problems in these five areas across 32 possible combinations of the five variables within their dichotomous format. With respect to multiple problems, in the Durham (Duke) and Cleveland studies, 12.5% and 10% of the samples, respectively, had problems in three or more of the areas listed, and, of these, 86% of the Durham and 73% of the Cleveland cases with three or more problems had ADL noted as one of the problem areas.[55(p65)]

Long-Range Evaluation System (LRES)

The Long-Range Evaluation System (LRES) reported by Granger is a functional-assessment method designed, tested, and used in clinical settings, including hospital inpatients in medical rehabilitation programs, outpatients, clients in day-care and home-care programs,[37(pp14-17)] and residents of long-term-care facilities. It is a measuring tool for describing areas of service need, severity of handicap, change in individuals over time, and the comparative status of groups of individuals treated at different times and in different locations. Basic profile dimensions are based upon the following areas:

active motion of limbs
verbal communication
hearing ability
visual ability
self-care ability

mobility
intellectual and emotional adaptability
adequacy of home setting
level of social interactions or dependency
level of support from family unit
financial resources
educational or vocational status

The data-collection forms are precoded for computer entry. Data are collected by clinicians serving the patient. Mutually exclusive definitions have been developed for the descriptive criteria, thus rendering a high degree of inter-rater reliability. Educational material has been developed, and workshops are conducted regularly to teach the uniform criteria. Scores generated by the assessment according to the Barthel index and PULSES profile are used to represent physical dependence. These scores have been shown to be valid measures of independence in personal care. Level of social support is measured by the ESCROW profile. It is a newer scale and its reliability and validity are still being tested.

The modified Barthel index used in LRES was studied in two sets of client populations. When administered at the time of discharge to ten stroke clients, it had a high interjudge reliability of .97 (two different nurses made judgments on the same client). When administered at admission to 100 rehabilitation clients, there was a high internal consistency reliability (an alpha coefficient of .92) indicating good scalability of the items in the index. The total score was found to be discriminating and valid, and changes over time were deemed to be a reliable measure of observed functional change.[56] In another study using modified versions of the PULSES profile and the Barthel index, the scales highly correlated with each other from rehabilitation hospital admission to discharge and to followup. Test-retest reliability was high at .87 and .89, respectively, and intercoder reliability was above .95 on both scales.[39(pp145–146)]

These Barthel index reliabilities are particularly encouraging in that workers with experience in collecting clinical data regard an interjudge reliability coefficient of .85 or better as acceptable. Further, they find it rather easy to train and attain the criterion of .85 reliability for measures of physical functioning, including the Barthel index, compared with greater difficulty in attaining this criterion level using measures of psychosocial functioning.[57]

Further study of the Barthel index scores in a hospital rehabilitation program for stroke clients showed that an initial score over 40 defined a population with a greater proportion of discharges home than those below 40. Clients with an initial score over 60 had a shorter length of stay than those below 60. A score of 60 appeared to be a pivotal point, at which almost all clients were independent in the very basic skills of feeding, bowel and bladder control, and grooming, and one-half were functioning with assistance in dressing, transfers, and ambulation.[58]

The Barthel index, as modified by Granger, has also been used as one of the key components in a number of service-planning studies conducted by HRCA for community and institutional groups.[27(pp64–65),37(pp14–17),59,60,61,62] In these applications, distinct subgroups of long-term-care clients were developed, and "ideal" service packages were suggested for each of the functionally homogeneous subgroups. In these studies, functional status proved to be a key overall determinant of the service packages required by various subgroups of persons, with other factors such as orientation, depression, communicative skills, and personality factors taking on important, but more limited definitional roles. These analyses, while demonstrating the general importance of functional status and the utility of the items listed in the Barthel index, also pointed to areas where more specificity would enhance the utility of the scale. For example, it was noted that definitions of an individual's need for human help in any of the categories was not sufficiently precise. Some of these individuals required only sporadic assistance, while others required considerable or highly intensive assistance. While the Barthel index has been primarily used in the LRES instrument for its total score, in the types of applications used by HRCA, particularly in areas such as bathing, dressing and mobility, it will be necessary to further define or to separate the with-assistance category into those who need little human assistance from those who need considerable human assistance. On an operational level, this categorization would relate to need for heavy lifting as well as the number of hours of assistance required or else the number of days during which assistance is required during the typical week.

In addition to including the Barthel index, the LRES has several features that are unique: there are a series of descriptive modules that are plugged in or left out as appropriate to the informational needs relevant to the particular population being evaluated; the method has been computerized to provide feedback summaries for incorporation into the client's clinical record; the data stored in the computer are used to compile a variety of management reports that reflect the characteristics of the population on whom the data have been collected; each record entered into the system has been designed for the particular encounter for which it is used and is time-oriented with respect to date of entry and whether it represents an admission, an interval, a discharge, or a followup report; the system is designed to track individuals over time through a series of facilities, whether inpatient or outpatient; and a method of program evaluation is accommodated, whereby results or outcomes of care can be compared with predetermined standards in measurable terms.

The Burton Approach

A more limited approach to the problem was envisioned by Burton, Granger, Greer, Morris, and Sherwood in their rather comprehensive attempt to relate functional status to the design criteria for housing for the physically handicapped.[63] The following variables were cited, along with the suggestion that one measure current performance, current capacity, and future potential (with rehabilitation) for functioning:

- static anthropemetric characteristics of various body systems
- physical functioning characteristics of various body systems
- cardiorespiratory and metabolic limitations
- visual limitations
- olfactory and gustatory limitations
- body sensitivity
- cognitive characteristics
- social characteristics

The above listing is more specific than would be required in the type of planning envisioned here but does suggest the need to be aware of the goals to which the services to be recommended will be addressed. To further clarify the extent to which this drawing of relationships may be amplified, Table 5-4 attempts to relate physical dysfunction to architectural design features.

Comprehensive Assessment System for Seniors (COMPASS)

The specification of distinct client characteristics and the translation of these characteristics into service goals were the objectives of a system designed by Morris and Mor in conjunction with the Volunteers for Services to Older Persons (VSOP) program in California. The services were then tested and modified by VSOP staff (including the design of their instrumentation: Comprehensive Assessment System for Seniors—COMPASS).[64] The crucial features of the COMPASS assessment system and the associated goal structure are the use of a systematic language of service goals; the enumeration of some 20 service goals addressing deficits in the elderly person's quality of life and system of support provision; the specification of critical-problem profiles based on client-assessment data indicative of a needed service goal (that is, a pattern of deficits in terms of the person's life functioning is conceptually linked to a goal that might be met through a variety of different service-implementation strategies).

The key to the system is the scoring of the client within each of 20 different descriptive profile elements or domains. The domains have been found by HRCA to be clinically meaningful in other long-term-care planning studies and were selected in an attempt to provide a comprehensive picture of the status of the

Table 5-4
Correlation between physical dysfunction and architectural design elements

User Functioning Category	Probable Related Dysfunctions	Related Architectural Elements

Physical functioning characteristics (other) than sensory and cognitive)
 head and neck
 trunk
 hands
 arms
 legs
 reflex activity
 reaction time
 continence
 aids (e.g., prostheses)
	Inoperable body parts
	 Reduced or excessive range of motion of body parts
	 Coordination disabilities
	 Absent, slowed, or random reflex activity
	 Slowed reaction time
	 Increased incontinence
	 Presence of aids (mechanical hands, lifts, electronic devices)
		Site location
		   transportation availability, access, and adjacency
		 General living and workplace Layout
		   workplace environment
		   workplace arrangement
		   work area layout
		   aisles and passageways
		   inclines
		 Furniture and workspace
		   seating
		   beds
		   general furnishing dimension
		   desks, table, work area
		   equipment arrangement
		 Equipment Design
		   design of control areas
		   grouping of controls
		 Control Design
		   buttons
		   switches
		   knobs
		   foot levers and handles
		   operating controls
		   physical efficiency of controls
		 Electrical considerations
		   interference
		   support
		 Aid accommodation and storage

individual. For each domain, the presence, partial presence, or absence of a problem is defined on the basis of the client's responses to precoded assessment questions. In some cases, there are varieties of "paths" or patterns of responses, which result in the decision that there is a problem, whereas for others there is only a single means for determining the presence of a problem. Obviously, not each domain, or profile element, is equally important in describing the individual's functioning and needs. In addition, in some cases the absence of a problem is in fact indicative of an important asset, whereas in others it is merely a neutral fact. Although the establishment of "cutting points" as to what does and does not constitute a problem is, of course, arbitrary, it was originally based on clinical experience in the successful use of such a system, as well as on substantial amounts of empirical evidence concerning the distribution of responses to the questions used in the scoring system across a variety of vulnerable and frail elderly populations. Since its original development, the VSOP project has further refined and validated the instrument, utilizing a variety of empirical and informed-expert standardization procedures. The areas measured in the COMPASS instrument are as follows:

functional status
behavioral problems
psychological problems
emotional problems
present life satisfaction
loneliness
interpersonal incompetence
acute recuperative state
social contact
economic status

One of the principal reasons for developing the instrument was to suggest a uniform conceptual framework for understanding all clients. Each client's situational problem set is unique, as would be the strategy for solving or ameliorating those problems. Nonetheless, it is possible, for conceptual purposes, to categorize problems into types and, in so doing, to discuss clients in terms of their patterns of problems. At the same time, it is recognized that a person is more than a string of unrelated problems. The person also has positive assets that any good service planner would take into consideration in developing and implementing a service plan to deal with the problems that do exist.

Although the development of a COMPASS client-problem profile provides a uniform manner of describing clients, it still leaves unstructured the determination of what the goals of a service intervention would be. The language of service goals, objectives, and strategies often becomes very confusing, and it is often impossible to maintain the distinctions between goals, objectives, and strategies as one proceeds to develop a service plan. In order to partially systematize this process, a model was developed to proceed logically from the client's characteristics through to the recommendation of service-intervention goals. This model also allows for the specification of measurable service-program objectives that

Chapter 5: Assessing and Meeting the Needs of the Long-Term-Care Person / 121

could be used to monitor the service strategy and to subsequently make adjustments. Table 5-5 presents the model, displaying the various components that are operational within the COMPASS System.

A set of 20 goals, into which most of the service needs of the vulnerable elderly can be subsumed, has been *tentatively* established. On a client-specific basis, the decision as to whether or not the client has a need in a given goal area is made by reviewing his or her COMPASS client-problem profile. Each goal is considered

Table 5-5
Goal-oriented service-management model

Client Problem Profile	Consideration of Goal Structure via Critical Client Profiles	Develop Service Strategies to Meet Goals	Service Objectives
Energy level	Accept dependence	A one-to-one service-to-goal correspondence is not required. One service can be geared to addressing multiple goals. It is advised that for each service the goal or goals being addressed should be recorded.	Such objectives should be estimates of the degree to which each goal will be met realistically in a given frame. It is suggested that the goal be expressed in terms of the client-problem profile elements—that is, movement from "severe" to "moderate" problems in IADL, or movement from a "moderate" to "no problem" in informal support provision.
Medical	Improve PADL		
Personal-care activities of daily living (PADL)	Improve IADL		
Instrumental activities of daily living (IADL)	Improve communication		
Institutional path	Improve orientation		
Competence	Improve economics		
Housing	Improve stamina		
Informal support provision	Improve caretaker skills		
Informal network reliance	Reduce isolation		
Informal network communication	Reduce inappropriate behavior		
Agency supports	Reduce network pressure		
Behavioral disturbance	Relieve distress		
Psychological disturbance	Improve emergency links		
Emotional state	Improve network communication		
Life satisfaction	Provide IADL help		
Loneliness	Provide nutritional advice		
Interpersonal incompetence	Provide health service		
Acute condition	Provide legal help		
Social contact	Provide appliances		
	Provide housing help		

independently. A series of goal-determination rules has been formulated for each goal. That is, if the client is characterized by one of a series of "critical profile patterns" (on the basis of the COMPASS client-problem profile), she or he is considered as either included or excluded from consideration of the particular goal. Basically, this method imposes a fairly rigid, but reasonable structure on the otherwise totally intuitive process of setting service goals. It entails the worker's asking a defined set of questions about the client in considering the possible recommendation of each of the 20 goals independently. For the most part, these questions about the client refer directly to the client-problem profile. However, some of the goals are such that additional information (also gathered in the assessment instrument), sometimes single questions, must be considered. At the present time, the translation rules to move from the problem profiles to the goal structure are the most tentative part of this system. The VSOP staff in California is working on this problem using a variety of clinical procedures and experiences, including a Delphi validation with experts in the field. For purposes of understanding, a partial write-up of the definitional procedures for one of the goals is given in Figure 5-1.

It should be observed that each of the assessment systems described above encompassed a large number of measurement areas. Other comprehensive functional assessment scales are under constant development.[65,66] For further background, the reader is referred to an updated summary of functional assessment scales and bibliography that appear in a recent publication, *Functional Limitations: A State of the Art Review*.[67]

Methods for describing functional limitations and disability are often not well developed, understood, or accepted and are infrequently used in practice. Functional limitations and residual abilities of an individual are identified by systematically taking an inventory of the repertoire of skills that are considered necessary to fulfill expected social roles or provide a satisfactory quality of life. Such lists can be literally endless and hopelessly detailed, on the one hand, or else too skimpy and insufficiently comprehensive, on the other hand. Instead of "laundry lists," it is more useful to employ a conversion to a numerical scoring method for representing defined domains in the continuum between intactness and deficiency. Disability is represented by the sum of interactions between the person and her or his environment that fail to meet expected social roles. Thus, functional assessment concentrates on displaying the presence or absence of key performances and behaviors within those domains that define expected social roles. These performances and behaviors are usually translated to mean an individual's basic strengths and weaknesses, which are then presented in a concise and synoptic format.

We would caution potential users of the various existing measurement systems to consider those systems that assess the needs of the long-term-care client most comprehensively. For some, this may mean a simple implementation of the existing assessment systems. Others may find the need to modify through expansion

---

DEFINITIONAL PROCEDURE

GOAL: *Improve Instrumental Activities Skills*

Description: This goal addresses teaching, training, or otherwise increasing the client's capacity to perform the instrumental activities of daily living (IADL). Such activities range from cooking, shopping, and doing housework to making change, using the telephone appropriately, and calling for a taxi for transportation. Improvement in this area can range across all such activities or be limited to one and can have as an objective complete independence in one or all activities or be directed at increasing the client's helping participation in even a minor instrumental activity that is otherwise performed by another person.

Rationale: The goal is suggested largely to enable the client to participate as much as is appropriately possible in the provision of his or her daily needs. It has the purpose of limiting excess dependence by training the client to do for himself or herself as much as is desirable and feasible.

Inclusion/Exclusion Logic: Anyone with a deficit in IADL should be initially included for consideration. Then, persons fitting any *one* of the critical problem profiles listed (not given in this example) should be *excluded* from consideration of the goal. Exclusion from the goal is warranted under those circumstances in which the client is so physically and/or mentally impaired that training is not realistic. Additionally there may be some circumstances in which, while the client is not totally impaired, the pattern of support received and his or her own satisfaction with the status quo make it inadvisable to disrupt the existing homeostasis by instituting a training program.

Figure 5.1. Definitional Procedure for a Service Goal

or contraction of one or more of these systems. In making a choice one should be aware of, and try to achieve, the following:

- comprehensiveness of coverage
- operational clarity
- ease and cost efficiency of use
- reliability and validity of goal-translation mechanisms
- intergoal care-planning relationships
- over-time utility as a tracking and monitoring system

At the same time, it must be noted that there are many scales being developed and proposed for use in assessing the types of care needed that do not adequately take into account the psychological and social aspects of quality of life of the long-term-care person, either in terms of configuration of psychological or social needs or in terms of the associated levels of service interventions required. It appears, therefore, that considerable efforts are needed to impress on those involved in the public-health field that, in developing means for assessing client needs and client outcomes, it is extremely important to consider the *total individual*, including the social and psychological quality-of-life components. It can be freely admitted that developing reliable and valid scales concerning the quality-of-life aspects is not an easy task. Certainly it is easier to measure physical functioning states through direct observation than it is to measure feelings or inner states of the individual. But classification systems that take into consideration the values, feelings, and desires of the individual—particularly those which take into consideration the client's own perceptions—are necessary if we, in fact, want to give more than lip service to the concept of promoting the quality of life and feelings of well-being of the elderly and chronically handicapped.

Spectrum of Long-Term-Care Services and the Need for Knowledge

Having described the long-term-care client and various ways of measuring the needs, how should he or she be served? There is an increased awareness of the need for a complete spectrum of long-term-care services, of which day care is one type. Weissert has asserted that

> services could be designed to take advantage of community, family and visitor involvement in care and could mitigate the problems of inappropriate placement in nursing homes by providing a broader array of placement choices.[68]

Data are being accumulated that indicate that at least some types of persons previously seen as needing around-the-clock supervision offered in institutions can function successfully in less protective settings, and that community service programs, when properly organized and implemented, can prevent institutionalization. But a great deal more knowledge is needed concerning which types of interventions will have desirable effects on different subgroups of the population. Knowledge concerning the potential benefits of innovative programs in long-term care, including differential effects on persons with different characteristics, is insufficient. It is particularly important that such programs be studied from their inception and that an experimental framework be employed. By studying the relationships between service interventions and the living conditions, health, and well-being of various subgroups of the physically impaired and aged long-term-care clients, more efficient patterns of delivery and utilization of health and social services can be developed.

Impact research is of particular importance in the case of rehabilitation studies of the physically impaired and the elderly. Without it, an intervention program may be considered a failure when in reality it is successful. Very often, the best we may expect to achieve is a slowdown in the degenerative process. Thus, if we merely study the "before and after" behavior of elderly persons being served by a program, we may be observing a downward pattern and assume failure when, in fact, the intervention may have been successful in slowing down the rate of deterioration. Unfortunately, many of the current innovative service programs assume rather than test for positive program impact. As pointed out by Anderson and Stone in their discussion of research findings concerning quality of nursing home care,

> In an examination of standards, that is, assumptions about what quality is, it becomes apparent that attention has focused mainly on ... characteristics which might be considered resources appropriate to the provision of good care, rather than on ... how that care affects ... conditions. ... Evaluating the quality of ... care then becomes a task of relating the care actually given an individual to some statement ... of ... goal achievement potential. Then quality could be measured, not in terms of *input* (facilities, staff, and other resources) or in terms of *output* (what programs and activities are undertaken or participated in), but in terms of *outcome*: is the patient restored to and maintained at the best level of functioning possible.[69]

Necessity for a Continuum of Long-Term-Care Services

The national testing of a system of long-term care would be greatly enhanced if there were a unified national policy and operational program mix for meeting long-term-care needs in the community.[70] To begin the discussion, we must first ask whether such a system does in fact exist. Unfortunately, the answer is no. There is no comprehensive, multifaceted program for meeting the needs of the long-term-care population. In its place there are numerous fragments of programs that tap discrete service needs with duplication, competition, and, in some cases, intentional confrontation based upon the separate, categorical funding of programs aimed at the same problem areas. One type of response has been a proliferation of less comprehensive, more focused services, such as transportation to outpatient clinics and other ancillary services, visiting-nurse services, homemaker services, mail-delivery systems, telephone checks, emergency "hot-line" provisions, and information, referral, and counseling services. Recent years have seen the development of some preliminary, but still severely limited, attempts at more comprehensive programs, such as (1) day hospitals and day care; (2) sheltered community-living arrangements, such as specialized apartments for the impaired and elderly, intermediate housing,[78] and foster care; and (3) community-based, individualized, coordinated programs of home care, such as Project Triage in Connecticut and the home-care demonstration programs under way in Georgia and in Monroe County, New York.[32(pp283-292), 71-79] The extent of this program confounding can be seen by the Orkand Corporation study conducted in 1977, indicating a minimum of 115 federal programs alone that provided cash, in-kind resources, and services to meet the needs of the elderly population.[80] Note of this situation was taken by A. Fleming:

> Although wide ranges of in-home and community based services are available to maintain older persons in their homes, most of these services are fragmented, financed under different Federal programs with differing eligibility requirements, income levels, and sometimes conflicting regulations.[81]

In the absence of a coordinated system of care, there is information on various components of such a system. There is a hope that a system could arise in which adult day care, institutional care, domiciliary care, sheltered congregate housing, and home care could all be integral components along a continuum of care. What then is the key to developing a continuum of long-term-care services? Is it some combination of formal services or must we look elsewhere for the cornerstone of good-quality community care? The answer, as will be discussed below, is that any systematic approach to delivering a continuum of care for the long-term-care population must rest on the informal support system. The complexities of support for the elderly provided by spouses, family, and friends that influence the ability of elderly to avoid institutionalization have been widely studied.[82-86]

Dependence of Highly Vulnerable Elderly on Relatives

The consensus is that the ability of vulnerable elderly to live in the community depends as much on personal isolation and effective helpers as it does on level of functioning.[87] The GAO Cleveland study, for example, on the basis of a small sample, showed that few institutionalized people had a spouse or lived with their children at the time they were institutionalized and that over three-quarters lived alone.[88] This finding of the institutionalized as previously living alone has been reported in many studies including, for example, the Kraus study using a Canadian elderly population. In the Cleveland study, family and friends provided 50% of the services received by older persons of all impairment levels, but over 70% of the services received by the greatly or extremely impaired group.[25] In an HRCA study of the needs of Massachusetts elderly, of those judged as not being able to live in the community without supports, 79% were assessed as likely to be institutionalized if the informal support services they were receiving were terminated.[10] It is interesting to note that these higher-risk people were functionally impaired, more likely not to have a spouse, and much more likely to be living with their offspring. They were also less likely to have close friends, daily phone contact, or daily contact with anyone living outside of their household. It can be hypothesized that the homes of their offspring provided immediate and highly personal health structures, and that the systems in which they live are undoubtedly responsive to their needs. In addition, on the basis of clinical judgment and the self-report of these elderly people, about 90% of the high-risk group indicated that the help they received would in all likelihood continue into the future.

The importance of supports received by vulnerable elderly living in the homes of their relatives in unquestioned, although the actual proportion of persons with such environments and the means through which they entered these environments is largely unknown. The distribution of elderly in various living arrangements is somewhat difficult to estimate from available data without making assumptions about who is the head of the household. As of the 1970 census, for example, some 7.4% of males 65 years of age or older and 22.8% of the females were living with someone other than a spouse.[89] Another figure of interest is that, in 1975, 3.7% of aged males and 12.7% of aged females were living in families in which they were noted as a relative, although no data are available on the nature of the dependence of the relationship. However, given the earlier estimate of population vulnerability and the Massachusetts findings regarding residential care, we can assume that the majority of persons listed as "other relatives" in the 1975 current population survey are receiving some type of supportive care from their families.

In an HRCA study of a random sample of elderly tenants living alone in age-integrated housing in Boston, when these elderly were trichotomized into severely handicapped, moderately handicapped, or not-handicapped strata, the severely handicapped were most likely to be receiving some type of formal service support across a wide variety of support areas.[90] Given the fact that they were living alone, one might expect the informal support system to be *unimportant*; however, the help provided by informal sources to these severely handicapped persons was judged by the HRCA staff to have played a *critical* role in maintaining a full one-third of these people in the community setting. Thus, not only are the severely handicapped persons more likely to receive formal agency services, but the informal help that they do receive is more important to their continued community maintenance than it is to the other two groups. Perhaps an even more interesting finding is the fact that the severely handicapped persons reported the highest level of confidence in the ability of their informal helpers to continue providing apparently crucial supports, even if their need for assistance were to increase. The self-perceptions of these severely handicapped persons are also borne out by the clinical impressions of the HRCA interviewers. Evidence of this commitment can be seen in the fact that the supporting persons who are in contact with the severely handicapped group were more likely to have initiated the contact themselves. Furthermore, the severely handicapped group was more likely than members of the other two groups to have daily contact with supporting persons. The qualitative difference in relationship that presumably emerges from this frequent contact may very well be interpreted by the sample member and the interviewing clinician as a sign of general resilience of the helping network, playing a crucial role in keeping these people in the community. Nonetheless, with respect to research findings, Lowenthal and Robinson report that relatively little is known about the degree to which friends and neighbors fill instrumental roles in the absence of or in lieu of family members.[86] Additionally, little is known about the prevalence of helping networks that combine both the more intensive support provided by family with that available from friends and neighbors. Addressing this issue, data have recently been presented regarding the helping patterns within a high-rise facility for the elderly in St. Louis.[61] In this instance, the most prevalent type of informal helper was an adult offspring, with 42% of the sample identifying an adult offspring as their primary source of support. Even more dramatically, of those persons with children within a one-half hour drive, 73% named an offspring as their most important helper. Neighbors entered the helping picture as secondary helpers. Thirty-one percent of the tenants had helped a neighbor in the past six months (most often with grocery shopping), and an additional 8% indicated that a neighbor would ask them for help if it was required. It can be seen from these data that almost 40% of the tenants enter into secondary supporting roles, providing assistance to other residents of this particular high-rise facility. This 40% figure is particularly impressive in light of the fact that one-half of the tenants had no needs that would have required help from others.

A final point regarding the strength and importance of informal helping networks can be made on the basis of an analysis of the Kent/Hirsch Survey of Needs of Black and White Aged in Philadelphia. In the HRCA analysis of these data, the most important finding to emerge is the near-total ability of service resources, both formal and informal, to meet the needs of those requiring assistance.[90] Some 70% of the sample members required assistance in at least one of 29 support areas. The average number of areas in which assistance was required was nine. Of those having needs, only 39% had any residual unmet needs once the help that was being received was taken into consideration. More importantly, the average number of unmet needs was only about one. What this means is that 93% of the overall needs found in this sample are being met, and although the black elderly had a significantly higher number of areas of need (with a mean of 9.4% needs as opposed to 8.6% needs), there was no difference by race in terms of the extent to which these needs were being met. The manner in which these needs were being met is comparable across the two racial groups—that is, blacks and whites had equivalent numbers of need areas met by informal and formal sources.

From the perspective of the problems faced by the vulnerable elderly, it can be seen that the management of these individuals becomes a lifelong commitment. This commitment has been largely taken up by the informal support systems of these people. It is the formal system that provides most alternative community services, and it is with this resource that much work needs to be done in the future. From the formal service perspective, it is clear that the aim of intervention should be to maintain and optimize the functional ability of the long-term-care person and also to optimally and maximally reinforce the informal support system. However, in all too many instances, many community programs have failed to incorporate these fundamental rehabilitation components, which would allow individuals and families to maximize autonomy and self-actualization. Many persons are simply being served by their informal system with some formal help in areas in which the elderly person is no longer able to complete a function. It is interesting to note that there is no real philosophical base, theoretical basis, or even causal model that would say that community programs have as one of their primary goals client rehabilitation to maximum possible functional status. In the absence of such an emphasis, we may be putting undue pressure on the informal support system, and this fact may prove in the long run to be an important explanation for premature institutional placement.

In this regard, it is interesting to note that there are other industrialized countries, such as England, in which minimal use has been made of long-term institutional alternatives. Community options have been tried, although the literature does not show with any finality the extent to which these options have achieved the types of success that are being sought within this country.[70]

The community housing and service system in the United States, as previously indicated, is composed of a wide variety of disparate parts. Many studies have appeared documenting needs and suggesting alternatives—for example, the estimate that the current supply of personal-care homes, sheltered-living arrangements, and congregate housing (including domiciliary care) was between 0.3 and 0.8 million in 1977 and that the demand was closer to 1.5 to 1.9 million persons,[20] a most shocking finding, if true, but who is to take up the challenge, what is the system that is to respond? In point of fact, how many persons involved at the various levels of service planning and delivery are even aware of this finding?

Community Demonstration Projects:
Successes and Failures

What follows is not a comprehensive description or review of the long-term-care system, but rather a discussion of some of the indicative studies relating to parts of this system. These studies demonstrate both the possibility for positively affecting the long-term-care client and the problems that can be involved in seeking to accomplish this task. The studies have immediate relevancy to adult day-care assessment because they point out the real potential that community programming can have for meeting the needs of the long-term-care client. Adult day care must still find a place within the long-term-care spectrum of services and these findings indicate some of the problems that should be anticipated, including questions that should be included in any assessment effort.

It should be obvious that institutional residency is to a large extent unacceptable to the elderly, although they can come to accept, rely, and want such placement. This does not mean that institutional placement is not appropriate in many instances. What it does mean is that for many individuals approaching the institutional setting, prior to having made the commitment to enter, some type of resocialization process probably takes place. In a recently completed study carried out by the Foundation for Health Care Evaluation (the PSRO agency in Minneapolis) in conjunction with HRCA, preadmission interviews with several hundred applicants for SNF (skilled-nursing facility) and ICF (intermediate-care facility) nursing homes revealed an overwhelming desire to return to the community.[91] These persons had neither accepted the inevitability of their long-term-care placement nor given up on their own potential for independent functioning. If elderly are indeed upset with the dependency effects of debilitation and do not want to give up their independent existence, then alternatives to institutionalization may very well have considerable effects. As a matter of fact, in an early study of waiting-list applicants to the Hebrew Rehabilitation Center for Aged, it was found that, by offering minimal contact and referral services, it was possible to have massive positive effects on the future rate of institutionalization. At the same time, with respect to functional health, there were no effects—the program neither benefited nor harmed the experimental group. The latter statement relative to harm is particularly important, in that the reduction in institutional placements was not accompanied by any concomitant differential losses in other health areas.[29]

Another community study conducted by HRCA in a transitional area of Boston focused on individuals who exhibited considerable fears concerning their changing neighborhoods.[92] The service component consisted of a referral system with individual case supports, without the types of direct resources that have been found in some of the more recent Medicare and Medicaid waiver studies that have been and are being conducted. This study resulted in differential institutional placement. In this instance, the random experimental and control groups experienced similar levels of out-migration from the transitional area. However, what is of importance is that there was significant experiment/control difference in the nature of the residential change. Forty-three percent of the controls who moved went into an institution, while only 22% of the experimentals who moved went into an institution. In addition, clinical judgment made at the time of pretest relative to the appropriateness of various placement options found that four times as many experimentals who were placed in institutions (42%) as compared with controls who were institutionalized (10%) were appropriately placed.

A third major study that HRCA recently completed involved a long-term followup of elderly and handicapped individuals who went into a sheltered-housing facility in Fall River, Massachusetts as an alternative to nursing-home placement.[76] The Fall River facility can be seen as an option to long-term-care-facility placement, and the goal of the study was to test the therapeutic potential of an environmental modification in conjunction with certain support services. Within this experiment, there were massive effects on various health variables, including, in this instance, death, with the experimentals experiencing reduced death rates. There were also significant reductions experienced by the experimentals, as compared with their matched controls, in institutionalization, and, when a cost-benefit comparison was made, very high benefit-to-cost ratios were observed. As was true in the previously discussed studies, there were no effects on functional health. For all intents and purposes, experimentals and controls had comparable levels of physical functioning problems over the five-year period during which measures were gathered.

The various components of a potential long-term-care system have not always been proven as beneficial as the examples cited above. Long-term-care service components can fail for any number of reasons, and we must be prepared to learn from these failures. In a recently completed study of the potential of discharging nursing-home clients, who were clinically judged to have the potential for discharge into community-care (or domiciliary-care) homes, there was an overwhelming lack of movement.[26] This program effort was carried out by the Vermont PRSO, making use of indigenous resources, and with a heavy emphasis on voluntary-provider (nursing-home) participation. The institutional subjects had been residents for an average of about two years, and some 75% were resistant to discharge. These subjects were not prepared to address the possibility of community residency, and these data would indicate that, in the absence of a concentrated motivational program, both the residents and facility staff were unwilling and/or unable to even initiate the discharge-planning process.

This finding of consumer resistance to a new intervention effort is common to many different programs, including adult day care.[93] One can design the best possible program, remove the financial and bureaucratic hindrances, and still fail because the clients are not adequately prepared for, or simply refuse to believe that they require, the designated service. In a recently completed study of a unique electronic medical monitoring system in the community, a concentrated program to overcome consumer resistance to the free service was implemented.[94] The program included mailings, one-to-one contact, extensive personal followups, and the involvement of formal and informal helpers of the long-term-care client whenever possible. Even with these efforts, a full 30% of the sample refused the service, and there were very few clients who changed their minds from negative to positive once having stated an opinion. Thus, even in the presence of a relatively sophisticated "selling" program, refusals occurred, and they appear to have been relatively unchangeable. On the positive side, more of the "higher-need" clients were found to accept the service, and, when procedures were instituted that removed any potential threat to the person's informal support system, acceptance rates increased. Thus, on the basis of this experience, we would conclude that the initial presentation of the program was crucial, that the informal support system should not be threatened (such as by putting pressure on for involvement in the particular service intervention), and that persons with the greatest need appear to sense this fact and are more likely, therefore, to participate in the program.

Another example of a program that failed to achieve its stated objectives is the Foundation for Health Care Evaluation PSRO long-term-care review system.[95] In this evaluation, all new admissions to a sample of Minneapolis long-term-care facilities were reviewed by means of a standardized questionnaire. The interviews were implemented on a delegated basis by the staff of the facilities. The major hypothesis being tested was that the new information would cause the facilities to act in the best interest of the clients, implementing programs to maximize both the most appropriate levels of care and functional independence of the clients. Unfortunately, there were no such results. Clients were systematically placed at too-high levels of care, levels of care that were governed by the bed availability of the facilities to which the clients were making application. In the absence of a total systems approach, the facilities appear to have "misinterpreted" the data and to have acted within limited institutional definitions of appropriate care.[91]

Another example of a program that failed was the Massachusetts implementation of an experimental home-care program in Worcester, Massachusetts making use of Medicaid funds to provide enriched services.[96] To understand the findings from the Worcester Home Care study, one must recognize the importance of getting the correct sample into the program, as was the case in many of the studies previously cited. Individuals who are in need and who are likely to be at risk unless services are provided must be identified, for they must be the ones served. In the study of home care conducted by the state of Massachusetts in Worcester, it was HRCA's feeling that the finding of a lack of effects was based primarily on the type of population selected. The state-supported screening unit identified, to a large extent, persons who did not have appropriate levels of need, and the existing community resources were equally as successful in meeting the needs of the controls as the program was in meeting the needs of the experimentals. Because of the small number of high-risk, vulnerable people identified, the chances of affecting these people to begin with were greatly reduced.

In the earlier-mentioned study of the electronic medical monitoring system and in a National Center for Health Services Research experiment involving a concentrated day-care program, extensive outreach programs were employed to identify persons at risk of institutionalization.[74,75] In both instances, impact data were reported indicating significant positive effects on the rate of skilled-nursing-facility utilization. Unfortunately, the magnitude of the effects was quite small. Weissert reports that "day care patients averaged 4 days per year of skilled nursing facility inpatient care, but control group members averaged 9 days."[75(p14)] The implications of this low level of nursing-home utilization are twofold: First, the persons who were, in fact, on a path toward an institution went unrecognized, and thus needless institutional placements were not prevented. Second, the comparative social cost of providing the service (the cost to the experimentals) was much greater than the costs for the controls. Weissert, with respect to cost, states that "day care patients averaged $2,692 more than the control group over a one year period."[75(p19)]

In several currently ongoing studies of community alternatives, a great deal of emphasis is being placed on identifying vulnerable individuals within more comprehensive programs. In the Monroe County Long-Term-Care Program study, for example, where it is possible to offer community-service alternatives based on a Medicaid waiver, all people applying to long-term-care facilities are being screened, and only those individuals who would have been appropriately placed in a domiciliary-care facility or institution and who would not be able to stay in the community without additional supports are receiving the Medicaid-waiver services. Unfortunately, the nature of the evaluation of this program being supported by the state of New York will seriously limit the lessons we will be able to learn from this program, in that there is no comparable "control" group. However, several preliminary comments are warranted, based upon the early impressions of the local evaluation committee, of which one of the authors (JNM) is a member, and the outside evaluator (MACRO Systems, Inc.). First, it has been possible to institute this program in a service-rich and highly competitive community. Large numbers of clients have been screened and placed in the community, and many of the program clients are deemed to need skilled nursing care. On the negative side, there have been difficulties in role definitions and, to some extent, with interagency cooperation. The problems in bringing the various actors together, within a voluntary planning and service-coordination effort, have been considerable.

Efforts such as that in Rochester are trying to work within the constraints of the existing service systems. It is apparent from this example that there is a need, and the client population can be screened and placed in the community. There are difficulties inherent in these types of nonsystematic voluntary participation efforts. The Congressional Budget Office study of long-term care for the elderly and disabled listed the problems as follows:

> To provide home care, it might be necessary to obtain income assistance from the welfare department, homemaker services from a Title XX funded social service program, and health care from the visiting nurse association with each agency insisting on its own review of the patient's eligibility. If one element of the package should fall through, the patient could not remain at home.[20]

Summary

Along with an individualized approach to long-term care, it is important to match an individual's need with an appropriate environmental setting and level-of-service support and to monitor and make appropriate corrections over time. Even apart from the issue of fair allocation of services in light of scarce resources and rising costs, it is generally assumed that the better the "fit" between the individual and the level of services received, the more likely it is that the desired outcome, including effects on the quality of life, will be achieved. Unfortunately, as noted previously, hard evidence is not yet available to differentiate clearly among community programs in terms of which are more or equally effective in providing rehabilitation and/or life enrichments for different types of persons requiring long-term care. Nor, for that matter, is information available that would permit the matching of individual needs to existing housing stock, so as to optimize the well-being of the person attempting to live independently under current community arrangements.

It is interesting to note, as Kahana and Coe do, that much of the focus of community programs for the elderly is usually on the provision of environmental supports of one sort or another, and this would, to a large extent, include adult day care.[87] However, to the extent that we do get into restorative and preventive programs, it will be necessary to better understand some of the dynamics that might lead to an individual actually experiencing a shift in functioning ability. Work in this area, at least within community alternative programming, is largely for the future. Kahana and Coe go so far as to say that the "utilization of home care programs for preventive purposes has been almost non-existent in the community, while at best, home care may serve to bring needed professional help into the homes of the incapacitated. At worst it provides simply a crutch to marginal survival." It should be clear that with many of the environmental options, including sheltered housing, domiciliary care, and service-oriented environmental programs, such as adult day care and day hospitals, an emphasis can reasonably be placed on prevention and restoration.

If we were to categorize some of the presently operational demonstration programs with respect to their specification of models for affecting health status, at least in terms of physical functioning, the casual models simply are lacking, even in such studies as Project Triage, the Monroe County Long-Term-Care Program, and the Georgia Alternative Health Service Project. For example, in the Georgia demonstration, it is indicated that physical independence is an outcome area to be measured, by three different measures: ADL, walking, and instrumental activities. However, there is no clear explication of why the program should effect this particular set of outcome dimensions. This does not mean that hypothesized casual models are always missing. Mitchell, in a comparison of community and institutional Veterans Administration (VA) programs, proves an explanation of why functional health may improve, based on the hypothesis that the elderly will prefer community residences even in the case of serious disability.[97] The person may, therefore, be more motivated to maintain or improve a certain level of physical functioning so as to facilitate their staying in the community, all other things being equal. Unfortunately, the groups being compared were not comparable at pretest, and the study of effects is therefore problematic. In this instance, the multiple regression procedures used showed there to be almost no relationship between the program status and change in functional health.

From a more comprehensive perspective, Conly has reviewed (as of June 1977) 25 community long-term-care research projects funded by the federal government, including adult day care.[93] Conly indicated that there was a major preoccupation in these studies with changing functioning and preventing unnecessary institutionalization. However, the aims were really not carried out, largely because of research failings. At the time of her review, and it should be noted that some of the studies that she reviewed were not complete at that time, she indicated that design and implementation problems meant that, to a large extent, the projects provided insufficient testing of the models that they were trying to look at. In this review, Conly is particularly interested in institutionalization as a health-outcome variable, and she indicates that since "there are no quantified models relating debility state, socioeconomic status, and personal characteristics, including personal references to the probability of institutionalization it is possible that the options tested will be relevant to only an inconsequential portion of the institutionalized or potentially institutionalized population."

In this review, we have attempted to point out that we have not gone very far in looking at community programming for the long-term-care client. It is obvious that there are studies in the field today that have the potential for answering many of the questions. Unfortunately, many of the studies have research designs that are sorely lacking, and the answers that they produce may not be conclusive. Impact evaluation, at this point in community programming, is a necessity. Peterson, in a editorial commenting on these issues, states that "the worst mistake we could make would be to rush to provide more ambulatory and domiciliary services as if we knew what to do. If we did, we would end up with more services, whether effective or ineffective, and add more expenditures to an already oppressive national bill. The first logical step is to perform a series of randomized clinical trials to ascertain which ambulatory or home services, if any, are effective in maintaining persons with chronic disease, especially the frail and elderly in their homes and communities."[98] We are in agreement with these comments. This is the challenge. Impact evaluation is a very difficult but important information-generation procedure for health-care and long-term-care policy formulation. If we intend to prolong life, reduce unnecessary institutional placements, and maximize functional independence, we had better be sure that the programs we are suggesting do, in fact, have the chance of achieving those goals. It is obvious today that there are great restrictions on program expansions, and this would seem to be a good time to take a firm look at which programs should be supported and which should fall by the wayside.

The Administration on Aging (AOA) has recently funded several such multiprogram comparison efforts. A large number of community-service programs are now operational and are about to be analyzed. These programs include Project Triage in Connecticut, the Domiciliary Care Program in Pennsylvania, the Monroe County Long-Term Care Program, the Georgia Alternative Health Service Project, the VSOP program in Los Angeles, the Wisconsin Community Care Organization Project, the "222" Analysis of Homemaker Services, and the analysis of various institutional and community programs in Delaware, just to mention a few. The potential for a considerable increase in the available knowledge is there. Let us hope that methodological problems and political decisions do not prevent our learning the answers.

References

1. Brotman HB: The fastest growing minority: The aging. *Am J Pub Health* **64:** 249–252, 1974.

2. Federal Council on Aging: *Annual Report to the President—1976.* DHEW Publication No (OHD) 77-2095. US Government Printing Office, 1977.

3. *Acute Conditions, Incidence and Associated Disability.* DHEW, PHS Publication No (PHS) 78-1548, Series 20, No 120. US Government Printing Office, 1978.

4. Ryder CF: The doctor's dilemma—Updated, in Katz AH, Felton JS (eds): *Health and the Community.* New York, The Free Press, 1965.

5. *Health United States 1978.* DHEW Publication No (PHS) 78-1232. US Government Printing Office, 1978.

6. Sherwood S: Long-term care: Issues, perspectives and directions, in Sherwood S (ed): *Long-term Care: A Handbook for Researchers, Planners and Providers.* New York, Spectrum Publications, Inc, 1975, pp 3–79.

7. *Health United States 1978.* DHEW Publication No (PHS) 78-1232. US Government Printing Office, 1978.

8. Nagi SZ: An epidemiology of disability among adults in the United States. *Milbank Memorial Fund Quarterly* **54**(4), Fall 1976.

9. Comptroller General of the United States: *Report to Congress: The Well-Being of Older People in Cleveland, Ohio.* US Accounting Office, 1977, p 10.

10. Sherwood S, Morris JN, Gutkin C, et al: The needs of elderly community residents of Massachusetts. Final contract report, supported by research contract with the Survey Research Program, University of Massachusetts, in connection with AOA Grant #90-A-641/01. Boston, Department of Social Gerontological Research, Hebrew Rehabilitation Center for Aged, 1977, p 103.

11. LaVor J: *Long-Term Care: A Challenge to Service Systems.* Office of the Assistant Secretary for Planning and Evaluation, DHEW, 1976.

12. AOA. *Some Prospects for the Future Elderly Population.* DHEW, OHD, AOA, National Clearinghouse on Aging, DHEW Publication No (DHDS) 78-20288, January 1978, pp 125–178.

13. Ruchlin H, Levey S: An economic perspective of long-term care, in Sherwood S (ed): *Long-Term Care: A Handbook for Researchers, Planners and Providers.* New York, Spectrum Publications, Inc, 1975.

14. Sherwood S (ed): *Long-Term Care.*

15. Palmore E: Total chance of institutionalization among the aged. *Gerontologist* **16:** 504–507, 1976.

16. York S, Calsyn R: Family involvement in nursing homes. *Gerontologist* **17:** 500–505, 1977.

17. Zappolo A: *Characteristics, Social Contacts, and Activities of Nursing Home Residents.* DHEW Publication No (HRA) 77-1778, Rockville, Md, DHEW, PHS, HRA, NCHS, 1977.

18. Barney J: The prerogative of choice in long-term care. *Gerontologist* **19**: 309–314, 1977.

19. Hammerman J, Friedsam HH, Shore H: Management perspectives in long-term care facilities, in Sherwood (ed): *Long-Term Care,* pp 179–212.

20. Congressional Budget Office, Congress of the United States: *Long-Term Care for the Elderly and Disabled.* Wash DC, US Government Printing Office, 1977.

21. National Health Survey: *Characteristics of Residents in Nursing Homes and Personal Care Homes.* US Publication, June/August, 1969, Series 121, No 19, HSMHA, National Center for Health Statistics, 1973.

22. Gottesman LE, Brody E: Psycho-social intervention programs within the institutional setting, in Sherwood (ed): *Long-Term Care,* pp 455–509.

23. Townsend P: The effects of family structure on the likelihood of admission to an institution in old age: The application of general theory, in Shanas E, Streib G (eds): *Social Structures and the Family.* Englewood Cliffs, NJ, Prentice-Hall, Inc, 1965, p 174.

24. Gottesman LE: Nursing home research project. Report to respondents. Philadelphia Geriatric Center, Fall, 1971, pp 1–21.

25. Kraus AS, Spasoff RA, Beattie EJ, et al: Elderly applicants to long-term care institutions. I. Their characteristics, health problems and state of mind. *J Am Geriatric Soc,* **24**: 117–125, 1976.

26. Sherwood S, Morris JN, Gutkin C: Impact of the VPSRO discharge planning program, in *HRCA, A Comprehensive Examination of the Characteristics and an Evaluation of the Dischargeability of a Select Group of Patients in Vermont Long-Term Care Facilities.* Boston, Department of Social Gerontological Research, Hebrew Rehabilitation Center for Aged, 1979.

27. Morris JN, Gutkin C: A comprehensive examination of characteristics and an evaluation of dischargeability of a select group of patients in Vermont long-term care facilities. Boston, Hebrew Rehabilitation Center for Aged, 1979, p 31.

28. Kahn K, Hines W, Woodson A, et al: A multidisciplinary approach to assessing the quality of care in long-term care facilities. *Gerontologist* **17**: 61–65, 1977.

29. Sherwood S, Morris JN: A study of aged applicants to a long-term care facility: A final report. Mimeo. In connection with DHEW/BHSR Grant HS00470. Boston, Hebrew Rehabilitation Center for Aged, 1974, pp 42–45.

30. Sutton JF: *Utilization of Nursing Homes.* DHEW, PHS, NCHS, DHEW Publication No (HRA) 77-1779. US Government Printing Office, 1977.

31. Fielding J: *Health Data Annual 1976.* Boston, Massachusetts Dept of Public Health, 1977, p 100.

32. Greer D, Sherwood S, Morris JN, et al: *An Alternative to Institutionalization.* Cambridge, Mass, Ballinger Publishing Co, 1979, pp 85–104.

33. DHEW, ICD: *Eighth Revision, International Classification of Diseases.* Adapted for use in the United States. DHEW (PHS) Publication No 1693, 1968.

34. Sherwood S, Morris JN, Barnhart E: Developing a system for assigning individuals into an appropriate residential setting. *J Gerontol* **30**: 331–341, 1975.

35. Goldfarb AI: The evaluation of geriatric patients following treatment, in Hoch P, Zubin J (eds): *Evaluation of Psychiatric Treatment*. New York, Grune & Stratton, Inc, 1964, pp 288–293.

36. Granger CV: *Medical Rehabilitation Research and Training Center Number Seven Annual Progress Report*. Boston, Tufts University School of Medicine, 1974, p 299.

37. ———: Functional assessment and the long-term care patient, in Kottke F (ed): *Handbook of Physical Medicine and Rehabilitation*. Boston, Tufts University School of Medicine, 1979, pp 45–61.

38. ———, Greer D: Functional status measurement and medical rehabilitation outcomes. *Arch Phys Med Rehab* **57**: 103–109, 1976.

39. ———, Albrecht G, Hamilton B: Outcome of comprehensive medical rehabilitation: Measurement by PULSES profile and the Barthel index. *Arch Phys Med Rehab* **60**: 145–154, 1979.

40. ———, Sherwood CC, Greer D: Functional status measures in a comprehensive stroke care program. *Arch Phys Med Rehab* **58**: 555–561, 1977.

41. Linn M, Linn B, Stein S: Ratings of impairment and functional status in prediction of mortality. *Psych Rep* **37**: 36–39, 1975.

42. Jones EW, McNitt BJ, McKnight EM: *Patient Classification for Long-Term Care User's Manual*. US Dept of Health, Education and Welfare, Dec 1973, pp 1–13.

43. Kahn R, Pollack M, Goldfarb AI: Factors related to individual differences in mental status of institutionalized aged, in Hoch P and Zubin J (eds): *Psychopathology of Aging*. New York, Grune & Stratton, 1961, pp 100–131.

44. Kastenbaum R, Sherwood S: VIRO: A scale for assessing the interview behavior of elderly people, in Kent DP, Kastenbaum R, Sherwood S (eds): *Research, Planning and Action for the Elderly*. New York, Behavioral Publications, 1972, pp 175–181.

45. Katz S, Downs TD, Cash R, et al: Progress in development of the index of ADL. *Gerontologist* **10** (1, pt 1):20–30, 1970.

46. ———, Ford AB, Downs TD, et al: *The Effects of Continued Care*. US Government Printing Office, DHEW Publication No (HSM) 73-3010, 1972, pp 36–59.

47. Lawton MP: Assessing the competence of older people, in Kent DP, Kastenbaum R, Sherwood S (eds): *Research, Planning and Action for the Elderly*.

48. Mahoney F, Barthel D: Functional evaluation: Barthel index. *Md State Med J* **14**: 61–65, 1965.

49. Pfeiffer E: Generic services for the long-term care patient, in Murnaghan J (ed): *Long-Term Care Data, Report of the Conference on Long-Term Health Care Data. Medical Care:* **14**(5), Supplement: 160–163, 1976.

50. Rosow I, Breslau N: A Guttman health scale for the aged. *J Gerontol* **21**: 556–557, 1966.

51. Wylie C: Measuring end results of rehabilitation of patients with stroke. *Public Health Reports* **82**: 893–898, 1967.

52. Weiler P, Rathbone-McCuan E: *Adult-Day Care: Community Work with the Elderly*. New York, Springer Publishing Co, 1978, pp 134–136.

53. Weed L: Medical records that guide and teach. *New Eng J Med* **278**: 593–600, 652–657, 1968.

54. ———: Medical records. *Medical Education and Patient Care*. Cleveland, Case Western Reserve University, 1969, pp 26–61.

55. Maddox G, Dellinger DC: Assessment of functional status in a program evaluation and resource allocation model. *The Annals* **438**: 59–70, 1978.

56. Tufts Medical Rehabilitation, Research and Training Center RT-7 Annual Progress Report. Boston, 1975–1976.

57. Mor V, Sherwood CC, Wieners C: Developing inter-rater reliability among social workers and public health nurses in the assessment of long-term care need. Boston, Department of Social Gerontological Research, Hebrew Rehabilitation Center for Aged, 1977, p 4.

58. Granger C, Dewis L, Peters N, et al: Stroke rehabilitation: An analysis of repeated Barthel index measures. *Arch Phys Med Rehab* **60**: 14–17, 1979.

59. Sherwood S, Mor V, Morris JN, et al: Final report: The clinical assessment of interviewable Rhode Island state mental health clients. Boston, Department of Social Gerontological Research, Hebrew Rehabilitation Center for Aged, 1977, pp 1–82.

60. Sherwood S, Morris JN: A program for meeting the needs of nursing home applicants who have intact communication skills. Boston, Department of Social Gerontological Research, Hebrew Rehabilitation Center for Aged, 1979, pp 3–6.

61. Morris JN, Sherwood S, Kasten S, et al: Parkview Towers resident typology. Boston, Hebrew Rehabilitation Center for Aged, July, 1979, p 6.

62. Sherwood CC, Sherwood S, Morris JN, et al: The clinical assessment of interviewable Rhode Island state chronic hospital patients. Boston, Department of Social Gerontological Research, Hebrew Rehabilitation Center for Aged, 1976, p 12.

63. Burton D, Granger C, Greer D, et al: Population description and identification. *Final Report: Residential Environments for the Functionally Disabled*. Wash DC, Gerontological Society, 1977, pp 26–33.

64. Morris JN, Mor V: HRCA assessment instrument and associated goal specification model description. Boston, Hebrew Rehabilitation Center for Aged, 1978, pp 1–10.

65. Breckenridge K: Medical rehabilitation program evaluation. *Arch Phys Med Rehab* **59**: 419–423, 1978.

66. Grauer H, Birnbom F: A geriatric functional rating scale to determine the need for institutional care. *J Am Geriatrics Soc* **23**: 472–476, 1975.

67. Muzzio TC, Burris CT: *Functional Limitations: A State of the Art Review*. Falls Church, Va, Indices, Inc, 1979, p 53.

68. Weissert WG: Long-term care: An overview, in DHEW: *Health United States 1978*, Hyattsville, Md, DHEW Publication No (PHS) 78-1232, 1978, p 99.

69. Anderson NN, Stone LB: Nursing homes: Research and public policy. *Gerontologist* **9**: 214–218, 1969.

70. Weilder P: Geriatric care abroad. *Forum*, pp 33–35, 1979.

71. Cosin LZ: The organization of a day hospital for psychiatric patients. *Proceedings Royal Soc Med* **49**: 237–239, 1956.

72. O'Brien TD, Roberts J, Breckenridge GR, et al: Some aspects of community care of the frail and elderly: The need for assessment. *Gerontologia Clinica*, 1968, pp 215–227.

73. McDonald RD, Neulander A, Holod O, et al: Description of a non-residential psychogeriatric day care facility. *Gerontologist* **11**: 322–327, 1971.

74. Robins EG: Therapeutic day care: Progress report on experiments to test the feasibility for third party reimbursement. Paper presented at 27th Annual Scientific Meeting of the Gerontological Society, Portland, Oreg, 1974, p 7.

75. Weissert WG, Wan TH, Livieratos BB: *Effects and Costs of Day Care and Homemaker Services for the Chronically Ill: A Randomized Experiment*. Hyattsville, Md, DHEW Publication No (PHS) 79-3250, NCHSR Publication and Information Branch, August 1979, pp 26–28.

76. Urban Systems Research-Engineering, Inc: *Evaluation of the Effectiveness of Congregate Housing for the Elderly—A Final Report*. US Government Printing Office, stock 023-000-00378-3, Oct 1976, pp 229–262.

77. Thompson MM: *Housing for the Handicapped and Disabled*. National Association of Housing and Redevelopment Officials, 1977, pp 11–21.

78. Brody EM: Service-supported independent living in an urban setting, in Byerts TO (ed): *Housing and Environment for the Elderly*. Gerontological Society, 1973, pp 191–197.

79. Hicks B, Raisz H, Segan J, et al: The Triage experiment in coordinated care for the elderly. *Am J Pub Health* **71**: 891–1003, 1981.

80. Orkand Corporation: *Final Report on an Inventory of Federal Outlays for the Elderly*. Report No TR-76-W-071, prepared for AOA, DHEW, 1977.

81. Fleming A: U.S. Congress, Subcommittee on Health and Long-Term Care: *New Perspectives in Health Care for Older Americans*, 94th Congress, 2nd Sess, 1976.

82. Shanas E: Measuring the home health needs of the aged in five countries. *J Gerontol* **26**: 37–40, 1971.

83. Maddox G: Social determinants of behavior, in Hine F, Pfeiffer E, Maddox G, et al (eds): *Behavioral Science: A Selective View*. Boston, Little, Brown, 1972, pp 233–260.

84. Jackson JJ: Comparative life styles and family and friend relationships among older black women. *Family Coordinator*, 1972.

85. Neugarten BL, Hagestad GO: Aged and life course, in Binstock RH, Shanas E (eds): *Handbook of Aging and the Social Sciences*, New York, Van Nostrand Reinhold, Co, 1976, pp 47–52.

86. Lowenthal MF, Robinson B: Social networks and isolation, in Binstock RH, Shanan E (eds): *Handbook of Aging and the Social Sciences*. New York, Van Nostrand Reinhold Co, 1976, pp 447–450.

87. Kahana E, Coe RM: Alternatives in long-term care, in Sherwood (ed): *Long-Term Care*, pp 516–519.

88. Comptroller General of the United States: *Home Health—The Need for a National Policy to Better Provide for the Elderly*. Report to the Congress, US Government Printing Office, HRD-78-19, December 30, 1977, pp 425–440.

89. Siegel JS: *Demographic Aspects of Aging and the Older Population in the United States*. US Government Printing Office, DHEW Publication No (HRA) 77-1232, 1976, p 152.

90. Progress Report, AOA Grant #90-A-129H. Boston, Hebrew Rehabilitation Center for Aged, Department of Social Gerontological Research, 1978, pp 80–85.

91. Morris JN, Sherwood S: Program for meeting the needs of nursing home applicants who have intact communication skills. Boston, Hebrew Rehabilitation Center for Aged, Department of Social Gerontological Research, 1978, pp 9–10.

92. Sherwood S, Morris JN: The Roxbury-Dorchester Experiment: A study of persons living in a transitional area. Boston, Hebrew Rehabilitation Center for Aged, Department of Social Gerontological Research, 1975, pp 23–25.

93. Conly S: Critical review of research on long-term care alternatives. Wash DC, Office of Social Services and Human Development, Office of the Assistant Secretary for Planning and Evaluation, DHEW, 1977, pp 21–22.

94. Sherwood S, Morris JN: Draft report of Lifeline evaluation study. Boston, Hebrew Rehabilitation Center for Aged, Department of Social Gerontological Research, 1979, pp 46–48.

95. Hendrickson M, Gustafson J: An integrated approach to review: A demonstration and evaluation of a long-term care program. Minneapolis, Foundation for Health Care Evaluation, 1979.

96. Sherwood S, Morris JN, Sherwood CC, et al: Final report concerning impact of services on health and well-being. Boston, Hebrew Rehabilitation Center for Aged, Department of Social Gerontological Research, 1975, pp 59–63.

97. Mitchell J: Patient outcomes in alternative long-term care settings. *Medical Care* 16: 439–452, 1978.

98. Peterson OL: Geriatrics: The need for science and policy. *Ann Int Med* 89: 279–281, 1978.

ID

The Adult Day-Care Experience

6

The History of Adult Day-Care Programs

Carole Lium O'Brien, RN, MS

Introduction

It is widely recognized that not only are older adults more often ill and/or disabled than younger persons, but they have less income and are less able to care for themselves. Coupled with these facts are sky-rocketing hospital and nursing home costs and the feeling that the whole system of long-term care as presently organized is unresponsive to human needs. Therefore, experts in the field of gerontology now agree that what is needed is more than marginal improvements in nursing-home-care quality. Indeed, long-term care must be viewed as a continuum ranging from home care and ambulatory care to institutional care.

One ambulatory-care option is the adult day center. In order to better understand the potential of adult day care as a community-based option in ambulatory care, it is helpful to review historically the progress made in this area, both within the United States and other countries.

The purpose of this chapter is to give the reader some background information about the adult day-care movement from its earliest beginnings in Russia through the psychiatric day hospital to its present adult day-care movement in the United States.

Historical Review of the Psychiatric Day Hospital

When and where did the day-hospital movement originate? Dzhagrov reports that a day hospital associated with the First Psychiatric Hospital in Moscow was created in 1933.[1] While this day hospital was unknown and probably had little or no effect on future day centers in Europe, it is accurate to say that it was the first organized day hosital for individuals with severe mental illness.[1(p96)]

The reason for the development of this day hospital was to decrease the acute shortage of hospital beds. The goal was to increase hospital-bed turnover by discharging clients earlier. In implementing this concept, the hospital authorities realized that adequate followup services were needed, so they instituted a setting similar to the hospital, where clients could come during the day, yet return home at night. Thus, the day hospital was born.

It was not until 1945 that the first psychiatric day hospital was established in the United States, at Adams House in Boston.[2] According to Cameron, psychoneurotics attended the Adams House under the directorship of Dr. J. M. Woodall.[1(p37)]

In 1938, the literature gives reference to Dr. Helen Boyle, who admitted day clients to the Lady Chester Hospital in Hove, England.[1(p78)] Aside from these few forerunners who used day services, the first organized day hospital in the western hemisphere for severely ill psychiatric participants was established in April 1946 at the Allan Memorial Institute of Psychiatry in Montreal, Canada.[3] The first in England was established at the Institute of Social Psychiatry in the mid 1940s.[4(p98)] In his monograph on the day hospital in England, Brierer reports that, although the idea first took shape in January 1947, its operation didn't begin until 1948.[4(p96)] In that same year, a day plan was set up at the Yale Psychiatric Clinic, and, in 1949, a day hospital took shape at the Menninger Clinic.[1(p38)]

From these early beginnings of the psychiatric day-hospital movement in the western world came the day-hospital movement in England, which directed its focus to the population "at risk" of institutionalization because of chronic illness.

Overview of the British Day-Hospital Movement

England began using day hospitals for disabled adults, many of whom were elderly,[5] and found that many participants could be discharged from an acute-care hospital earlier if they were able to continue with their necessary treatments on a day basis. Besides receiving their necessary treatments, day hospital participants could be better assessed for additional community-service needs once they were back in their own homes. In addition, long-term-care arrangements in institutional settings could be arranged more appropriately when necessary.

Brocklehurst defines the British geriatric day hospitals as follows:

> A day hospital is a building to which patients may come, or be brought, in the morning, where they may spend several hours in therapeutic activity and whence they return subsequently on the same day to their own homes. The building is generally, although not always, within the curtilage of an ordinary hospital. It may be no more than a single room especially adapted, or a whole purpose-built structure of many varied rooms. Geriatric day hospitals provide facilities for physiotherapy and occupational therapys, for medical examination and nursing treatment, and usually for various other activities including investigation, speech therapy, dentistry, chiropody and hairdressing. The building and its facilities may be used entirely for day patients coming from their homes, or it may be used by in-patients as well, who come over from the wards in the morning and return in the afternoon.*[6(p101)]

The first hospital in the English system to include geriatric participants with physical disabilities was the Cowley Road Day Hospital in Oxford, England.[7] By the 1960s, this model of care was being used extensively. The emphasis in these hospitals was on participants relearning activities of daily living, receiving various therapies, being part of a social-activity program, participating in group work, and receiving good nutrition. Advantages of this model were that (1) it enabled participants to go home earlier; (2) it continued assisting participants as needed; and (3) it provided respite for the elderly person's relatives.[8] By the end of 1970, there were 119 geriatric day hospitals in Great Britain,[9(p23)] in comparison with 15 day health centers functioning in the United States at that time.[9(p26)]

In 1971, the English Department of Health and Social Security devised guidelines for the operation of their day-hospital system. They suggested at this time that these day hospitals be considered an integral part of the continuum of services offered to the elderly. They also defined the participants who would best be served by these hospitals. An appropriate participant population was defined as those who were "at risk" of institutionalization, those who needed close followup upon discharge from the hospital, and those who were awaiting hospital admission.[10]

Once the day-hospital model took hold in England, there appeared to be a need for another model of day care. This model would include those elderly persons who were not in need of such a concentrated rehabilitation regimen and was called the day center.

Brocklehurst defined the day center in England as follows:

> Day centres provide social facilities—company, a cooked meal, possibly a bath and chiropody, but none of the medical services found in the day hospital. Day centres are usually run by local authorities or voluntary bodies (often both together coordinating their work through the old people's welfare committee). Nevertheless, transport is an essential part of both the day centre and the day hospital.[6(p116)]

---

*Reproduced from *The Geriatric Day Hospital*, by JC Brocklehurst, 1970. This and all other quotations from this source are reprinted by kind permission of the publishers, King Edward's Hospital Fund for London.

In essence, the differences between the day hospital and day center are (1) the services offered; (2) the client population; (3) the expected outcomes; and (4) the staffing pattern. As mentioned before, the day hospital in England focused on rehabilitation and treatment. The clients attending a day hospital were expected to benefit from both of these services and either gain in their optimal level of functioning or at least maintain their current level of functioning. The day center's focus was on social kinds of services (that is, group work, activities programs, and field trips). The participants of such programs were considered "the frail" elderly rather than "at risk" population, who needed little physical assistance but more peer support and socialization programs.

When those participants attending the day hospital achieved their maximum level of functioning, they could be transferred to an adult day-care center, where they would receive the necessary supervision to maintain their current level of functioning. This network of services in England does seem to offer a comprehensive continuum of services that continues to be lacking in the United States today.

Day Hospitals in Israel

While the proportion of elderly in Israel is now relatively small, a marked shift in the makeup of the population is anticipated. This shift is due in part to the large numbers of elderly persons migrating to Israel. Estimates for the 1980s show that the number of persons over 65 years of age will double.[11(p3)] Therefore, a high priority is being given to the development of home-health services and day hospitals.[11(p4)] Currently there are nine day hospitals in Israel.[11(p5)] All of these are based on the British model of day hospitals and are located directly in or on the grounds of the parent hospital. According to Dr. Silberstein, the director of Chronic Illness and Aging, the day hospital has as its major objectives "the shortening of hospital stay by providing treatment without the hotel services, and the prevention or postponement of inpatient care."[11(p5)] In some instances, the day hospital also provides diagnostic workups.

In Israel (as in other countries), there is a growing need for adult day care for the socially isolated, "frail" elderly as well as for the population now being serviced through day hospital. However, at this point in time, the adult day-care model is still in its formative stage.

Canadian Adult Day Care

Whether inspired or spurred by such developments as day hospitals and adult day-care centers in England and the burgeoning use of this form of care in the psychiatric field, the adult day-care concept was picked up quickly and enthusiastically in Canada by Jewish Homes for the Aged. The Baycrest Jewish Home of the

Aged is thought to be the first adult day-care center in Toronto.[12(p9)] The firm but gentle pressure of the Home's board of directors pushed the professional staff into investigating the need for adult day-care services in the summer of 1958. By June of 1959, a program was started with eight day residents.[12(p10)] The primary purposes of this program were (1) to provide a coordinated activities program; (2) to provide a safe environment for the "frail" elderly; (3) to provide a balanced diet; (4) to relieve family tensions and give the family some respite; and (5) to serve as an adjustment phase from community living to residential nursing-home living. Therefore, it followed a model like the English adult day-care center.

> While the idea of a Day Care Center Program was greeted with much enthusiasm in Canada a survey conducted in 1962 of some thirty eight Jewish Homes revealed that seventeen offered Day Care Center Programs, but significantly only eleven of these programs were in actual use. Of these eleven, four programs had two or less persons participating and one program was obviously a Drop-In Center rather than a true Day Care Center Program. Thus six homes, not including the Jewish Home for the Aged in Toronto, had Day Care Center Programs operating with appropriate usage.[12(p10)]

The day hospital at Maimonides Hospital in Montreal was established as a pilot psychogeriatric project in 1966 with 10 participants.[13(p3)] By 1974, as day-hospital studies were completed, it became clear that there were long-term-maintenance participants and short-term participants within the structure of the day hospital. The goal for both these types of participants at Maimonides Day Hospital was to provide therapeutic services aimed at keeping the elderly person independent and functioning in the community for as long as possible in order to prevent premature institutionalization. Thus, their focus was on the "at risk" population.

The Maimonides program provides comprehensive services for persons suffering "quite severe physical and mental disorders and who are too emotionally and physically deteriorated to use existing social clubs and recreation centers."[14(p18)] The day hospital serves 53 persons, with an average daily attendance of 25. Hours are from 9 A.M. to 5 P.M., Monday through Friday. A chartered bus is used in bringing participants to and from home. The Maimonides Hospital is a chronic-disease hospital and consequently provides a broad range of supportive medical services in addition to an array of therapeutic social and recreational opportunities. Medical services include cardiology, dermatology, gynecology, neurology, opthalmology, orthopedics, physical therapy, dentistry, urology, speech therapy, podiatry, and diagnostic radiology.

To be accepted as a Maimonides Day Hospital participant, applicants must be ambulatory, able to travel by bus, and able to cope with most requirements of daily living. The average participant age is 73.

> On the basis of ... clinical assessments, 15 patients or 6 percent of the total 250 patients treated to date (1970) in the day hospital have been referred to institutional care. Two hundred and thirty five or 94 percent have been able to continue maintaining themselves in the community, a fact that seems related to the diminution of the social isolation to which these patients were subjected before their admission into the day hospital program.[14(p19)]

It is interesting to note that Maimonides and the Jewish Home programs differ considerably. Maimonides Day Hospital fits the British model of the day hospital, whereas Baycrest Jewish Adult Day Care Center fits the British model of the social day-care centers.

Although there were three day hospitals in Winnepeg, Canada in 1973, adult day-care centers had not yet been started there.[15] Therefore, in 1973, a pilot study began at the Luther Home for the purpose of demonstrating the use and value of an adult day-care center in a personal-care home.[15] Its main objective was to enhance social functioning through supportive services.

In looking at the various Canadian programs, one can see that Canada has been working with the day-hospital model as well as the adult day-care-center model, where those participants can go when they no longer need day-hospital services, but are still unable to attend centers for the well aged.[13(p4)]

European Adult Day Health Programs

Both Denmark and Sweden have ongoing day-care programs that are covered under their national health-insurance plans. Similarly, these countries have followed both British models of the day hospital and adult day-care centers. Yet, there are some significant differences within their systems.

In Denmark, the day nursing home, like the British day hospital, provides a higher level of care than the social day center. Like its British counterpart, the social day center maintains both the physical and mental health of the participants through activities, occupational therapy, social gatherings, and field trips. In addition, the social day center provides home visiting and facilities for hairdressing. Unlike the British model, however, these adult day centers involve participants who are considered "well" elderly along with the "frail" elderly.

Although adult day centers in Denmark have been in operation for only a decade, they are fairly well established, whereas those in Sweden are not very well developed. In fact, it is only in the last few years that priority has been given to long-term care in the Swedish health-care system.[16] The most used adult day-care center program in Sweden is the "ward." It is very similar to the British model of the day hospital, with the main thrust being toward physical therapy.

One interesting contribution of the Swedes to the adult day-care movement is their use of levels of care within the day ward. These levels of care are designated in the following way: (1) level one—much emphasis is placed on physical therapy; (2) level two—self-training and group training are encouraged; and (3) level three—participants continue visiting after discharge on a monthly basis. These three levels of care show that Sweden has a system that tries to encourage movement out of adult day care when not needed and that it also emphasizes placing services where the need exists.

The Adult Day-Care Movement in the United States

Background

Until recently, the United States has perpetuated a model of long-term care that provides services for the disabled and elderly primarily in institutional settings. The nursing home as one type of institutional setting began to develop rapidly during the 1930s.[17(p12)] One reason for this rapid development was the enactment of the Social Security Act of 1935, in which federal funds were made available to the needy aged. As a result, the number of proprietary boarding and nursing homes increased and flourished, and the number of public almshouses subsequently declined.[17(p13)] In 1965, with the enactment of Medicare and Medicaid, once again reimbursement for institutionalization was reinforced. This policy has continued to date to encourage the use of institutional models for long-term care.

In 1975, about 5% of the United States population 65 and over resided in nursing homes.[18(p7)] This population is composed of primarily the very elderly; 75% are 75 years or older. A greater percentage of nursing home residents are female than male, white than other races, and widowed than other marital status.[18(p8)] For the most part, nursing-care and related homes are evenly located throughout the United States, with the North Central region having the greatest concentration.[18(p8)] In 1971, the number of beds in nursing homes had more than doubled since 1963.[18(p8)] Of the more than 20 million Americans over 65 years of age, 80% report one or more chronic illnesses that require medical supervision.[18(p10)] However, only 5% require long-term care in such institutions as the nursing home.

Studies show that there are clients in such institutions who do not need the services provided in these facilities and would not be there if other alternatives were available to them.[19] There are about 41% of nursing-home residents who receive intensive medical and nursing care and 32% who receive routine medical and nursing care–for example, blood-pressure readings.[18(p10)] Few residents receive any therapy: 15% receive recreational therapy, 10% receive physical therapy, and 6% receive occupational therapy.[18(p11)]

Such data enforce the words of M. Delar Carter in the following statement:

> There is a consensus among health care authorities that a significant number of the patient population are treated in facilities equipped for care beyond those patient's needs. The health care system is oriented primarily toward treatment of the acute phase of illness and does not offer a complete spectrum of health care by providing available alternatives and educating physicians and patients in the use of acceptable alternatives. This problem becomes even more significant for the elderly, because there is no incentive or reimbursement to keep the patient well in the present system.[20]

Health-care options for the elderly or disabled group who can no longer completely care for themselves have been similar throughout the nation:

1. Institutionalization in a nursing home, rest home, or chronic care hospital:

> People with relatively minor illnesses who could well be taken care of at home, or with little outside help could be managing on their own, are too often automatically dispatched to a nursing home. And too often this is the wrong answer.[21]

2. Moving in with other family members, frequently adult children:

> For some ... this is a good arrangement. For others, it is not. The older person loses his independence, is often a financial burden, and the lifestyle of both the older person and the younger family are disrupted. A typical problem is that care for the older person interferes with or prevents a family member's employment. All of this in turn puts stress on family relationships.[5(p12)]

3. Remaining at home with maximum possible reliance upon home care services, volunteer helpers, social workers, and the like:

> But the services are often limited in size, scope and lack connection to other vital needs.[5(p13)]

Searching for Alternatives: Federal Studies

Within the last ten years, there has been federal and state involvement in a search for alternative approaches to the institutional long-term-care model. Several approaches have been suggested, and legislation has been introduced in Congress for researching these measures. Among them is adult day care, which is described as a coordinated program of services provided in ambulatory settings.[22(p2)] Federal interest in adult day care has been characterized by various initiatives aimed at developing demonstration programs to explore adult day care as an alternative to institutional care for the disabled and chronically ill elderly.

In June 1974, a preliminary analysis of 15 programs was prepared for the Division of Long-Term Care by Eloise Rathbone McCuan, Ph.D., Muriel G. Rose, M.S.W., and John Bland, M.S.W. of the Levindale Geriatric Research Center in Baltimore, Maryland. The major effort of this report was to define, describe, and compare the major program elements of these 15 selected adult day-care centers. This report served as a descriptive prelude to the Transcentury Report, which was completed in 1975.

In response to Section 222 of Public Law 92-603, which provided congressional authorization for experimental adult day-care programs, HEW awarded four research and demonstration grants to evaluate the cost effectiveness of this service and to determine the feasibility of expanding service coverage through the Medicare and Medicaid programs.[23] A 1975 directive outlining HEW's short- and long-range strategy for developing alternative-care settings called for the limited expansion of experimental programs by encouraging state Medicaid agencies to establish similar demonstration programs. All experimental programs in the demonstration project were expected to carry out the services as defined by these definitions and guidelines. They begin with the following definition:

> Guidelines and Definitions for Day Care Services
> To Be Carried Out in Experiments and Demonstrations
> Authorized Under P.L. 92-603, Section 222 (b).

Definitions:

(a) "Day Care" is a program of services provided under health leadership in an ambulatory care setting for adults who do not require 24-hour institutional care and yet, due to physical and/or mental impairment, are not capable of full-time independent living. Participants in the day-care program are referred to the program by their attending physician or by some other appropriate source such as an institutional discharge planning program, a welfare agency, etc. The essential elements of a day-care program are directed toward meeting the health maintenance and restoration needs of participants. However, there are socialization elements in the program which by overcoming the isolation so often associated with illness in the aged and disabled, are considered vital for the purposes of fostering and maintaining the maximum possible state of health and well-being.

(b) "Impaired adult" means a chronically ill or disabled adult whose illness or disability may not require twenty-four hour inpatient care but which, in the absence of day care services, may precipitate admission to or prolonged stay in a hospital, nursing home or other long-term facility.[24]

As a result of Public Law 92-603, the Department of Health, Education and Welfare hired the Transcentury Corporation to study ten already existing adult day-care programs.[22] Although some adult day-care centers began as early as 1957 in the United States, this was the first attempt in describing the adult day-care movement as it existed in the United States.[22] In these adult day-care programs, services ranged from the provision of cheerful daytime environments with emphasis on arts, crafts, and good fellowship (that is, a strong socialization component) to programs of comprehensive health care and rehabilitation services (that is, a strong health component).

The summary of findings from the Transcentury Report showed two distinct models of adult day-care programs. Model I is characterized by its relatively heavy emphasis on health services.[22(p51)] It has a high ratio of professional personnel and participants who have recently suffered serious illnesses and need rehabilitative care.[22(p52)] This is the rehabilitative model similar to England's day hospital. Model II emphasizes daytime supervision for the generally less impaired person. It has fewer professional personnel, and its participants are suffering from infirmities of old age and in less need of rehabilitation.[22(p54)] This is the social model much like the English adult day center.

After the Transcentury Report, the next federal study to be conducted was by William Weissert in 1978. In this National Center for Health Services Research Project, six demonstration sites were selected. The establishment of these sites was under Section 222 projects. The purpose of the study was to look at the costs and effectiveness of adult day care and homemaker services.[25(p1)] These services were reimbursed by Medicare funds. Findings from these experiments show that those who used adult day care had either sustained or increased levels of contentment, mental functioning, and social activity and had reduced rates of institutionalization.[25(p14)] Although these outcomes are favorable, they cannot be generalized to participants in all adult day-care settings because the participants in this experiment were not randomly selected and, therefore, were not representative of all participants who would become eligible for these services.

The effects of adult day-care services and costs were mixed. Though existing Medicare costs were reduced by a decreased utilization of other Medicare services, total costs for adult day-care services were higher for participants in these programs.[25(p28)] Further information relative to the Weissert report and cost implications can be found in Chapter 14.

Congressional Hearing 1980

Since the publication of this report in 1979, no other major federal studies have been initiated. However, on April 23, 1980, a congressional hearing was planned in Washington by Representative Claude Pepper, chairman of the Select Committee on Aging. The House Select Committee on Aging was formed in October 1974 by the Committee Reform Amendments of the 93rd Congress. It received wide support by a 323 to 84 House floor vote. The purposes of this committee are to

(1) STUDY PROBLEMS: to conduct continuing comprehensive study of the problems of the older American, including income maintenance, housing, health,

welfare, employment, education, recreation, and participation in family and community life;
(2) ENCOURAGE POSITIVE PROGRAMS: to study the means of encouraging the development of public and private programs and policies to assist the older American in taking full part in national life and to encourage the utilization of his knowledge, skills, special aptitudes and abilities to contribute to a better life for all Americans;
(3) DEVELOP COORDINATION POLICIES: to develop policies to encourage the coordination of both governmental and private programs designed to deal with problems of aging; and
(4) REVIEW RECOMMENDATIONS: to review recommendations mady by the President or by the White House Conference on Aging relating to programs or policies affecting older Americans.

The committee carries out these responsibilities by informing the House on problems of the older American; advising those House committees which have legislative jurisdiction (i.e., to which bills are referred for action); overseeing Executive Branch to ensure that the laws having applicability to problems of aging are properly executed. Primarily a fact-finding body, the select committee has no legislative responsibilities.[26]

When reviewing these purposes, the hearing called by Representative Pepper would seem to relate most to purpose number two. Thus, on April 18, 1980, the Representative released the following statement:

Pepper Calls April 23 Hearing to Explore
Effectiveness of Day Care for Elderly

Washington, D.C., April 18—House Aging Committee Chairman Claude Pepper (D-Fla.) today announced the first Congressional hearing on day care for the elderly. The hearing will be conducted by the Subcommittee on Health and Long-Term Care on Wednesday, April 23, at 10 A.M. in Room 210 of the Cannon House Office Building.

'Adult day care can be an exciting discovery for the family trying to care for an impaired elderly relative at home,' said Pepper. 'Contrary to the prevailing thoughts, families want to keep them at home. In spite of this desire, it can be a tremendous burden for families to provide 24-hour care for an older person who needs professional services. The cards are stacked in favor of nursing home placement. Day care gives these families a break, while allowing elderly persons to remain in the community, outside an institution.

'The beauty of day care is that it can be molded to fit the needs of the individual. Services can be predominantly medical, or social, or somewhere in between,' he continued.

Witnesses at the hearing will include a stroke victim who is a 'graduate' of adult day care; family members of adult day care clients; directors of various 'models' of adult day care programs; state officials; and a panel of HEW officials associated with programs which provide support for day care.

'Adult day care, a concept unique to most Americans, has been used successfully in other industrialized countries for many years, but it is a relatively new approach in the United States,' observed Pepper. 'Our Subcommittee will examine this form of care for the promise it holds not only for enriching the lives of the elderly, but for holding down health costs by delaying or preventing institutionalization,' he concluded.[27]

On April 23, 1980, the following opening statement was presented by Representative Claude Pepper:

It is my pleasure to convene this hearing—the First Congressional Hearing devoted exclusively to an examination of Day Care for the elderly.

By all accounts Adult Day Care is an idea whose time has come. In 1974, there were only some 15 programs in the United States. Today, there are over 600. This rapid growth has come about without Federal policy, without a mandate to the States, and without a unified funding source.

In my book, this qualifies Adult Day Care as something of a phenomenon. What created the momentum for this kind of expansion? I believe the answer is that day care grew from grass roots—with community efforts responding to community need.

Popular opinion would have us believe that many American families don't care about their elders—that they are content to dump their mothers and fathers and aunts and uncles into institutions and leave responsibility for their care to others. That kind of mentality is dangerous, and it's misleading.

The fact is that most American families don't have the resources to provide 100 percent of the care an impaired older relative might need to stay out of a nursing home. The complexities of our increasingly mobile and impersonal society make it difficult to keep a household running smoothly.

The needs of an impaired older relative who requires special care can compound the difficulties. For lack of alternatives, this situation far too often results in the nursing home placement.

This does not mean that families don't wish to care for their elderly. To the contrary, it often means that all other doors are closed. We want to open those doors. Our Committee has devoted years of work to making home health care available to the elderly. Our task is by no means completed, but we have achieved considerable progress. Home care and day care should go hand-in-hand as components of a continuum of community-based care for the elderly.

In our hearing today, we want to learn what day care means to families. We want to know how the various programs work. We want to discuss the costs of day care. And we want to know exactly what the Federal Government is doing in this area.

A principal concern has been the lack of a policy focus in day care. Some 16 potential sources of funding have been identified. We have distributed a survey to all the states which we hope will prove beneficial in getting a better idea of the extent of day care around the country.

Encouraging day care does not just mean a few dollars. It might mean a reorganization of the haphazard financing structure. We know that of the 600 programs in existence now, well over 300 receive Title XX Social Service funds; over 100 receive funds under Title III of the Older Americans Act; and 125 receive reimbursement under Medicaid. The remainder of day care support comes from a hodge-podge of public and private sources, area agencies on aging and others. Moreover, a large number of persons—as many as one-half of the participants in some programs—pay their own way.

We have much to learn today. I want to welcome each of you to this hearing. We are especially pleased to have with us a number of members of the National Institute of Adult Day Care of the National Council on the Aging. Your concern and your expertise are welcome, and I want to encourage you to work with our Committee in the Development of long-term care policies which will enhance the lives of elderly Americans now and in the future.[28]

During the hearing, several persons testified as stated in the above announcement. In the next section of this chapter, a few of these testimonies will be presented: the first by Horace Woods, a former adult day-care participant; the second by Daniel Driscoll, a representative from the National Council on Aging; the third by Kathryn Morrison, a representative from the Administration on Aging; the fourth by William Weissert of the National Center for Health Services Research; and the fifth by Anne Klapfish of the Massachusetts Department of Medicaid.

Testimony of Horace Woods

What follows is my testimony in support of the continued need for Senior Day Care Centers throughout the country:

Because it filled a void in my life, I have the fondest regard for the Woods Adult Day Care Center.

Three years ago, while recuperating from a stroke, the Health Department Therapist suggested that I attend an adult day care center for continued maintenance therapy, both physical and mental.

Thank God, in November, 1976, I was accepted by the Woods Adult Day Care Center in Severna Park, Maryland. At that time, despondency and a feeling of uselessness prevailed in my life. Usually in the case of senior illness or handicap, he/she experiences a traumatic shock when they discover their inability to function as well as before.

Prior to my stroke, I worked with retarded adults in work training at the Providence Center in Annapolis, Maryland for five gratifying years. Married, I lived with my wife in my own home.

On acceptance at the center, consideration of my physical limitations were dealt with (being paralyzed on my left side). The therapist from the Health Department followed me at the center during this transition time and provided a physical fitness program for the center staff to follow in my maintenance routine. Also, I participated in the center's activities, learning to make tapestries—using a punch needle with one hand, and later teaching others how to perform with one hand also. An aide encouraged me in creative writing and, much to my surprise, I found myself developing my latent talent in writing. These associations renewed my usefulness, sense of purpose, and hope for the future. I regained my confidence in my ability to assist and train.

It was quite a relief to get out of the house for a few hours daily to meet new friends and socialize with peers. While my attendance at the center was without fee, my home was at a great distance and I had to pay for my own transportation. Unfortunately, it was so expensive I could only afford to attend two days a week.

The counseling and training at the center taught me to live more independently, strengthening family ties, as President Carter has advocated, and to remain in my community—dispelling my fears of institutionalization. At the same time, my presence at the center allowed my family to fulfill their daily obligations, content in the knowledge that their loved one was adequately being cared for during the day.

Now a widower, I graduated from the day care center and attended a senior center closer to my home. While transportation remains a problem, I have been able to maintain my own home and use the Meals on Wheels Service.

Physical, mental and social rehabilitation, the prerequisites for a full life, in our waning years is available at the day care center through their counseling, activities and associations—again, I have a feeling of self-worth.

> 'I have a new lease on life
> Adult Day Care Centers are a Godsend.'

During my three years at the center, I witnessed some dramatic changes in center participants. Those who had withdrawn into a shell became actively involved in activities and relationships, and those who had been rejected, looked forward to the center as a haven, "a Home Away From Home," all due to the atmosphere and the knowledge that someone cared.

> With a waiting list backlog
> The need for day care expansion is there
> What's needed now is for all society to care.[29]

Testimony of Daniel Driscoll

Mr. Chairman, and distinguished members of the House Subcommittee on Health and Long-Term Care:

I am Daniel Driscoll, Director of Special Care Services at the Waxter Center for Senior Citizens in Baltimore, Maryland, and serve as Chairperson of the National Institute on Adult Day Care (NIAD), a program of the National Council on the Aging (NCOA).

This morning I would like to briefly describe the Waxter Center's Day Care Program and highlight some of the concerns and recommendations of NIAD.

The Waxter Center is a large, municipal, multi-purpose senior center located on the fringe of downtown Baltimore. The Center opened its doors in 1974 and now operates seven days a week as a focal point of service to Baltimore's senior citizens, serving a current membership of over 15,000 persons. It offers a full range of services designed to keep the elderly well, active and independent.

As a component of the Waxter Center, the Day Care Program is a structured rehabilitative program for the impaired elderly. It is designed for those persons who are disabled emotionally, physically or socially to such a degree that they are unable to function independently. The Program participants present a variety of problems ranging from severe and chronic physical and mental handicaps to an array of multiple social and health-related problems. It is to be noted that this population is significantly more impaired and different from the membership served through the regular senior center programs and activities. The Program serves an average of 18 persons per day with a total enrollment of approximately 40 different persons.

The prime objective of Waxter's Day Program is to assist those elderly persons who impairments prohibit living independently without support services, to reach and/or maintain their maximum potential for independent living as an alternative to inappropriate institutionalization.

The Program is designed for a number of purposes:

(1) to reduce isolation and immobility
(2) to stimulate interests in leisure activities
(3) to provide opportunities for socialization
(4) to enhance activities of daily living with instruction in self-care, health maintenance, consumer protection and referral to other community services as needed
(5) to improve health status by maintaining necessary liaison with providers of health care, and
(6) to coordinate care and counseling with the family, providing support and assistance to these caregivers.

Admission to the program is based on a comprehensive, professional assessment, including evaluation of physical and mental health status, and of the person's environmental and social situation. A functional assessment is completed, drawing a profile of the participant's performance in tasks of daily living. An individualized care plan is developed outlining the needs of the participant and, is refined and revised as needs change.

A wide range of activities are offered in a protective setting within the center that promote the highest level of independence possible. The careful professional assessment provides for the type of care needed by each individual, taking care not to over or under service. As a part of the senior center system, the full range of Waxter's facilities, services and resources are available to day care participants.

Discharge from the Program is a possible goal considered even at the point of admission. In those cases where progress to greater independence seems indicated, on-going planning for discharge is made with the participant.

As a component of the senior center, the day care program is unique in its ability to bring the impaired older person into contact and relationship with well peers. This experience provides incentive and motivation toward improvement for the disabled day care participant.

From the national perspective, there are several issues which I would like to highlight.

In this era where the key words are coordination and cost containment, Adult Day Care is beginning to show many exciting ways to approach these problems. It is an important component of the continuum of services, perhaps most strikingly indicated by the very fact that day care has *not* developed from the top down. Rather, it has been a grass roots movement, born out of a real community need and sponsored by a wide variety of public and private sources. The number of day care programs has increased significantly during the past several years, with only minimal assistance and direction from the Federal sector. To encourage continued development of this needed service National Institute of Adult Day Care would like to recommend the following:

(1) Legislative and executive action to remove the barriers to the integrated use of Medicare, Medicaid and Title XX social service dollars to support day care programs. Federal Mechanisms are needed to encourage the increased use of funds for the expansion of day care as a service option and effective implementation.

(2) Uniform standards be developed to serve as a model for the delivery of quality day care services. An exploratory survey conducted by NIAD has confirmed that standards of operation vary tremendously among the states. While 30 states have established standards, over half are designed for funding purposes only and do not adequately address the programmatic and quality control factors of service delivery. In the historical framework of the senior center field and Vocational Rehabilitation Services, it is further recommended that practitioners be intimately involved in this process. Workers in the field are sensitive to the needs of day care clients and can serve as a vehicle for standards development.

(3) Additional and expanded evaluation of day care be undertaken. We must look at what is currently being done, what are the variations in practice and what is the potential of this service option. Policy cannot be made on existing limited data. There has been a tendency to "compare apples and oranges" instead of what the real costs would be to society if adult day care participants had to receive all these services available at the Center through some other source. Day care is currently operating in 43 states which suggests there is already sufficient experience to confirm that it is a viable and needed service. This delivery of service should not be interrupted for the sake of research but rather evaluation should be designed for the further development and refinement of day care.

(4) Finally, we recommend the designation of a single Federal agency which will have responsibility for the evaluation and development of this rich service option. Coordination of activities in regard to day care must be effected to better enable practitioners to negotiate the labyrinth of acronyms in their efforts to deliver services to the most vulnerable segment of the aging population.

I would like to thank the Committee for the opportunity of testifying this morning. This hearing is a milestone in the day care movement, for which we are appreciative.[30]

Testimony of Kathryn Morrison

Mr. Chairman, and Committee members, I am Kathryn Morrison, Deputy Commissioner for the Administration on Aging, and I am pleased to respond to your invitation to discuss Adult Day Care on behalf of Commissioner Robert Benedict. Adult Day Care is well recognized as a service that can prevent, shorten or delay the need for institutional care or expand care choices available to families.

The AOA supports Adult Day Care in several ways. Under the Older Americans Act, it provides Title III-B funds for support Adult Day Care Services. It provides funds for the operation of senior centers in which many Adult Day Care programs are located. In some instances, Adult Day Care residents participate in congregate nutrition programs.

Currently, 45 states report that they have Adult Day Care funded either through Title XIX or Title XX or Title III dollars. Of these, 19 states report using Title III dollars. For example, there are 69 day care centers supported by Title III in the states represented by the members of this Committee. Thrity-four of those are in senior centers.

Mr. Chairman, I would like to report on some of the more important and innovative projects that the AOA has supported. Let me describe for you, an example where Title III funds (together with other Federal resources) are playing a significant role in assisting day care. In Dade County, Florida, there are currently seven day care centers, four of which are sponsored by the Dade County Elderly Services Division and use Title III funds. These four centers serve 270 clients a month. Of the older persons who receive such services, 90% are at or below the poverty level. In some cases, older persons volunteer in each of these centers to help those who are less able. Families are involved as volunteers as well. Each center provides hot meals, transportation services, health screening and education and family counseling. When an individual condition improves enough, the Elderly Service Division has a special assistance effort entitled the "Impact Program." Under this program if an individual declines in his or her physical condition, the Elderly Service Division provides for home visits. This is an example where Title III funds provide an important care choice for older persons and their families.

The AOA has invested $4.2 million in model day care projects between 1972 and 1980. These model projects cover a range of day care concerns. Let me cite just a few: The Burke Rehabilitation Center Project, a day hospital, was funded to determine the reasonableness of a day hospital as a means of providing rehabilitative services for the chronically ill or the physiacally disabled older adults. This demonstration has shown the value of this setting in encouraging participants to renew their interest in themselves and others, by group activities which require interpersonal communication.

A grant awarded to Case Western Reserve University in Cleveland, Ohio, focused on both physically and mentally impaired older persons. This project not only provided services to the frail elderly, but also to the family and to older volunteers to activate mutual help. The On Lok Senior Health Services Program in San Francisco, California, is a pioneer in the field of Adult Day Care designed to adapt to the ethnic and cultural backgrounds of Filipino, Chinese, and Italian older persons.

A Lockport, New York, project demonstrated the feasibility of integrating severely and moderately impaired older persons within the structure of a multi-purpose senior center program. A project in Wichita, Kansas, has shown that Adult Day Care services can be provided in rural areas, by using an existing nursing home. Public and private replication of these models has contributed to the growth from 15 programs nationally in 1974 to an estimated 600 in 1980.

There remain a number of questions about the provision of day care, including issues of funding, cost of services, and variety of service models and the mix of services. The AOA is currently investing research dollars in identifying answers to some of these problems. For example, we will receive in the next few months an assessment of the cost of alternative levels of care, and a comparison of benefits received in day care centers, day hospitals, nursing homes and domiciliary care arrangements.

Additionally, AOA provides funds for training service providers and state and area agencies personnel involved with providing Adult Day Care.

The 1978 amendments contain a new provision, Section 422, special projects in comprehensive long-term care. The AOA together with the Health Care Financing Administration is launching a major demonstration program this year which will include Adult Day Care as an important service element.

Mr. Chairman, this concludes my prepared remarks. I would be happy to answer any questions you may have.[31]

Testimony of William Weissert

Mr. Chairman and members of the Committee, thank you for the opportunity to present the findings from a recently completed study of the effects and costs of Adult Day Care. The study was conducted by the National Center for Health Services Research in response to a congressional mandate contained in Section 222 of Public Law 92-603, the 1972 amendments to the U.S. Social Security Act. The purpose of this study was to determine whether or not day care services would improve patient outcomes or reduce costs. It began in 1974 and ended in 1977. Data were analyzed in 1978 and 1979.

Services were provided by four day care programs which were reimbursed through Medicare waivers granted under the special authority of Section 222. The Programs operated in Syracuse and White Plains, New York; Lexington, Kentucky; and San Francisco, California.

The programs studied were of the health oriented type rather than the social type of day care which has become more prevalent in the U.S. Health oriented meant that patients received nursing supervision, meals, transportation, social work services, and health services such as physical therapy, occupational therapy, or speech therapy, if they needed it.

Six hundred forty-four patients participated in the study. They were all Medicare eligible, their average age was 74, and about half the patients were 75 years old or older. The majority was female, 80 percent were white, three-fourths lived with family or others, more than half were severely dependent, almost a third were only minimally dependent, three-fourths came from the community rather than from a hospital, and circulatory disorders and injuries due to fractures were the most prevalent diagnosed conditions suffered.

Patients were referred to the study by their physicians, hospitals, community service agencies, welfare departments, and their families. Of course only those who wanted day care were studied, since it would not be possible or worthwhile to provide day care to patients who didn't want it.

All patients were assessed by day care staff teams which included physicians, nurses, social workers, and sometimes one or more therapists.

If the team felt the patient might benefit from day care, the patient either was enrolled in day care or assigned to a control group which didn't receive day care and was used for comparison purposes.

Each quarter, the two groups' health and social status and use of health services were compared.

Results showed that day care patients did no better than the control group on most measures, including physical functioning, mental functioning, contentment, activity level, or hospitalization. Those in day care did have a lower rate of nursing home use and lower death rates, but when more sophisticated statistical techniques were used, it became evident that these benefits were almost totally due to small initial differences in diagnoses, sex, age, living arrangements, race, and dependency level, between the day care and control groups rather than any benefit of day care.

Cost findings were no more encouraging. For the day care group, Medicare reimbursements were almost three-fourths more than the control group.

Two other findings are important:

(1) Each day care program had a difficult time getting enough patients. Intake periods had to be extended several times; and
(2) The rate of nursing home use in the study was low: Only less than one-fifth of all patients entered a skilled nursing facility. This indicates that most patients who used day care were using it as an add-on to existing services rather than as a substitute for nursing home care.

One important limitation on the applicability of these findings to the whole day care question you are considering should be noted: As I indicated, this was a study of the health oriented type of day care not social day care. Health oriented day care is more expensive and usually serves sicker and more dependent patients than social programs. In a study I did in 1974 and 1975, I found that social day care programs were considerably less expensive than health-oriented day care. I concluded then that day care might be cheaper than nurisng homes, if it could serve the right patients. In other words, unless day care can be shown to reduce use of other expensive services, it will always be more expensive, regardless of what it costs. What we found in this study was that for most patients it did not substitute for existing services and so it cost more. Nor were these extra costs offset by beneficial effects on patients.

In summary, we used a sophisticated research methodology, in most cases, we used experienced day care providers, and we assessed a large number of potential benefits of day care, but we found no significant benefits, while we did find high costs.

Of course, this is one study. As a responsible researcher, I would urge the committee to seek additional research before drawing conclusions.

Finally, this study has been published by the National Center for Health Services Research and is about to be published by some of the leading scientific journals. Copies are available from my office.[32]

164 / Part II: The Adult Day-Care Experience

Testimony of Anne Klapfish

Opening my discussion I will describe briefly the state network of adult day health programs in Massachusetts. I will then discuss William Weissert's report on the effects and costs of day care, both in terms of the report itself and in comparison with findings in Massachusetts. In conclusion, I will offer a recommendation to this committee calling for Federal initiative and action to ensure that Adult Day Care secures its rightful place in the long-term care continuum.

Ironically, as I implore you today for recognition of Adult Day Care as a viable and integral component of the long-term care continuumn, six years ago it was the Federal government through the Department of Health, Education and Welfare, that implored Massachusetts and other states to recognize the need for the establishment of alternatives to long-term institutional care. Adult Day Care was recommended as one such alternative.

Due to Federal prompting and great interest on the part of state policy makers and practitioners, the Massachusetts' Medicaid program in 1975/76 awarded six contracts to nursing homes, hospitals and community providers to operate Adult Day Care programs in a one-year pilot study.

Although Federal guidelines and various experts in the field suggested that Adult Day Care was divided into three distinct models of care: a therapeutic/rehabilitation model; a health maintenance model; and a social model, Massachusetts opted for a different route. From a demographic, client need and cost efficiency stand point, it was felt that a merging of these models would be more appropriate.

In 1977, the six pilot programs were evaluated. The evaluation demonstrated that Adult Day Care was indeed a deterrent to institutional placement, that it was cost efficient, that there was a high degree of client and family satisfaction with the program, in short, that it was a workable and necessary service option in Massachusetts.

The evaluation study resulted in a commitment by the state to expand Adult Day Care services. This commitment went beyond a dollar commitment from the Medicaid program. An inter-state agency committee was formed to input into major policy decisions and to, along with Health Systems Agencies and Area Agencies on Aging, review incoming Adult Day Care proposals. In addition, Area Agencies on Aging and several local communities contributed the necessary seed money for day care development.

The net result is that today in Massachusetts we have forty-five approved Adult Day Care programs and expect by the fall to have over fifty programs.

The major components of the Massachusetts Adult Day Health Programs are: health restoration, monitoring and supervision, social service counseling to clients and caretakers, therapeutic recreation and social interaction, personal care services, nutrition and transportation services.

The staff of each program, in a ratio of one staff person per every six clients, is comprised of full-time health professionals, social services professionals, a therapeutic recreation director, aides and physical, occupational and speech therapy consultants.

Programs are reviewed quarterly for regulation compliance and quality assurance.

In Massachusetts, we are currently serving over 1800 people ranging in age from 24–99. It is *significant* that at the point of admission to the program all clients are deemed by nursing review staff to be both eligible for and in risk of intermediate or skilled nursing home placement.

It is also significant that the per diem rate for Adult Day Care services is currently $16 per person. In addition to the per diem rate, Medicaid pays for transportation and direct therapy costs. The total average cost for Adult Day Care services in Massachusetts is $23–24 per person per day for a highly health-oriented program.

It is obvious that the findings in Massachusetts differ greatly from the glaring conclusions drawn in Mr. Weissert's report; those conclusions most notably being that the average cost of a health oriented day care program is $52 per day and that Adult Day Care is not a substitute for nursing home placement.

These conclusions, although certainly devastating to Adult Day Care through their visibility, are not, however, the major sin of the Weissert report. The sin is the *thrust* of the *only* major study in Adult Day Care to be undertaken by the Federal government.

First, the report compares the impact of day care on the cost and usage of skilled nursing home care from a Medicare focal point.

Experience in Massachusetts indicates that day care clients, percentage wise, are most likely to enter or be at risk of intermediate nursing home care. Intermediate care facilities are largely paid with the Medicaid dollar not the Medicare dollar. To look at the potential cost savings of Adult Day Care in comparison with institutional care from the focal point of the federal health care dollar one must examine Medicaid costs in relation to day care before conclusions can be drawn.

Secondly, the selection of programs studied in the Weissert report ensured that the average cost figures for health oriented day care would be higher than representative in other health oriented programs nationwide. These programs were gilded with a range of professional services and staff higher than the norm and inevitably more costly than typical. In addition the programs as part of a Medicare demonstration project were only liable for reporting costs and were given no incentives to contain costs.

In terms of the add-on versus substitute issue raised in the report the conclusions are again not surprising, given that clients would be more likely to enter an intermediate care facility rather than a skilled facility. Also, there was no evidence that clients in either the experimental or control group were assessed to be at risk of institutional placement upon entering the program or the study.

It is unfortunate that the thrust of cost savings and substitute service issues would be the more positive aspects of the Weissert report. For example, the report states that 'higher proportions of day care experimental than control group patients improved or maintained in levels of contentment, mental function and social activity.' In addition, the report suggests that those in the day care experimental group were kept alive longer through the program.

It's bad that not only quality of life but length of life also becomes a secondary issue to the dollar. Medicare decided not so long ago that providing life was worth $600–$700 dollars a day for renal dialysis patients. Now we are arguing that $52 is too much to prolong life for Adult Day Care clients when even the $52 is inaccurate.

In conclusion, I offer the following recommendation to the committee for consideration:

I recommend the establishment of a federal office on Adult Day Care whose function would be:

— to establish policy standards that would ensure a basic nationwide uniformity and understanding of Adult Day Care yet be flexible enough in these standards to allow for demographic and client need differences.
— to explore ways of integrating or channelling the multiple funding sources now being used for Adult Day Care thereby easing for practitioners and clients a major barrier in the development, continuation and use of Adult Day Care.
— to ensure equitable funding for the broad range of persons appropriate for day care services to make day care not just a program for the rich and or the poor.
— to act as a coordinator of and clearing house for the wide range of existing material in the Adult Day Care field.
— to provide leadership and technical assistance in the further development of Adult Day Care.

Day care is an essential and cost efficient program. It deserves your utmost attention and I hope after careful weighing of the testimony you will initiate action to ensure that Adult Day Care becomes an accepted and expected integral component of the long-term care continuum.[33]

This hearing on adult day care was the first congressional hearing since 1976 and the only congressional hearing to be held since that time relating solely to adult day care. Professionals in the field feel that the hearing was an important step in the continuing interest of the federal leaders relative to adult day-care programs.

Proposed Federal Legislation, 1980

One of the newest pieces of legislation (HR6194) that would impact on adult day-care services is the Medicaid Community Care Act of 1980. In this bill, Representative Pepper and Senator Waxman have attempted to broaden Medicaid's emphasis to encourage the development of more appropriate and available community programs for the population of elderly and disabled at risk for institutionalization.[34] For those individuals at risk of institutionalization in a long-term-care facility, the bill will increase the federal contribution match for community services by 25% under the following conditions:

1. The state provides a comprehensive medical and social assessment of each person who may require nursing home care. The assessment would encompass all factors relating to the person's ability to live in the community.
2. The state provides an expanded range of home and community-based services for those persons at risk who can and who choose to remain in the community.
3. The state provides these services under financial limits established by the Secretary [of Health and Human Services], at a rate not to exceed nursing home care in that state.

4. The state coordinates community-based services for this population with similar services provided under Medicare, Title XX, the Older Americans Act and other related programs.[34]

The author refers the reader to Appendix A for the text of the bill.

Clearly, the intent of this bill was to develop a continuum of long-term-care, community-based services, which would include adult day-care programs. This legislation is a much-needed beginning in changing the focus of Medicaid reimbursement from nursing homes to people's homes. As of this writing (August 1981) the bill had not passed into law. It will be interesting to follow any new bill like it in light of the present administration's budget cuts.

A second bill (HR3900) introduced in Congress was the Medicare Amendments of 1980. This legislation was written by Representatives Raugel, Carman, Vanik, and Ford and incorporates provisions of legislation authored by Congressman Pepper (HR2567) to expand home health care under Medicare.[35(p4)] In addition, services that are now received under home care and offered in adult day-care programs would be reimbursed through adult day care if the person preferred to receive them there. Under the proposal, the prior-hospitalization requirement under Part A of Medicare, the $60 deductible under Part B of Medicare, and the 100-visit limit under both Parts A and B of Medicare would be eliminated. The bill also expands mental-health care by tripling the outpatient reimbursement limit from $250 to $750, reducing the coinsurance obligation from 50% to 20%, and providing reimbursement for psychological care. Moreover, Medicare would reimburse all services provided by a community mental-health center (CMHC).

On March 4, 1980, the Commerce Committee reported out a slightly different version of HR3990, which places more restrictions on CMHC personnel authorized to perform reimbursable services. At this time (August 1981), the bill had not been passed.[35(p4)]

State Involvement

At present, 34 states have standards for adult day-care centers, whereas 9 states have no standards. Both the states of Massachusetts and California have been leaders in the field of adult day care in developing statewide Medicaid programs. In Massachusetts, legislation (H-2476) was introduced in 1975, directing the Department of Public Health to establish rules and regulations for certifying long-term-care facilities to provide adult day-care services.[36] Although this bill was voted down, the Department of Welfare, Medicaid Division, went on to develop a pilot study relative to adult day-care services in the same year. Because of the success of these programs and the state's interest in developing long-term-care alternatives to the nursing home, Massachusetts under the state's Medicaid program began its adult day-care services package. At that time, services could be offered within a nursing-home setting or through a free-standing community agency. The services were reimbursed at $12 a day, inclusive of transportation costs. Over the past five years, the services are still being offered in both types of settings, are health-oriented, and being reimbursed at $16 a day, exclusive of transportation costs. The number of programs has expanded to 47 statewide.

In California, the signing of AB1611, the California Adult Day Health Care Act and Adult Day Health Medi-Cal Law, by Governor Brown effective January 1, 1978, meant a statewide adult day-care program was mandated.[37] A further discussion of this legislation is found in Chapter 9. Since its enactment, California has established, to July 1979, 11 licensed adult day-care programs.

As forerunners in the development of statewide Medicaid programs, both California and Massachusetts have received and continue to receive many inquiries from other states for their guidelines and procedures. One of the states that recently fashioned their program from these two examples is New Jersey. Clearly, the trend for states to study and implement Medicaid-reimbursement adult day-care programs continues to grow. It is only through such developments at the state level that standards and criteria can be developed and effectively evaluated. Therefore, it is encouraging to see this trend spread.

American College of Nursing Home Administrators Survey

Although most of the adult day-care centers for the elderly that were surveyed are social in nature, adult day programs with strong health components were being established as extensions of long-term-care facilities. Such programs may eventually be the most practical approach to attending services for the disabled and elderly populations. Interestingly enough, Mr. Harvey Wertlieb and Ms. Melinda Dee, writing for the American Nursing Home Association, state:

> A.N.H.A.'s members have come to realize that day care is, or could be, an extension of the services delivered in the long-term care facility. A day care program can be set up as a distinct part of the existing facility, using a ward or wing for the participants.[37]

Two surveys conducted by the American College of Nursing Home Administrators, Department of Education, Research, and Development in the fall of 1976 (1) determined the level of interest among college members in adult day care and (2) gathered data about states' regulations, standards, and licensing procedures concerning adult day care.[38(pp30–34)]

The results of the level of interest among college members in adult day care are given in Table 6-1. One notes that almost all of the 200 respondents indicated that they would be interested in starting such a program and also attending a series of seminars on the services provided by such a program.[38(p30)]

The second survey's results are found in Table 6-2.

Of the 50 states that responded, 15 have instituted formal regulations and

Table 6-1
Adult day-care survey of American College of Nursing Home Administrators membership (200 respondents)

	Yes %	No %	Not Sure %	No Response %
1. Do you feel that the nursing home is an appropriate setting in which to offer adult day care?	96.0	2.5	1.5	
2. Do you feel that adult day care is an appropriate modality of care for older people who are somewhat independent?	97.0	0.5	2.5	
3. Given the opportunity, would you be interested in participating in a seminar series on adult day care?	96.0	3.0	1.0	
4. Does your facility currently operate an adult day-care program?	10.0	90.0		
5. If no, have you considered starting an adult day-care center in your facility?	84.5	9.5	0.5	5.5
6. To your knowledge, are there any adult day-care centers presently serving your community?	25.0	75.0		

Reprinted from Volume V, Number 1, 1977 of *The Journal of Long-Term Care Administration* published by the American College of Nursing Home Administrators, Inc.

standards covering adult day care (Alabama, California, Idaho, Kentucky, Louisiana, Maryland, Massachusetts, Minnesota, Nebraska, New Jersey, New York, North Carolina, Oregon, Rhode Island, and Utah).[38(p30)]

Ten states require facilities for the elderly be licensed (California, Kansas, Kentucky, Massachusetts, New Hampshire, New Jersey, New York, Oregon, South Carolina, and Utah).[38(p32)] Seven of the 10 states have an adult day-care licensure procedure that is distinct from that of nursing homes (California, Hawaii, Kentucky, New Hampshire, New Jersey, South Carolina, and Utah).[38(p31)]

Of the 33 states that do not have special licensure procedures for adult day-care programs, 12 indicated that they do intend to create such procedures in the near future (Arkansas, Connecticut, Georgia, Maine, Maryland, Mississippi, New Mexico, North Carolina, Rhode Island, Washington, Wisconsin, and Wyoming), and 3 states (South Dakota, Tennessee, and Texas) are presently considering the matter.[38(p33)] Two states (Illinois and Indiana) indicated that they know of no such plans, and 3 states (Louisiana, Minnesota, and West Virginia) made no response to this question.[38(p34)]

Table 6-2
Adult day-care survey of state departments of health

States () = State Not Responding	States with Day Care Regulations and Standards	States Requiring Day Care Licensure	States Requiring Licensure District from Nursing Home License	States Planning to Create License Procedure for Day Care Soon
Alabama	*			
Alaska				
Arizona				
Arkansas				*
California	*	*	*	
Colorado				
Connecticut				
Delaware	being developed			*
D.C.				
Florida				
Georgia				
Hawaii	*		*	*
Idaho	*			
Illinois				
Indiana				
(Iowa)				
Kansas		*		
Kentucky	*	*	*	
Louisiana	*			
Maine				*
Maryland	*			*
Massachusetts	*	*		
Minnesota	*			
Michigan				
Mississippi				*
(Missouri)				
Montana				
Nebraska	*			
Nevada				
New Hampshire		*	*	
New Jersey	*	*	*	
New Mexico				*
New York	*	*		
North Carolina	*			*
North Dakota				
Ohio				

Table 6-2 *(continued)*

States () = State Not Responding	Regulations & Standards — States with Day Care Regulations and Standards	Licensure Procedures — States Requiring Day Care Licensure	States Requiring Licensure District from Nursing Home License	States Planning to Create License Procedure for Day Care Soon
Oklahoma				
Oregon	*	*		
(Pennsylvania)				
Rhode Island	*			*
S. Carolina	being	*	*	
S. Dakota	developed			
Tennessee				
Texas				
Utah	*	*	*	
Vermont				
Virginia				
Washington				*
W. Virginia				
Wisconsin				*
Wyoming				*
Guam				
Puerto Rico				
(Virgin Islands)				

Reprinted from Volume V, Number 1, 1977 of *The Journal of Long-Term Care Administration* published by the American College of Nursing Home Administrators, Inc.

Types of Adult Day-Care Programs in the United States

As of spring, 1980, there were 608 adult day-care programs in the United States, with more opening each day. Of the 608 programs, about 300 were funded by Title XX funds (social-oriented); 100 by Title XIX funds (health-oriented); and 120 by Title III funds (social- or health-oriented).[40] Discussion of these funding sources and their implications in adult day-care programming can be found in Chapter 9. However, the facts and figures in this chapter are results of analyzing the 1977 Adult Day Care Directory and will probably be outdated when the 1980 directory becomes available.

Clearly, the concept of adult day services applies to any service provided during the day when participants return home at night. One unique feature of the adult day-care movement in the United States is that it cannot only meet the long-term needs of participants, but also takes into account the individual needs. For example, services in these programs are tailored specifically for each participant so that they can be rehabilitated to a higher level of functioning, maintained at a current level of functioning, or prevented from incurring illness that would alter their present level of functioning. Within the expansion of the United States movement, states have developed programs according to the funding sources available. These programs range from purely social to a mixture of social and health services, to a high degree of health and restorative services. Because of these trends, Edith Robins in 1975 proposed four models of adult day-care services. More recently, she claimed that these models were not mutually exclusive.[40] Further, she stated that a blending of models and overlap of program models can and do occur.[40] When referring to the table, one should keep in mind the above-mentioned blending and overlap of the models.

Table 6-3 outlines four models currently being used in adult day-care programming.

As the table shows, candidates for adult day-care services range from those persons who are socially isolated and needing social activities to those who are living with family and need some continued support services, such as nursing or physical therapy, to those who would remain inpatients without daily intensive restorative services. Thus, one can see that adult day-care services are oriented toward primary, secondary, and tertiary levels of prevention.

A more intense and detailed presentation of models is given in Chapter 10. The reader is referred to this chapter for further information on models, types, and the differences between each. In addition, an expanded explanation of considerations needed to decide on a specific model is presented in Chapter 10.

National Institute on Adult Day Care (NIAD)

At the National Council on Aging (NCOA) convention in Washington, D.C., April 20–24, 1980, the members of that organization voted to adopt a National Institute on Adult Day Care (NIAD) under the auspices of the National Council on Aging. A task force had been developed in 1978, which had requested the NCOA to accept NIAD as an institute under the NCOA. With acceptance granted, interim procedures were adopted by the NIAD affiliates of NCOA's 1979 annual conference. Over the year (from the 1979 to the 1980 annual conference), the NIAD Development Committee diligently worked to develop more comprehensive operating rules. These rules are shown in Figure 6-1.

With the growth and development of the NIAD under the National Council on Aging, it is anticipated that the goals of those working in these programs will

Table 6-3
Adult day-care-service models

Model Type	Services	Type of Participant	Facility
I.	Intensive restorative, medical and health services (medical nursing and therapies, activities)	Persons who are in active phase of recovery and otherwise would remain inpatients	Extended care facility or hospital
II.	Time-limited, restorative, medical and health services (nursing and therapies, activities)	Persons with chronic problems who are post extended-care or hospital care	Nursing home
III.	Long-term health-maintenance services (nursing and other support services, activities)	"At risk" persons who would be prematurely institutionalized	Nursing home or freestanding community center
IV.	Preventive health services (psychosocial activities in protected environment)	"Frail" persons needing psychosocial activities	Freestanding community center, multipurpose senior center, or nursing home

Adapted from the four modules of adult day care defined by Edith Robins in "Operational Research in Geriatric Day Care in the United States," paper presented at the 10th International Gerontological Congress, Jerusalem, Israel, June 1975. With the permission of the author.

be unified. Furthermore, it is felt that a national body representing adult day-care programs will enhance communications with our federal leaders. This ongoing and frequent exchange of ideas and information will hopefully influence the legislators in favor of such programs.

Summary

It is encouraging to view the international growth of the adult day-care movement since its inception in Russia in 1942. Clearly, this growth has initiated the very recent developments within the United States, particularly in the past few years when the federal government has placed a greater focus on serving the "frail" and disabled elderly. Long-term-care planners and providers firmly believe that the adult day-care movement within the United States is a viable option within a continuum of long-term-care services. In addition, they see it as coordinated with other service components, such as home care, institutional care, drop-in centers, and home health care. Indeed, it is one innovative option that can add to, help organize, and blend the more traditional health- and social-service delivery systems in the United States for meeting the needs of our disabled adults and infirmed elderly.

1980
Rules of Operation
of the
National Institute on Adult Day Care
A Program of
The National Council on the Aging

PREAMBLE

The increasing number of people who live to advanced years and whose functional level is impaired has created a need for a broad range of community services to assist older people to remain in the community. An adult day-care program provides a gamut of services in a congregate setting, enhancing the daily lives of its participants and supporting their continued involvement in the community. Adult day care is a generic term that applies to a variety of programs offering services that range from active rehabilitation to social and health-related care. Various terminology is applied: day care, day treatment, day health care, psychiatric day treatment, partial hospitalization, and day hospital care. Adult day care is coordinated with, and relates to, other agencies and services such as senior centers, in-home services, and institutional and hospital care. It is an innovative way to organize and blend traditional health and social services for the disabled older person. The National Institute on Adult Day Care is established within the framework of the National Council on the Aging in order to provide the most appropriate vehicle for communication and action for all who work in adult day care.

ARTICLE I—NAME

The name shall be the National Institute on Adult Day Care (NIAD).

ARTICLE II—PURPOSE

1. To promote the concept of adult day care as a viable community-based option for disabled older persons within the larger continuum of long-term care.

2. To collect, prepare, and disseminate information on all aspects of adult day care.

3. To provide assistance and guidance to adult day-care programs and to those seeking to establish new programs through consultation services, publication of instructional materials, and the formulation of standards.

4. To provide opportunities for the exchange of information and expertise related to the organization, operation, and services of adult day care by means of national and regional conferences and seminars.

5. To assist in improving and extending adult day-care programs by working closely with the national, state, and local organizations and governmental agencies.

6. To improve adult day-care services through the stimulation of research projects to enable adult day-care providers to formulate new concepts and encourage documentation.

7. To encourage adult day-care programs to participate in local area health planning activities in order to coordinate and enhance the effectiveness of adult day care.

8. To encourage the training of personnel to work with disabled older people and the establishment of appropriate personnel standards and practices.

9. To develop social and public policy positions related to the needs and interests of adult day-care programs and their target population and to stimulate action on legislative, public policy, and service delivery issues.

Figure 6-1. Rules of Operation of the National Institute on Adult Day Care. (From *Rules of Operation of NIAD,* by the National Institute on Adult Day Care, Wash DC, National Council on Aging, 1980.)

ARTICLE III—RELATIONSHIP TO THE NATIONAL COUNCIL ON THE AGING

Section A. The Institute shall be an integral part of the National Council on the Aging, which shall assign appropriate staff to carry out the purposes of the Institute. The Institute shall be consulted on all matters pertaining to adult day-care programs.

Section B. The elected chairperson of the Institute shall serve on the NCOA board of directors during his/her term as chairperson.

Section C. NCOA shall be the sole financial agent of the Institute. All grants and contracts of the Institute shall be administered through NCOA.

ARTICLE IV—MEMBERSHIP

Membership in the National Council on the Aging is a prerequisite for affiliation with the Institute. Such affiliation shall be open to all members of the NCOA, individuals, and agencies who so indicate. They shall be entitled to all services offered by the NCOA and NIAD.

ARTICLE V—NATIONAL STEERING COMMITTEE

Section A. There shall be a governing body of the Institute called the National Steering Committee composed of fifteen (15) members, of whom three (3) shall be officers, two (2) shall be at-large representatives, and ten (10) regional representatives subject to the provisions set forth in Section D of this Article V.

Section B. A chairperson, chairperson-elect, and a secretary, all of whom shall be elected for two-year terms by the total membership of the NIAD, shall serve as the officers of both the Institute and of the National Steering Committee. None is eligible for re-election to the same office.

Section C. The two (2) at-large members of the National Steering Committee shall be elected by the total NIAD membership, shall serve a two-year term and may be re-elected for one (1) additional consecutive term.

Section D. The ten (10) federal government regions shall constitute the regions for the NIAD. Each region shall elect one (1) representative to serve for a two-year term on the National Steering Committee as set forth in Article X, Section A. A representative may be re-elected to serve for one (1) additional consecutive term. To provide for continuity of the work of the National Steering Committee the ten (10) regions shall be divided into two (2) blocks, each composed of five (5) regions. Each block shall elect its representatives in alternate years beginning in 1980.

Implementation of the full regional representation on the National Steering Committee shall take place in two steps. Following the election of the officers at the Institute's April 1980 meeting, the officers shall determine by lot which of the five (5) regions shall constitute each block and which of these blocks shall elect representatives to the National Steering Committee in 1980; the second block to elect its representatives in 1981. Within ninety (90) days of the 1980 meeting, the five (5) 1980 representatives shall be selected as established under Article X, Section A. Thereafter whether the regional representatives are elected by regional organizations or selected by the Selection Committee as outlined in Article X, Section A, the process shall be completed prior to the NIAD annual meeting.

Figure 6-1. *(continued)*

Section E. Officers shall be persons involved in the provision of adult day care and be members of the NCOA. Their duties shall include:
1. Chairperson: Act as liaison between the board of directors of the NCOA and the Institute; officiate at meetings of the Institute and of the National Steering Committee; represent the Institute in official business.
2. Chairperson-elect: Shall carry out the duties of the chairperson in his/her absence and be the regional coordinator.
3. Secretary: Maintain minutes of Institute and National Steering Committee meetings and assure communication to affiliate members of the Institute.

Section F. If the chairperson should become unable to fulfill the duties of that office, the chairperson-elect shall assume the duties of chairperson. This shall not affect the assumption of the office of chairperson in what would be the normal order of succession. The National Steering Committee shall appoint a replacement for the office of secretary should the position become vacant.

Section G. A quorum of the National Steering Committee shall be a majority of its members.

Section H. If a question arises as to the qualifications of a National Steering Committee member or the adequacy with which a member is fulfilling the responsibilities of office, the chairperson of the Committee shall determine whether or not the existence of a vacancy on the Committee shall be declared.

Section I. The National Steering Committee is empowered to act on behalf of the total membership of the Institute in all matters pertaining to the Institute during the interval between membership meeting.

Section J. The National Steering Committee shall meet on the call of the chairperson but a minimum of two (2) meetings annually shall be held. A meeting may also be called at the request of eight National Steering Committee members.

ARTICLE VI—NIAD MEETINGS

There shall be an annual membership meeting of the NIAD which shall be held, when possible, in conjunction with a national or regional meeting of NCOA.

ARTICLE VII—COMMITTEES

Section A. The standing committees of the Institute shall include: Publications and Research, Standards and Guidelines, Social Policy and Action, Conference and Training, Public Relations and Organizational Liaison. Other standing committees may be established as deemed necessary by the National Steering Committee. Duties of the standing committees shall be determined by the National Steering Committee.

Section B. All standing committee chairpersons must be members of the National Steering Committee. They shall be appointed by the chairperson of the Institute with the approval of the National Steering Committee.

Section C. The chairperson, or the National Steering Committee, may establish ad hoc (special) committees as are required to fulfill the purposes of the Institute. The chairperson of any such committee need not be a member of the National Steering Committee but may be invited to attend meetings of the National Steering Committee.

Figure 6-1. *(continued)*

Section D. Members of standing and ad hoc committees may be selected from the total membership of the Institute.

ARTICLE VIII—NOMINATING COMMITTEE

Section A. A Nominating Committee, for the purpose of preparing a slate of nominees for the appropriate officer and at-large positions, shall be composed of three (3) regional representative members of the National Steering Committee. The Nominating Committee shall be elected at the first meeting of the National Steering Committee held following the NIAD annual meeting.

Section B. The Nominating Committee shall elect its own chairperson.

Section C. A quorum for the Nominating Committee shall be two (2) members.

ARTICLE IX—NOMINATIONS AND ELECTIONS

Section A. Following the election of 1980, during the month of January of each even-numbered year, members of the Institute shall be requested to submit the names and qualifications of those persons believed by them to be appropriately qualified to serve as officers and at-large members. Such recommendations shall be considered by the Nominating Committee as it prepares a slate of candidates. All candidates for elected positions must be members of the Institute.

Section B. The Nominating Committee shall prepare a slate of a minimum of two (2) and a maximum of four (4) candidates for each office and at-large position.

Section C. A ballot shall be mailed to all members of the Institute in good standing approximately four (4) weeks prior to the election. An election shall be held four (4) weeks prior to the NIAD annual meeting in each even-numbered year.

Section D. The chairperson of the Institute shall appoint an Election Committee composed of three (3) Institute members to tabulate the results of the election and make a written report to the chairperson of the National Steering Committee within one (1) week following the election deadline.

Section E. New officers shall be installed at the NIAD annual meeting.

ARTICLE X—REGIONAL ORGANIZATIONS

Section A. A regional adult day care organization shall be established in each of the ten (10) federal regions, with a minimum of one (1) representative from each state within a region. Each regional organization shall elect one (1) representative to the National Steering Committee as set forth in Article V, Sections A and D. Regional representatives to the National Steering Committee shall be members of the Institute.

Until such time as the regional-state pattern outlined above has been established the following arrangements shall pertain:

a. State associations set up as of April 1980 or at any time thereafter shall be invited by the chairperson of the NIAD to appoint a representative to the regional organization. In those states where no association has been established the chairperson of NIAD shall seek a suitable representative.

Figure 6-1. *(continued)*

b. A Selection Committee, composed of a chairperson and two (2) other members, shall be elected annually by the membership of the NIAD until such time as the ten (10) regional organizations have all been established. Its task shall be to select those persons who shall serve as the regional representatives on the National Steering Committee from a list of candidates proposed by the state associations and by the chairperson of the NIAD for those states that do not have such an association. As regional organizations are established, they will assume this responsibility for their respective region. To establish the procedures set forth in Article V, Section D, paragraph 2, the Selection Committee elected at the NIAD meeting in April 1980 shall serve in selecting the regional representatives for both 1980 and 1981.

Section B. The purpose of the regional organizations shall be to develop working groups at local levels to address local issues to enhance the efforts of the National Steering Committee and to promote the Institute.

Section C. All regional organizational plans shall be approved by the National Steering Committee, and nothing in regional operating procedures may contravene the operating rules of the Institute or Articles of Incorporation of NCOA.

Section D. Voting members of regional organizations shall be NCOA members in good standing.

Section E. Each region shall be encouraged to plan an adult day care conference, when possible in conjunction with a regional meeting of NCOA. Regions may combine to hold joint regional meetings and conferences.

Section F. Each regional organization shall be encouraged to have one meeting each year to conduct its business.

ARTICLE XI—PARLIAMENTARY PROCEDURES

In any matters or procedures not considered in these operating rules, the current edition of Robert's Rules of Order shall apply.

ARTICLE XII—AMENDMENTS

Section A. These operating rules may be amended in whole or in part at any national meeting of the membership of the Institute or by a mail vote of the membership. An affirmative vote of two-thirds (2/3) of the members voting shall be required. Any proposed change(s) shall be submitted in writing to the membership thirty (30) days in advance of the meeting or mail vote.

Section B. Proposed change(s) in the operating rules shall be submitted to the National Steering Committee of the Institute for review. The Committee shall determine if action is required immediately or can await the next annual meeting of the Institute.

Section C. Any proposed change in the operating rules of the Institute submitted to the membership shall be accompanied by a statement supporting or rejecting the said change, such statement to be prepared by the National Steering Committee and/or the member proposing the change.

Figure 6-1. *(continued)*

References

1. Kramer BM: *Day Hospital*. New York, Grune & Stratton, 1962, p 38.

2. Barton WE: *Administration in Psychiatry*. Springfield, Ill, CC Thomas, Publisher, 1962, p 23.

3. Cameron DE: The day hospital. *Modern Hospital* **69**: 16, 1947.

4. Brierer J: *The Day Hospital: An Experiment in Social Psychiatry and Synthoanalytic Psychotherapy*. London, Lewis Company, 1951.

5. Padula H: *Developing Day Care for Older People*. Wash, DC, National Council on Aging, 1972, p 4.

6. Brocklehurst JC: *The Geriatric Day Hospital*. London, King Edward's Hospital Fund, 1970.

7. Andrews J: A geriatric day ward in an English hospital. *J Am Geri Soc* **18**: 378–386, 1970.

8. Farndale J: *The Day Hospital Movement in Great Britain*. New York, Pergamon Press, 1961, p 44.

9. Trager J: *Adult Day Facilities*. Wash, DC, US Senate, 1977.

10. *Geriatric Day Hospitals*. London, Department of Health and Social Security, Reference F/G, 54/17, December 7, 1971.

11. Robins EG: *Report on Day Hospitals in Israel and Great Britain*. DHEW, October 15, 1973.

12. Survey of day care programs. Toronto, Canada, Jewish Home for the Aged, 1964 (unpublished paper).

13. The role of day hospital. Montreal, Canada, Maimonides Day Hospital, 1975 (unpublished paper).

14. Novick L: Day care meets geriatric needs. *Hospitals*, vol 12, 1973.

15. Lampe M: Adult day care: A planning paper. Winnipeg, Manitoba, Department of Health and Social Development, Sept 2, 1975.

16. Linder L: Factors to consider in long-term care. Upsala, Sweden, Sept 1974 (unpublished paper), p 7.

17. Division of Hospital and Medical Facilities: *The Nation's Health Facilities: Ten Years of the Hill Burton and Medical Facilities Program 1946–1956*. DHEW, PHS Publication No 616, 1958.

18. National Center for Health Statistics. *In Health, United States*. DHEW, Publication No 761232, 1974.

19. *Nursing and Long-Term Care: Toward Quality Care for Aging. A Report from the Committee on Skilled Nursing Care*. Kansas City, Mo, American Nurses Association, 1975, p 43.

20. Carter MD: Statement on options for health care services. Testimony presented to the Committee on Skilled Nursing Care, Colorado State Nurses Association. Denver, Colo, Sept 16, 1974, p 2.

21. Moss BB: *Caring for the Aged*. Garden City, NY, Doubleday & Co, Inc, 1966, p 107.

22. Weissert W, Hurd, G, Steinhardt B: *Adult Day Care in the U.S.: A Comparative Study*. Wash, DC, The Transcentury Corporation, June 30, 1975.

23. U.S. Division of Long-Term Care: *Preliminary Analysis of Select Geriatric Day Care Programs*. DHEW, 1974.

24. Definition of day care services. Public Law 92-603, Section 222 (G). DHEW, 1974.

25. Weissert W: *Effects and Costs of Day Care and Homemakers Services for the Chronically Ill: A Randomized Experiment*. Hyattsville, Md, DHEW, National Center for Health Services Research, 1977.

26. U.S. Congress: Purposes for House Select Committee on Aging. Newsletter, Select Committee on Aging, US House of Representatives, 1974.

27. Pepper C: Select Committee on Aging. Newsletter, US House of Representatives, April 18, 1980.

28. ———: Opening remarks at the adult day care hearing. House Select Committee on Aging, April 23, 1980.

29. Woods, H: Testimony: Adult day care hearing. Ibid.

30. Driscoll, D: Testimony. Ibid.

31. Morrison, K: Testimony. Ibid.

32. Weissert, W: Testimony. Ibid.

33. Klapfish, A: Testimony. Ibid.

34. Pepper C, Waxman H: Medicaid Community Care Act, HR6194. Congressional Record. US House of Representatives, December 19, 1979.

35. Select Committee on Aging. *Status of Major Legislation Affecting the Elderly in the 96th Congress as of April 14, 1980*. House Select Committee on Aging, 1980.

36. Bill No. 2476. House of Representatives, Boston, 1975.

37. VonBehren R: Adult day health services: A final report. Los Angeles, California Department of Health Services, 1979, p 8.

38. ACHNA's research book: Surveys on adult day care services. *J Long-Term Care Admin* 5:30–34, 1977.

39. Robins EG: *1980 National Directory of Adult Day Health programs*. Wash, DC, US Government Printing Office, Summer, 1980.

40. ———: Presentation at National Council on Aging Conference. Wash, DC, Apr 21, 1980, pp 1-6.

7

British Geriatric Day Hospitals: Implications for America

Vera Teyrovsky Goupille, MSc

Introduction

Britain is the leader of the adult day-care movement, with the oldest and most extensive system of day-care services. On any weekday, it has been estimated that 40,000 people attend 1000 day-care centers for the elderly.[1] These day units vary in their location, size, and function. Yet, they are important in extending care to some of Britain's 6.7 million citizens over the age of 65, who constitute over 13% of the total population.[2]

One of the earliest developments in day care is the geriatric day hospital. In its more than 25 years of operation in Britain, it has proved to be an effective alternative to institutional health care and more than satisfactory to the participants[3] and staff.[4(pp253-257),5] Today geriatric day hospitals are viewed as a necessary part of the National Health Service (NHS).

It is important to identify the factors that shaped the development of the day hospital service in Britain. The success of this service, to a large extent, can be explained by external forces. Key factors that will be explored in this chapter are historical forces, method of funding, and the general system of health care in Britain.

The day-hospital movement, as Farndale first coined the term in 1961, has undergone some changes since its beginning. The responsibilities of the day hospital have essentially remained the same, but its organization has and is still changing. The objectives of care in day hospitals was first outlined by Boucher:

1. to prevent or retard physical and mental deterioration
2. to give appropriate treatment and to permit after-care of clients discharged from hospital
3. to save hospital beds
4. to give relief to relatives by caring for clients during the day[6]

More recently, the functions by which these objectives can be met have been differentiated among rehabilitation, maintenance, and social care.[7] Debate has centered around the extent to which each of these objectives is met. The trend is increasingly toward specialization of functions, particularly differentiating between short-term rehabilitative care and long-term maintenance. Some day hospitals have gone as far as specializing only for stroke clients or orthopedic clients.

Staff have been able to focus on critical factors affecting the day-to-day operations of day hospitals in hope of improving the quality of care they provide. Major efforts have been put into developing the rehabilitative function of day hospitals.

As part of the National Health Service, day hospitals are linked to other services. Therefore, staff of day hospitals, in particular geriatricians, have been able to influence the development of other services that complement day-hospital care. Day centers are an example of such complementary services, and, in some cases, it was the geriatrician who influenced the development of more day centers. As part of a system of care, day hospitals are informed and affected by changes in other parts of the system. Local adaptations can sometimes be made so that day hospitals may function somewhat like a day center, and a day center situated in a residential home may more closely resemble a day hospital.

In any case, the development of day hospitals for the elderly in Britain has been steady. There is a "reasonably well understood agenda of priorities," states Carter.[1] Attention has yet been averted from the development of day hospitals and day-care services for the elderly to the pursuit of definition of a day hospital compared with a day center, as it has been in America.

It is important that America consider a number of factors influencing Britain's successful development of day-hospital care if it wants to achieve the same. It is not sufficient to look at the characteristics of a facility. It is time that America state its responsibilities toward the elderly, support its statement with adequate and consistent funds, and finally provide an organizational structure so that health and social services for the elderly may be coordinated.

Background

Britain has a long, bleak history of institutional care, beginning with the establishment of workhouses and asylums in Victorian times. The elderly had long been neglected.[8] With the National Health Service (NHS) Act of 1946, geriatrics was established as a new specialty in an effort to improve the care of the elderly and free hospital beds. However, after World War II, England was left in a poor financial state, and funding for the new NHS was strict. The new specialty of geriatrics had to make do with less than the more established specialties.

These factors encouraged the development of alternative forms of care for the elderly. Geriatricians had to establish a reputation for the new specialty and were in a position to actively implement new ideas. Today, as Bagnall commented, "community care is all the rage and the trend has swung against institutions. Institutions are seen as expensive to run, difficult to staff, especially at nights and weekends. . . . Day care is seen as the remedy for all these ills and rarely can any concept have pleased so many."[4(p261)]

Additionally, the central government in Britain has continually supported the development of day-hospital care. As early as 1957, the minister of health encouraged their development. In 1971, government policy recommended that two geriatric day-hospital places per 1000 persons aged 65 and over be established.[9] Similarly, two places per 1000 in psychogeriatric day hospitals were recommended in 1972.[10] These recommendations greatly encouraged the development of day hospitals.

The first geriatric day hospital was organized in 1952 within the main hospital at Cowley Road, Oxford. The day hospital moved into the first purpose-built facility in 1958.[11] Yet, Brocklehurst found 90 day hospitals in operation in 1969, and, by 1978, 302 day hospitals were open.[12] This rapid development is thought by many to be a testimonial to the need day hospitals fill.[13]

Day centers are a more recent development. Geriatric and psychogeriatric types of day centers may be provided by local authorities under the 1968 Health Services and Public Health Act.[14] Voluntary organizations have run numerous day centers prior to this; however, major developments in day care in Britain have occurred primarily since 1970.

In general, day-care centers and day hospitals cater to different client groups. Day-hospital clients are the most physically demanding of any group in day services. The average day hospital has 30 places, with the majority of clients attending twice a week; 89%–95% are brought to the hospital by special transport for rehabilitation, maintenance treatment, medical investigation, and social care.

The day-hospital facility is perhaps best described by Brocklehurst as:

> a building to which patients may come, or be brought in the morning, where they may spend several hours in therapeutic activity and whence they return subsequently

on the same day to their own homes. . . . It may be no more than a single room specially adapted, or a whole purpose-built structure of many varied rooms. Geriatric Day Hospitals provide facilities for physiotherapy and occupational therapys, for medical examination and nursing treatment, and usually for various other activities including investigation, speech therapy, dentistry, chiropody and hairdressing. The building and its facilities may be used entirely for day patients coming from their homes, or it may be used by in-patients as well, who come over from the wards in the morning and return in the afternoon.[7]

From the beginning, nearly all day hospitals have been situated on the premises of hospitals, either acute or geriatric long-stay. This arrangement has the advantage that facilities and staff can be shared with other hospital departments and is convenient for the medical and allied professions.

Unlike day-care centers, day hospitals are predominantly staffed by professionals. The most numerous are the nurses. Volunteers or unqualified staff predominate in day centers. The major program in day centers consists of arts and crafts and some social activity. The activities are organized for the group rather than the individual.

Woodford-Williams and Alvarez concluded that there are four types of clients who need day-hospital care:

1. those who could be cured and eventually could be discharged
2. those who were physically dependent
3. those who were emotionally dependent
4. those who attended to relieve strain on relatives[15]

Day hospitals offer an alternative to hospital care and yet provide more individual care than day centers. This form of medically orientated day care aims to serve frail elderly persons who might otherwise be hospitalized or, if already in hospital, would have no hope of discharge. Day hospitals can be said to be preventive when they defer or prevent institutionalization. In as much as they serve a participant group that is already frail and in need of support, they are not preventive in the first degree—that is, day hospitals are not preventing well elderly persons from becoming frail.

Service Characteristics

Day hospitals are defined as providing four major functions:

1. medical or nursing investigation
2. rehabilitation
3. maintenance treatment
4. social care

Medical or nursing investigation can be carried out at a slower pace in a day hospital. A physical examination or medical tests can be done over a period of hours, and the client can rest as necessary. Admission to a hospital, medical treatment, or admission to a day hospital may then be recommended.

Day hospitals have a multidisciplinary staff who assist in assessing clients at the time of admission, on an ongoing basis, and at the time of discharge. An occupational therapist assesses the client's ability to perform activities of daily living—that is, dressing, toilet and self-care, mobility, eating activities, domestic activities. A physiotherapist assesses the client's muscle strength, joint range, functional activities such as getting into bed, and mental state.

There is some evidence that the type of client attending geriatric day hospitals has changed over the last ten years. Brocklehurst and Brocklehurst and Tucker found the distribution of principal diagnoses shown in Table 7-1. The earlier study was conducted at five day hospitals and included 465 patients. In the more recent study, 30 day hospitals and 233 clients were included. This change is also reflected in the reasons given for attendance (see Table 7-2).

Reasons for Attendance

Since ultimate responsibility for a client resides with the geriatrician, it is the geriatrician who does the final assessment and determines the reason for attendance. Rehabilitation can be said to be provided in the prospect of improving physical disability to a point of maximum independence for a given client. Once maximum independence is achieved, maintenance treatment is provided in the

Table 7-1
Principal diagnoses of patients attending British geriatric day hospitals

Diagnosis	% of Patients 1970*	1979[†]
Arthritis or fractured femur	30	23
Stroke	30	37
Cerebral arteriosclerosis, dementia, parkinsonism, or other central nervous disorders	22	13
Depression	4	3
Circulatory disorders	—	7
Respiratory disorders	—	3
Other	14	14

*Data from *The Geriatric Day Hospital*, by JC Brocklehurst. London, King Edward's Hospital Fund for London, 1970.
[†]Data from *Progress in Day Care*, by JC Brocklehurst and JS Tucker. London, King Edward's Hospital Fund for London, 1980.

Table 7-2
Reasons for attendance in British geriatric day hospitals

Reasons	% of Patients 1970*	1979†
Rehabilitation	41	42.5
Physical maintenance	29	20.5
Social	6	13
Other	24	24

*Data from *The Geriatric Day Hospital,* by JC Brocklehurst. London, King Edward's Hospital Fund for London, 1970.
†Data from *Progress in Day Care,* by JC Brocklehurst and JS Tucker. London, King Edward's Hospital Fund for London, 1980.

prospect of improving physical disability to a point of maximum independence for a given client. Otherwise, elderly persons may deteriorate slowly once they are cut off from the stimulus of a geriatric department, states Brocklehurst. Therefore, day-hospital attendance for an indefinite period for some elderly persons ensures that the state of independence achieved is maintained. Social care is necessary when an elderly person needs companionship, yet is unsuitable for a social day center in which nursing care is not available.

Often dentists, chiropodists, and speech therapists visit a day hospital. Therapists' time tends to be limited, so nurses tend to provide the bulk of care by bathing, redressing wounds, and transporting clients from one therapy to another. The senior nurse tends to coordinate the various services, whereas the geriatrician sets the policies. Whatever the admission policies, client mix does not prove to be a problem in English day hospitals. Seldom are younger clients (under 50) mixed with older ones, just as the elderly mentally infirm are not treated in the same day hospital as those who are not mentally infirm. Only 10%–20% of the clients in geriatric day hospitals can be said to be mentally infirm. In most cases, it can be said that their mental states were not the cause of their admission, but rather were in addition to a multiple of physical ailments. Finally, only those who have no "socially undesirable traits" are admitted. This criterion is thought important for the morale of both clients and staff.

One controversial issue is the optimal size for day hospitals. The average day hospital has 30 places, but the range is from 6 to 120. As recently as 1975, the Scottish Hospital Centre (1973) recommended 30–50 places in a day hospital. In 1970, Brocklehurst found that one-third of day hospitals has less than 20 places, whereas 25% had 40 or more. Millard, in his study of three day hospitals, concluded that the smaller the day hospitals, the better, in terms of rehabilitation—that is, the 28-place day hospital retained patients for twice as long as the 12-place day hospital.[16]

Operational Problems

Day-hospital staff are most concerned with a number of operational problems that affect the quality of the service. Transportation, recruitment of professional staff, and timely client discharge are critical to the effective operation of day hospitals. These factors become more of an issue when day care is highly medical and serves frail elderly persons as in the United Kingdom.

The transportation service affects the amount of time clients are able to spend at the day hospital, the mood of the clients when they arrive at the hospital, and the drop-out rate. Day-hospital clients in the United Kingdom spend anywhere from one-half to two and one-half hours travelling a distance of 5–16 miles in an ambulance or special bus, which usually carries 6–12 persons. The service is expensive and is estimated to cost $6.50 (£3.20) per client per attendance. Since clients are often very frail, do not have their own means of transportation, or need to be assisted down stairs, most have to be specially transported to the day hospital. Most vehicles are inappropriate and difficult to staff. High turnover of drivers affects the quality of the transport service and patient satisfaction.

Recruitment of professional staff is particularly a problem in major cities, such as London, where day hospitals have to compete for staff. In suburban and rural areas, recruitment is not as much of a problem since many occupational therapists, physical therapists, and nurses are married women with children, who welcome part-time work near their homes.

Farndale found that the majority of the ten geriatric day hospitals studied were managed by therapists.[11] Brocklehurst found that nurses were most often in charge.[7] The government has now accepted this trend and recommends that geriatric day hospitals be managed by nurses. This recommendation reflects the difficulty with which professional staff are recruited to work with the elderly.

As in the United States, therapists working with the elderly are thought to be the least competent in their professions. Professionals just out of training who elect to work with the elderly may find it difficult to find a job later in a different branch of their profession. For example, a nurse trying to get into pediatrics from geriatrics may have some difficulty, even though her salary may have been higher in the geriatric field because of the salary bonus (geriatric lead-in) given in the United Kingdom for working with older persons.

Discharging from a day hospital requires much staff time. Often the client's reaction to the mere suggestion of discharge is to revert back to an earlier state of disability. Liaison between social services must constantly be maintained, as the majority of clients are referred to social-service day centers within six months of admission to a day hospital. For these reasons, some have suggested that discharge planning begin at the time of admission.

Other countries can learn from Britain's day-hospital service. Each change in the service brings a number of new problems. Before changing client groups, staffing arrangements, and the provision of services in day care, plans should be made to deal with the impact of those changes. It is likely that the operation problems encountered by Britain will occur elsewhere. Transportation is an important feature of any program that serves the frail elderly. The training and recruitment of staff should proceed or be in conjunction with the development of a service.

Policies and Trends

In Britain, day hospitals are increasingly specializing by function. Day hospitals are in the medical-care system, which is distinct from social services in Britain. Originally, day hospitals provided an alternative to inpatient hospital care in the broadest sense. Cosin in 1954 described his day hospital as breaking "a vicious circle in poor inter-personal family relationships."[17] Most clients were referred to the day hospital after inpatient treatment so as to facilitate their return home. Cosin spends much time discussing the necessary psychosocial climate. As day hospitals were primarily to keep clients out of hospitals, they were more willing to provide whatever was necessary to do so; that is, emotional support and social activities could be justifiable in day hospitals.

There are several reasons why clients with emotional disorders were so numerous in the early operations of the day hospital. First, these clients would be the ones least likely to benefit from hospitalization and would benefit most by remaining in the community. Second, they could be maintained in the community at less cost than the physically frail. In early post-1948 years, geriatricians had little financial support. Geriatricians have slowly amassed resources, such as acute-hospital beds, assessment wards, and day units, and all the supporting staff required to operate them. Lastly, social and emotional problems often take much longer to rehabilitate than physical ailments.

Other events have helped to free geriatricians' resources for the more physically frail elderly. Since the opening of the first day hospital for the elderly in Britain, geriatricians have encouraged local authorities (social service departments) to open day centers. Day centers are on the increase, taking responsibility for emotional support and social activities once provided by day hospitals, much to the relief of geriatricians. Thus, geriatricians are able to concentrate their resources on the physically frail elderly. Thus, more and more frequently, the client enters a day hospital for the expressed purpose of receiving some form of physical rehabilitation. When rehabilitation is completed, the client is to progress to a social service or voluntary day center.

Farndale defined three main types of day hospitals after studying 38 psychiatric and 10 geriatric day hospitals open in 1960.

1. where continued medical treatment is provided, and clients attend regularly ("in-clients with sleeping-out passes")
2. where clients attend for two or three days a week for intensive occupational therapy and physiotherapy, but no social activities

3. where day care is offered with infrequent attendance, sometimes only once a week[11]

Two streams of clients were identified: short-stay and long-stay, the latter requiring primarily maintenance treatment.

Increasingly, leaders in geriatrics in Britain, such as Pathy and Millard, are convinced that day hospitals are serving two primary purposes, which are inherently in opposition with each other. "Long-stay clients get in the way of those needing short-term treatment and in addition, consider that their presence in the same unit is detrimental to the needs of both groups. The key to admission to the day hospital is physical ill-health, but many day hospital activities generate togetherness rather than individual independence. Under these circumstances it is not surprising that some clients lovingly referred to the 28-place day hospital in our previous study as 'our club.'"[18]

More and more examples can be seen where at least the two functions of short-term rehabilitation and long-term maintenance are separated. In some cases the geriatrician has established two or three day hospitals in an area, each with a different responsibility. Woodford-Williams and Alvarez stated that one-half of the persons attending day hospitals in their area could equally well have attended a day center. One-third had attended for more than two years. Alvarez now manages three types of day hospitals. The intensity of medical therapeutic and nursing care varies in each. One is intended for more short-term rehabilitative treatment, with less emphasis on nursing care and group activities. Dr. Pathy also has three day hospitals, ranging from a highly therapeutic orientation to a social and emotional supportive one where "diversional therapy" is the main activity.

Both geriatricians conclude that these divisions of function make better use of scarce resources—that is, money, professional staff, facilities, and transportation—and encourage smaller day hospitals. No one model of day-hospital care is thought to be adequate. The need for separate geriatric and psychogeriatric day hospitals has long been accepted. Geriatric day hospitals are increasingly specializing in either maintenance care or some form of rehabilitative treatment. Yet, geriatricians are still reaching on for the answers to such questions as:

1. What is the full potential of day hospitals?
2. How much is maintenance care the responsibility of the health service versus the social services?
3. What type of staff should be employed?
4. How could clients be rehabilitated more quickly?

Method of Funding

Funding of day hospitals has been consistent in Britain. There is no means test, so that every person who is registered with the NHS is eligible. Day hospitals are funded at 100% occupancy. The effect of this method of funding is varied, but entirely to the benefit of the client. First, once funded, the day hospital need not vie for funding in order to maintain in existence. Staff can therefore channel their time into improving the service and rallying for more staff, and little staff time is spent filling out forms for reimbursement.

Second, under this method of funding, clients are selected according to need rather than to fill in empty places. When demand is low, a rate per attendance tends to encourage long-stay maintenance rather than a short-term therapeutic approach to care. This method of funding, whereby funds are consistent, thus does not encourage inadequate admissions and prolonged maintenance, as does the per diem method.

The average cost per client day was found to be $20 (£9.57) excluding transportation, which was $6.50 (£3.20) in 1978. However, the range of costs varied across the United Kingdom from a low of $10 (£5.00) to a high of $30 (£15.32), excluding transportation.

Martin and Millard have calculated the cost of salaries in the southwest region of England by estimating the hours worked per week by day-hospital staff.[16] Using midpoint salary scales of 1976, the average cost per attender per day was $10.* The range was from $7 to $35. They also found an inverse relationship of salary costs to size. The average cost per place in terms of salary was $1550, which ranged from $800 at the largest unit to $3500 at an 18-place day hospital. Therefore, salary costs per year in a 30-place day hospital were roughly $24,000–$60,000 in 1976.*

Day-hospital treatment is not inexpensive, and these costs are in addition to the cost of the secondary health and social services and the cost of living at home.[19] Little evidence is available that day care and day-hospital care are cheaper than inpatient care, but they appear to be more cost-effective.

Pathy and Peach, in a study of 40 closely matched day clients in Cardiff, found day care to be cost-effective.[20] Costs for support services, such as Meals-on-Wheels, home helps, and community nursing were included. Similar clients improved more quickly in day care so that even if treatment cost more in the short run—that is, for clients attending a day hospital four to five days a week—an episode of illness cost less in the long run. However, more evidence needs to be gathered so that the costs and cost benefits can be calculated and a final conclusion reached.

Within a System

Day hospitals form an integral part of the system of care for the elderly in Britain, unlike day-care programs in the United States. Day hospitals are not an isolated service. Other services, such as day centers, home helps, and community nurses

---

*It should be noted that salaries are approximately 50% lower than in the United States.

Chapter 7: British Geriatric Day Hospitals: Implications for America / 191

play an active role in the admission and discharge of clients. Coordination and cooperation are facilitated by clear points of entry and exit (see Figure 7-1). It is essential that service be coordinated if the elderly are to be maintained in the community. The elderly person who attends a day hospital twice a week in Britain in most cases also receives other forms of support.[21]

Thus, a client who attends a day hospital on Monday and Wednesday receives Meals-on-Wheels the remaining three weekdays and perhaps home help on Friday. A communication network needs to be arranged.

Having a multidisciplinary team, as day hospitals do, facilitates communication. Links with other community services are established so that a client can be supported in the community and eventually be discharged from the day hospital. Figure 7-2 illustrates how a client moves from service to service as necessary. Without the links, the participant usually drops out and reappears in an acute ward when a crises occurs or is inappropriately maintained in one service. Because the geriatrician is in charge of the day-hospital long-stay wards and geriatric assessment wards, he is in a better position to coordinate health services and use resources effectively. Obviously, he is familiar with the options of care.

Client recruitment is not a problem as it is in day-care centers in the United States; 40%–50% of patients are referred to the day hospital upon discharge as inpatients.[13] Thus, administrators do not have to spend their time promoting the service and recruiting clients as they have to in the United States.

The existing organizational structures in Britain for health services and social services facilitates the development of new day-care services in several ways. New services can begin functioning more quickly. Facilities can often be shared so that initial expenditures are minimal. Administrative costs are contained as few Medicaid/Medicare-type forms need to be filled out. And, finally, points of entry and exit are easily identifiable in Britain's system of care.

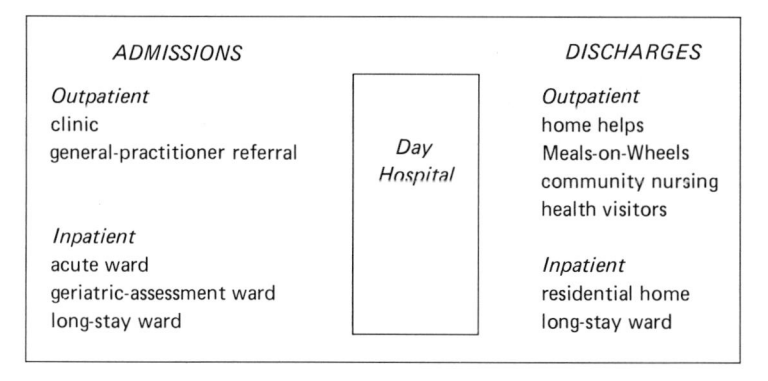

ADMISSIONS		DISCHARGES
Outpatient clinic general-practitioner referral	Day Hospital	*Outpatient* home helps Meals-on-Wheels community nursing health visitors
Inpatient acute ward geriatric-assessment ward long-stay ward		*Inpatient* residential home long-stay ward

Figure 7-1. Points of Entrance to and Exit from a Day Hospital

ADULT DAY CARE

Within a System — **Without a System**

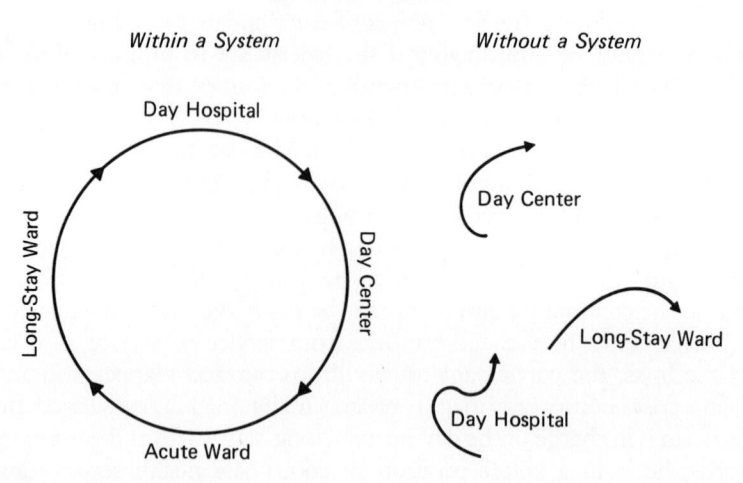

Figure 7-2. How a Day Hospital and a Day Center Appear Within a System and with No System

As Maddox concisely describes, in dealing with the complex, ever-changing needs of the elderly the absence of a comprehensive, coordinated system of care, the issue of community and home care as cost-effective remains unresolved.[22]

Summary

Day hospitals are a multidisciplinary service adapted to meet the complex needs of the elderly, whose health status can change easily and rapidly. The day hospital is not seen as the all-embracing day-care service, but rather as a medical model of day care. It can be provided in conjunction to institutional care prior to discharge or to the elderly in the community who are also receiving support from their family or from other support services, such as meals-on-wheels and home helps. It is the point at which hospital health services and community services meet.

The day hospital is an expensive service, which, if organized within a system of care, can be more efficient and effective. Its success in Britain hinges on the fact that it is not an isolated service.

The implication for the United States is that planning services for the elderly should begin at the national level so that an organizational structure for the development of day-care services can be designed. The method, consistency, and comprehensiveness of funding will affect not only the characteristics of the service but the direction in which the service will change over time.

In Britain, keeping the elderly in their own homes for as long as is safe and possible is a national policy.[23] Both the National Health Service and Local Authority Social Services are given the responsibility of helping the elderly remain independent. At times there is an overlap, but most see this as a system of checks and balances. The United States has such a system in its government, and now is the time that it extend such principles to the care of the elderly.

References

1. Carter J: *Day Services for Adults . . . From Where To Go.* London, George Allen and Unwin, 1981.

2. Office of Population Censuses and Surveys: *Population Projections.* London, Her Majesty's Stationery Office, 1976.

3. Peach H, Pathy MS: Evaluation of patients' assessment of day hospital care. *Brit J Prevent Soc Med* **31:** 209–210, 1977.

4. Bagnall MK: Day care and social needs. *Gerontologia Clinica* **16:** 253–257, 1974.

5. Peach H, Pathy MS: Evaluation of the day hospital in rehabilitation of the elderly. Unpublished.

6. Ministry of Health: A survey of services available to the chronic sick and elderly, 1954–1955. *Reports on Health and Medical Subjects*, Vol 98. London, Her Majesty's Stationery Office, 1957.

7. Brocklehurst JC: *The Geriatric Day Hospital.* London, King Edward's Hospital Fund, 1970.

8. Exton-Smith AN, Crocket GS: The chronic sick under new management. *Lancet* **1:** 116–118, 1949.

9. Department of Health and Social Security: *Hospital Geriatric Services.* DS329/71, Appendix B. London, 1971.

10. Department of Health and Social Security: *Services for Mental Illness Related to Old Age.* Memorandum accompanying HM 71. London, 1972.

11. Farndale J: *The Day Hospital Movement in Great Britain.* Oxford, England, Pergamon Press, 1961.

12. Brocklehurst JC, Tucker JS: *Progress in Day Care.* London, King Edward's Hospital Fund for London, 1980.

13. Pathy MS: Day hospitals for geriatric patients. *Lancet* **2:** 533–535, 1969.

14. Brocklehurst JC: *Geriatric Care in Advanced Societies.* Lancaster, England, MTP, 1975.

15. Woodford-Williams E, Alvarez AS: Four Years Experience of a Day Hospital in Geriatric Practice. *Gerontologia Clinica* **7:** 96–106, 1965.

16. Martin A, Millard, PH: The new patient index—A method of measuring activity of day hospitals. *Age and Aging* **4:** 114, 1975.

17. Cosin L: The place of the day hospital in the geriatric unit. *Practitioner* **172:** 552–559, 1954.

18. Martin A, Millard PH: Day hospitals for the elderly: Therapeutic or social. London, Geriatric Teaching and Research Unit, St. Georges' Hospital, 1978.

19. Ross DN: Geriatric day hospitals: Counting the cost compared with other methods of support. *Age and Aging* **5:** 171–175, 1976.

20. Pathy MS, Peach H: Cost-benefit study of a geriatric day hospital and in-patient ward. Unpublished.

21. ———: Social support of patients attending a geriatric day hospital. *Journal of Epidemiology and Community Health,* **32:** 33–37, 1978.

22. Maddox GL: The unrealised potential of an old idea, Exton-Smith AN, Evans JG (eds.): in *Care of the Elderly.* London, Academic Press, pp 147–161, 1977.

23. Department of Health and Social Security: *A Happier Old Age.* London, Her Majesty's Stationery Office, pp 215–218, 1978.

8

Community-Based Adult Day-Care Programs in Florida

Trudy B. White, MS

Introduction

Retirement to Florida where the sun shines and the weather is warm year round has become the trend for an ever-increasing number of older persons escaping from the long, cold winters in the North. This trend has established Florida as the only state in the United States in which the percentage of persons 65 and older has grown because of in-migration rather than because of out-migration of the young.[1]

This influx of older persons has swelled Florida's 65 and older population to approximately 1½ million persons or 16% of the total state population.[2] The tendency to relocate in particular areas in Florida has the elderly population in several counties approaching 40%.[2]

This influx of older persons into the state and their concentration in selected areas have caused a growing demand for social, economic, and medical services targeted at this group's specific problems and needs. The response has been the development of a variety of social-service programs, including that of adult day care.

Funding/Administration

At present, there are approximately 35 adult day-care programs operating in the state of Florida. They are funded and/or administered through a variety of means, including Title III, Title XX, and Community Care for the Elderly. All of these are funneled through Florida's Health and Rehabilitative Services Office and Area Agencies on Aging. Additional agencies providing support include the United Way, local citizen groups, city governments, the Jewish Community Centers, the Catholic Services Bureau, and others.

One source of funding that is fairly unique to the state of Florida is that of Community Care for the Elderly. In 1973, the Florida legislature passed the Community Care for the Elderly Act (CCE). The aim of the legislators was to prevent inappropriate institutionalization of the elderly in Florida by making provisions for community-support programs in the four areas of home-delivered services, multiservice senior centers, family placement, and adult day-care programs. In 1977, state general revenue funds were appropriated for seven demonstration projects throughout the state.

A recent state evaluation of these projects produced numerous positive results, of which the following three are but a few:

1. Even though CCE participants were frailer and poorer than the general elderly population in Florida, their rate of institutionalization was less than half that for the state's general elderly population.
2. Overall CCE participants improved in the physical, mental, and social dimensions of their lives. Particular gain was indicated in social adjustment.
3. Financially, these CCE participants who were maintained in the community instead of being institutionalized saved the state approximately $1000 per year per person.

In 1979, because of the success of these model projects, additional CCE funding was channeled into Florida communities for further development of CCE projects.

Fees

Because of extensive state and federal funding, Florida's adult day-care programs generally operate free of charge to the participants. Donations are accepted and encouraged and are funneled back into the programs through various means. However, appropriate adult day-care clients are not required to pay for services received.

Licenses

Prior to 1980 Florida had no comprehensive statewide guidelines or standards for the operation of all adult day-care programs serving the elderly. The various funding sources were mainly responsible for setting parameters within which programs functioned. Within those limitations, each program was free to select facilities, hire staff, and design activities and services based on the needs of the persons within the program's geographic service area.

This past year Florida's Health and Rehabilitative Services Office instituted licensing procedures for all adult day-care programs. The growth in the number of programs within the state has necessitated this step in order to assure program quality. To obtain a license to operate, each program must conform to prescribed regulations addressing services, facilities, and staffing.

Models and Goals

A variety of adult day-care models have evolved in Florida, including a social/recreational model, in which emphasis is placed on group interaction and socialization among clients; a medical model, in which the focus is on health and the medical restoration of the clients; and a mental-health model, in which emphasis is on the use of treatment and therapy to maintain or restore proper mental functioning. The majority of the Florida adult day-care programs are predominantly patterned on a social/recreational model, although all programs include elements of each model.

The following goals of adult day-care programs reflect this mix of concern for the mental and physical well-being of older persons:

1. to delay or prevent institutionalization of the elderly by providing an alternative
2. to prevent loneliness, isolation, and withdrawal of older persons
3. to eliminate the monotony of daily existence by returning a participant to productive activity and involvement
4. to improve the quality of life for the participant
5. to improve the participant's self-image

All adult day-care programs, regardless of individual emphasis, seek to provide a protective environment in which older persons receive preventative, remedial, and restorative services.

Participants

Florida's adult day-care centers predominantly cater to the frail elderly—those with physical handicaps due to a range of diseases such as strokes, Parkinson's disease, heart conditions, and the like, and those suffering from mild to moderate mental confusion.

Participants range in age from 60 years to as old as 100 years, with the average age being approximately 75. Participants in programs who are 75 years and older range from 45% to 90%, with the majority of the programs operating with approximately the same number below and above 75 years of age. The number of females in the programs ranges from approximately 50% to as high as 90%. However, most of the programs have approximately 60% females and 40% males.

Adult day-care participants are a part of a variety of living arrangements. By far the majority make their homes in some type of family situation with relatives or friends, as would be expected since Florida adult day centers are attempting to help maintain older persons in their family environments. Generally only a small number live alone or in group-living facilities.

The number of days that a participant attends a program ranges from one to five. However, the large majority accepted into programs are assigned to an average of three days each week, with many attending all five days. With the well-established adult day-care centers, waiting lists reflect the tremendous growth in need for these programs. Older persons and their families often have to wait several weeks before space is available. The average number of participant spaces is 30–35.

Facilities

Adult day-care programs are housed under a variety of roofs. Programs are functioning in facilities that are part of senior centers, nursing homes, and service organizations. Programs are also operating out of all types of separate physical facilities, including store fronts and churches.

Most programs have one large room that will accommodate all the participants for large group activities. Many of these programs also have smaller rooms, which are necessary for some of the therapy activities and private sessions.

Staffing

The majority of the adult day-care centers operate with two to four professional staff members who have college degrees and who serve in positions such as director/coordinator, social worker, nurse/licensed practical nurse, or activity coordinator. These persons plan and implement the program's activities and services.

Adult day-care centers also rely heavily on two other groups of persons. Nearly all programs have paid aides with high-school degrees. These persons provide the daily assistance required by day-care participants and help to implement many of the planned activities. Volunteers are another extremely valuable group in many programs. The extent to which volunteers are used appears to vary with the ability of the program to pay aides and the philosophy of the director/coordinator. Some adult day-care centers use a minimum number of volunteers, preferring to depend on paid staff. Many other programs utilize as many as 10 to 14 regular volunteers, feeling these persons' abilities and enthusiasm are vital to the program. In addition to professional staff, aides, and volunteers, a few programs have secretarial and transportation employees.

Provisions for in-service training for these staff members are made by each individual adult day-care program. Time invested in formal training sessions ranges from utilizing portions of monthly staff meetings, to planned seminars occurring several times per year, to attendance at regional and national conventions. The needs of individual programs determine topics, and presenters include staff members and professionals from the community.

Participant Assessment

Most of the adult day-care programs use similar assessment procedures. After receiving a referral from an agency or an inquiry phone call from a family, the social worker or coordinator will schedule a home visit with the prospective participant and family. During this visit, assessment/intake forms designed by the individual programs are used to gather information concerning the participant and family, and program requirements are discussed. Assessing the potential participant in the home is important for several reasons:

1. The participant and family are more likely to be at ease and thus provide more complete information.
2. It allows the social worker to assess disabilities and to evaluate more accurately how well the potential participant actually functions.
3. It allows the social worker an opportunity to assess more closely the participant family environment and interaction. This point is particularly important since many adult day-care participants come from family situations that are stressful to both the elderly individual and the family members.

Criteria for acceptance vary widely, but, in general, most programs will not accept participants who are

1. less than 60 years of age
2. totally disoriented and in need or constant watching by a staff member
3. potentially harmful to other participants
4. incontinent
5. living in a nursing home
6. capable of performing activities of daily living without aid

Most adult day-care centers will take individuals living alone. This type of support can help these persons maintain their independence within the community. A few accept participants who are incontinent and highly disoriented. Program facilities and philosophy are often the determining factors with this issue.

Direct Program Services

Transportation

Transportation, which is one of adult day care's most vital services, is also one of the most troublesome. In many programs, families must be relied upon to provide this important link with the program by arranging their schedules for delivering and picking up the elderly participants. Many programs accommodate the working family by opening prior to 8 A.M. and closing after 5 P.M.

A large number of appropriate participants live in circumstances that simply are void of any consistent sources for transportation. Some programs have been able to afford their own van and driver, thus creating reliable and steady transportation because of the program's control of scheduling. But, even at best, program-provided transportation is generally very limited because of such factors as small capacity of vans, time consumed in traveling within the geographic area served, and the time required to load and unload frail elderly.

For program-provided transportation, many adult day-care centers must depend on arrangements with outside transportation agencies. These sources often do not provide the consistent and caring service that is necessary for the transportation of the participants.

Nutrition

The noon meal is an important part of all adult day-care programs. The majority participate in the nutrition program provided through Title III-C of the Older Americans Act. Participants on special diets eat what is allowable from the regular lunch or they bring their own meal. Snacks are available in most programs, often provided through donations.

Social, Recreational, and Educational Activities

Social, recreational, and educational activities compose the bulk of the daily programming provided for adult day-care participants. With the goals of adult day-care programs as a basis, the aim of these activity programs is innovation within a structured environment. All the centers plan a variety of activities, including arts and crafts, music, exercises, movies, current events, discussions, health talks, information sharing, community-awareness groups, bingo, plant and gardening groups, outings, parties, games, dancing, and much more.

Therapy Activities

Only a small number of the programs are involved in extensive therapeutic activities, since the majority are essentially social/recreational models. However, several programs are utilizing reality-orientation and remotivation sessions with their confused participants. Others provide occupational therapists to augment arts and crafts programs and music therapists to implement musical activities.

Social Services and Counseling

All adult day-care centers provide individual participant counseling, basically on an "as needed" schedule. In some programs, participant group counseling and family counseling are available. When appropriate, as it often is, participants or families are provided with information about services that are available through other community agencies. When necessary, program staff actively aid participants in obtaining needed services.

Medical and Health Services

In general, medical services in adult day-care programs are fairly limited in scope. All programs require some type of a medical form describing a participant's state of health, and the majority have a nurse on staff and take responsibility for dispensing medications during the day. Within the parameters of present program activities and services, emphasis is on social and mental stimulation and not on directly serving a client's medical needs. Many programs provide health counseling for participants, alert families to health problems noticed by staff, and suggest potential medical resources.

Indirect Services

Through special arrangements, many programs have easy access to a number of services that are not provided by staff and that are not a typical and regular part of an adult day-care program. These services reach out from the program and link participants to services outside typical social-service agencies. These services are often available on a reduced-fee or no-fee basis. Participants with a variety of health problems are being referred to health-care clinics, or appointments are being made with medical doctors, dentists, ophthalmologists, and psychiatrists. Participants who need a lawyer are being referred to legal-aid services. When appropriate, participants have direct access to home health care and companion and homemaker chore services. Programs tend to use these indirect services sparingly, trying to reserve their use for those persons who have no resources of their own upon which to rely.

Summary

Florida adult day-care programs are still young. Most have been operating only a few years. They are evolving, changing, and striving to fill this important area of need that exists on a comprehensive continuum of health-care services for the elderly.

References

1. The elderly in America. *Population Bulletin*, vol 30, no 3. Wash DC, Population Reference Bureau, Inc., 1975.

2. Osterind CC: *Older People in Florida: A Statistical Abstract*. Gainsville, Florida, University of Florida, Center for Gerontological Studies and Programs, 1976.

9

Funding

Carole Lium O'Brien, RN, MS
Sarah J. Schiermeyer, RN

Introduction

The present regular funding sources used for adult day care are Titles XIX and XX of the Social Security Act and Title III of the Older Americans Act. Of the almost 300 programs listed in the May 1978 edition of the Directory of Adult Day Care Centers, 64 use Title XIX (Medicaid) for reimbursement for health care; 135 use Title XX for reimbursement for social services; and 63 Title III funds (see Figure 9-1). Also used, but less often, are Title XVIII (Medicare) of the Social Security Act, Titles IV, V, VII of the Older Americans Act, and Revenue Sharing. Additional funding from nongovernment sources is received by 166 programs. These sources are usually philanthropic, although increasingly, private insurance companies are calling adult day care a covered benefit and paying all or part of the cost.[1(pp1-5)] Table 9-1 gives a further breakdown of federal funding distribution for adult day-care programs by state.

Each of the government sources is limited by the kind of service it will cover, the amount of funds available for coverage, and eligibility requirements. Adult day-care programs therefore will frequently seek reimbursement from more than one government source. This process entails enormous amounts of paper work and an intimacy with government regulations, and, despite substantial govern-

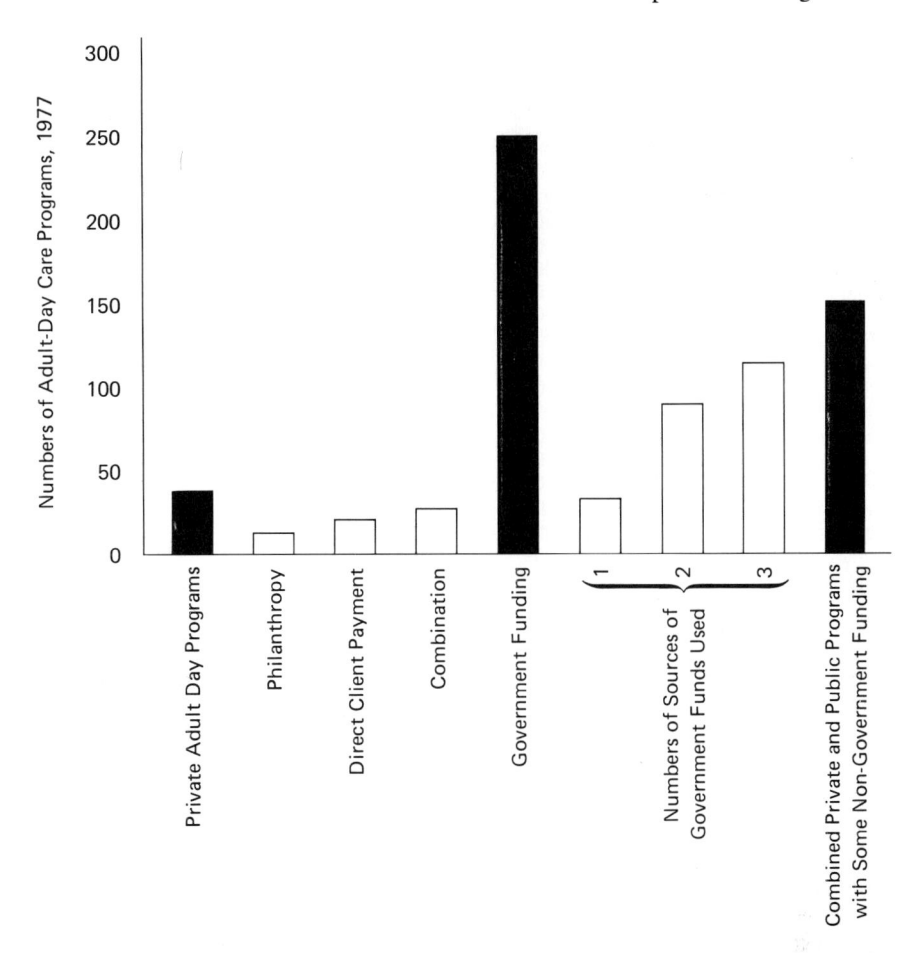

Figure 9-1. Funding Distribution of Adult Day-Care Programs, 1977 (Data from *Directory of Adult Day Care Centers*, by HEW Health Standards and Quality Bureau. Rockville, Md, US Government Printing Office, 1978.)

ment support, some centers have been threatened with closing because of insufficient funding.

In recent months, the *NEWS*, the newsletter of The Greater Boston Health Planning Council, has kept readers abreast of crucial health-planning budget deliberations in Washington. Whereas the outcome of this continuing debate most directly affects the future of the health-planning agencies, many other proposed funding changes will also have major impact on the people and programs with which we have worked closely in recent years. One of the most important of these funding changes is the "block grant" proposal.

Table 9-1
Department of Health, Education and Welfare grant funds, Program for Aging, fiscal year 1978

State	Nutrition Project	Title III Model Project	Title V Senior Centers
Alabama	$ 4,057,000	$ 45,000	$ 644,000
Alaska	1,238,000	18,000	200,000
Arkansas	2,423,000	476,000	392,000
California	21,999,000	2,831,000	3,645,000
Colorado	2,266,000	150,000	366,000
Connecticut	3,469,000	599,000	561,000
Delaware	1,238,000	25,000	200,000
District of Columbia	1,260,000	2,457,000	200,000
Florida	13,279	497,000	2,146,000
Georgia	4,684,000	18,000	744,000
Hawaii	1,260,000	154,000	—
Idaho	1,260,000	56,000	200,000
Illinois	12,153,000	855,000	1,964,000
Indiana	5,521,000	18,000	892,000
Iowa	3,688,000	185,000	586,000
Kansas	2,911,000	126,000	462,000
Kentucky	3,792,000	140,000	613,000
Louisiana	3,717,000	42,000	590,000
Maine	1,283,000	134,000	207,000
Maryland	3,748,000	158,000	606,000
Massachusetts	7,044,000	685,000	1,118,000
Michigan	8,848,000	319,000	1,405,000
Minnesota	4,434,000	85,000	717,000
Mississippi	2,624,000	18,000	417,000
Missouri	5,997,000	45,000	969,000
Montana	1,260,000	18,000	200,000
Nebraska	1,917,000	51,000	310,000
Nevada	1,260,000	141,000	300,000
New Hampshire	1,260,000	32,000	200,000
New Jersey	8,275,000	135,000	1,337,000
New Mexico	1,260,000	138,000	200,000
New York	21,731,000	1,590,000	200,000
North Carolina	5,374,000	45,000	868,000
North Dakota	1,238,000	44,000	200,000
Ohio	11,202,000	380,000	1,811,000
Oklahoma	3,449,000	132,000	548
Oregon	2,741,000	324,000	443,000
Pennsylvania	14,903,000	754,000	2,366,000
Rhode Island	1,238,000	80,000	200,000
South Carolina	2,580,000	18,000	410,000
South Dakota	1,260,000	127,000	200,000
Tennessee	4,712,000	195,000	748,000
Texas	12,384,000	180,000	1,977,000
Utah	1,248,000	41,000	200,000
Vermont	1,238,000	45,000	200,000
Virginia	4,755,000	45,000	755,000
Washington	3,875,000	32,000	616,000
West Virginia	2,271,000	18,000	360,000
Wisconsin	5,379,000	121,000	854,000
Wyoming	1,238,000	27,000	200,000

Data from *Geographic Distribution of Federal Funds in Summary*, Fiscal Year 1978, by Community Services Administration, US Government Printing Office.

The idea of the "block grant" proposal is to take almost all health and social-service programs, which up to now have been funded categorically and administered federally, and lump them into a few huge funding blocks to be administered by the states. Health and Human Services Secretary Richard Schweiker was recently quoted in *U.S. News and World Report* as saying that the Reagan team believes the block grants will "save $73 million in overhead costs . . . and give the states flexibility in allocating their resources."[2] Twenty-three health programs would be consolidated into two basic block grants, "health services" and "preventive health," budgeted at $1.1 billion and $260 million respectively. These figures are calculated to be 25% below current funding levels for the categorical programs.

The *services* block includes community health centers, black-lung clinics, migrant-health programs, home health services, maternal- and child-health services, hemophiliac services, sudden-infant-death-syndrome monitoring and research programs, emergency medical services, mental-health services, and alcohol- and drug-abuse programs. The *preventive* block consolidates family-planning clinics, genetic-diseases programs, health-incentive grants, risk-reduction education, health education, venereal-diseases prevention, immunization, fluoridation, adolescent health services, rat control, lead-based-paint poisoning programs, and environmental-hazards-control programs, and is responsible for approving or denying grant applications for many of these programs. As yet, there is no clear answer as to just which state agency would assume this function and the difficult task of ensuring that the monies are distributed fairly and spent properly.

One group adamantly opposed to the new concept is the National Association of Community Health Centers, which claims that the block grants would increase administrative overhead and bureaucracy within the states; eliminate the flexibility to respond to change on the national level; and eliminate meaningful oversight for program effectiveness and management.

Secretary Schweiker has said that, before spending any money, the states will have to publish a spending plan. At the end of the year, they will also have to publish a spending report, which will be audited independently. The audit will be overseen by the General Accounting Office and the inspector general will have the authority to investigate violations.[3]

In order for this new concept to become a reality, Congress must agree to it, and legislation authorizing the old categorical grant approach must be repealed. Under this approach, adult day care would be vulnerable to being overlooked and underfunded.

Federal support has helped adult day care to flourish as well as it has. Prior to 1973, when government support was in its infancy, there were fewer than 15 adult day-care programs in the United States.[1(p1)]

The following section discusses briefly each of the funding mechanisms mentioned. Emphasis is on covered services, eligibility, and congressional appropriations. Efforts have not been made to highlight inclusions and exclusions that apply to American Indians and residents of American protectorates. These areas of concern are specialized and are felt to be better dealt with elsewhere.

Government Funding Sources

Social Security Act

Title XVIII—Medicare. Medicare, signed into law in 1965, established a national program of hospital and medical insurance. It became and has remained the major source of security against the financial ravages of major illness for the majority of aged individuals over 65 in this country. Eligibility is extended to most members of the work force, and to some spouses upon turning 65; to certain disabled persons; and to those with terminal renal disease.

Payment under Part A of the Title will be made for

> inpatient hospital services for up to 150 days during any spell of illness minus one day for each day of inpatient hospital services in excess of 90 received during and proceeding spell of illness . . . ; post-hospital extended care services for up to 100 days during any spell of illness; and post-hospital home health services for up to 100 visits . . . after the beginning of one spell of illness and before the beginning of the next.[4(p407)]

Both skilled-nursing care and rehabilitation potential are required for eligibility for post hospital benefits. In addition, speech, physical, and occupational therapies are covered benefits under this requirement and can be provided in an adult day-care program, provided the services are given by licensed therapists.

The time limits and rehabilitation potential requirements have restricted the usefullness of this title for adult day-care-center reimbursement. However, in the fall of 1979, DHEW issued a grant to On Lok Senior Health Services for a comprehensive-use study in San Francisco, California. It will allow payment, under Medicare, for all medical and social services in an attempt to avoid crisis situations that could lead to premature hospitalization. If the study shows this use to be cost-benefit effective, Medicare coverage could possibly be extended to all adult day-care-center participants who qualify for Medicare.

Title XIX—Medicaid. The purpose of Title XIX is

> to enable each state as far as practicable under the conditions of such state to furnish (1) medical assistance on behalf of families with dependent children and of *aged, blind* or *disabled* individuals whose incomes and resources are insufficient to meet the cost of necessary medical services and (2) rehabilitation and other services to help such families and individuals attain or retain capability for independence or self-care.[4(p507)]

These services include care for almost all health-related problems and are unrestricted by time limits. They can thus be used for the provision of long-term-maintenance care and other forms of tertiary intervention.

Under this title, reimbursement for services, which are allowed in the State Medicaid program can be used to provide day care services.[5(pII-6)]

In health model programs ... medicaid reimbursement may be available [for medical, nursing, and social activities, rehabilitative and occupational therapies]. In social model programs, reimbursement may not be possible for the full complement of services; however, some health services for individuals can be reimbursed as individual medical services.[5(pII-7)]

Medicaid is a grant-in-aid program in which the state and federal governments share the costs of the program. By law, the federal portion may not be less than 50% nor more than 83% of the total expended. The state per centum is computed by the following formula:

$$\frac{(\text{state per capita income})^2}{0.45 \times (\text{national per capita income})^2}$$

The programs are administered by the states, and, therefore, there are essentially 50 Medicaid programs. The states are subject to broad federal standards and guidelines, but set their own reimbursement rates and some benefit and eligibility standards.

At present, reimbursement levels are generally considered unsatisfactory. Initially, in Massachusetts, for example, reimbursement for 1977 was set at $13 per day per participant, with no allowance for transportation, yet program costs ran from $17 to $22 per day. Currently, the rate is $13 per day, with additional money paying for transportation. A greater insufficiency is that reimbursement is made only for days attended, and yet the program must function at the same level, and overhead costs remain the same, whatever the census. Unanticipated absences are frequent because of the state of health of the participants and the variable reliability of transportation.[6]

The states and the federal government are looking for ways to lower expenditures and/or provide more cost-effectiveness and have therefore made a number of cost-analysis studies of adult day-care programs. The Levindale "Geriatric Day Care Center Research and Demonstration Project"[7] is an example of such a study.

AB1611—Medi-Cal. Significantly, after conducting several cost-effectiveness evaluations on demonstration programs, California passed landmark legislation specifying adult day care as a covered benefit under Medi-Cal (California Medicaid) and providing for its expansion, licensing, evaluation, and coordination. This legislation removes adult day care from the category "experimental" and ensures long-term funding and support. The initial appropriation (1977) for this legislation, Assembly Bill 1611, was $1,000,000, to be allocated for matching federal funds and used for adult day-care services and administrative costs.

California's definition of adult day care is in agreement with that of the authors:

> "Adult day health care" means an organized day program of therapeutic, social, and health activities and services provided pursuant to this chapter to elderly persons

with functional impairments, either physical or mental, for the purpose of restoring or maintaining optimal capacity for self-care. Provided on a short-term basis, adult day health care serves as a transition from a health facility or home health program to personal independence. Provided on a long-term basis, it serves as an option to institutionalization in long-term care facilities, when 24-hour skilled nursing care is not medically necessary or viewed as desirable by the recipient or his family.[8(p3)]

Further, the bill states succinctly what is hoped will be accomplished by its passage:

a) Assure that elderly persons are not institutionalized inappropriately or prematurely.
b) Provide a viable alternative to institutionalization for those older impaired persons who are capable of living at home with the aid of appropriate health care or rehabilitative and social services.
c) Establish adult day health centers in the community for such purpose, which will be easily accessible to all participants, including the economically disadvantaged older person, and which will provide outpatient health, rehabilitative, and social services necessary to permit the participants to maintain personal independence and lead meaningful lives.
d) Include the services of adult day health centers as a benefit under the Medi-Cal Act, which shall be an initial and integral part in the development of an overall plan for a coordinated, comprehensive continuum of optional long-term care services based upon appropriate need.[8(pp2-3)]

These outcomes correspond to outcomes believed by the authors to be appropriate to adult day-care services.

Additional provisions of the bill that merit comment are

1. Any facility that provides a specialized outpatient program of both medical and nonmedical services to the elderly must be licensed under adult day-care provisions and restrictions.
2. Adult day-care planning councils, at the county level, are to be established in counties that have adult day-care facilities, and the plans to be developed by these councils must be in accordance with guidelines established by the state adult day-care review committee.
3. All decision-making bodies substantially represent the elderly in their membership.
4. As of December 1, 1978, a uniform method of evaluation was adopted by the state for use at all licensed adult day-care centers. It seeks to measure
   a. compliance with regulations adopted pursuant to this chapter
   b. continued demonstrated community need
   c. conformity of the program to individual participants' assessed and reassessed needs and interests, with particular attention to visual, auditory, and equipment needs

d. suitability of program changes to the community and participants served
e. compliance with requirements of law pertaining to fire and life and safety[9(p9)]

Assembly Bill 1611 defines and reinforces the adult day-care concept as a legitimate and useful long-term-care option. It has not been possible, before this, to establish a sufficient number of adult day-care centers from which to gather the data needed to determine the full impact of adult day care on care of the elderly. The accumulation of this data could, in turn, influence the establishment of adult day care as a benefit under Medicare.

Title XX—grants to states for services. Title XX was enacted and funds appropriated

> for the purpose of encouraging each state, as far as practicable under the conditions in that state, to furnish services directed at the goal of
> 1) achieving or maintaining economic self-support to prevent, reduce, or eliminate dependency.
> 2) achieving or maintaining self-sufficiency, including reduction or prevention of dependency.
> 3) preventing or remedying neglect, abuse, or exploitation of children and adults unable to protect their own interests, or preserving, rehabilitating, or reuniting families.
> 4) preventing or reducing inappropriate institutional care by providing for community-based care, home-based care, or other forms of less intensive care, or
> 5) securing referral or admission for institutional care when other forms of care are not appropriate, or providing services to individuals in institutions.[4(p541)]

The covered services that are applicable to adult day care and satisfy the stated goals include, but are not limited to, day care for adults, transportation, food preparation and delivery, information, referral counseling, health support, and combinations of these as necessary to meet the special needs of the aged. Planning, administration, evaluation, and personnel training and retraining can also be financed under Title XX.

> FFP (Federal Matching) is not available for medical care, other than family planning services, except when it is an integral but subordinate part of a service described in the service plan and the medical care is not available to the individual under a state's approved Title XIX plan and to the extent the individual or provider is not eligible to receive payment under Title XVIII for the provision of service to the individual.[4(p40)]

Because of these restrictions, Title XX funds are used primarily for social programs.

Eligibility standards are set by both the federal and state governments. Federal regulations require that 50% of the funds must be used to provide services to individuals who are eligible for, or are recipients of, supplemental security income benefits under Title XVI. Payment may not be made for services to persons whose income exceeds 115% of the median income of a family of four in the state, and a fee must be charged, reasonably related to income, if income exceeds either 80% of the median income of a family of four in the state or the median income of a family of four in the nation, or when the size of the family exceeds four and adjustments for size indicate gross income to be below 115% and above 80% of the median income of a family of four in the state. There are no residency or citizenship requirements.

Federal expenditures, as they apply under this title to adult day-care programs are equal to 75% of the total cost of the program. "The appropriation is limited to $2,500,000,000 for each fiscal year after fiscal year 1979."[4(p542)] Beyond the state's allotment, the state is responsible for 100% of the costs of maintaining the programs. For the fiscal year ending September 30, 1979, Congress amended the limitation to be 107.407% of the appropriation. Prior to that, Congress had augmented the appropriation by 106.4% for fiscal year 1976 and 108% for fiscal years 1977 and 1978. The appropriation for 1979 was $2,700,000,000; thus, the 1980 appropriation represents a significant drop, in actual dollars and in spending power. This drop will require increased state expenditures to maintain existing programs. New startups and expansions will be evaluated very carefully by states that are seeking ways to cut state expenditures.

Older Americans Act

Title III—grants for state and community programs on aging.

> Title III authorizes the making of grants . . . for paying part or all of the cost of developing or operating statewide, regional, metropolitan area, county, city or community model projects which will expand or improve social services or otherwise promote the well-being of older persons.[9(p32)]

Areas of concern are housing, education, retirement planning, and special needs of physically or mentally impaired elders, such as special transportation, escort service, homemaker, home-health and shopping services, reader services, and letter-writing services. Emphasis is placed on the need to provide these services especially to those not provided for under other provisions of the Older Americans Act, as amended, such as low-income, limited-English-speaking, and rural elderly.

Title III specifically directs that the funds be used to assist the elderly to remain independent by

> providing financial assistance for the establishment and operation of senior ambulatory care day centers (providing a planned schedule of health, therapeutic, educational, nutritional, recreational and social services at least 24 hours per week, transportation arrangements at low or no cost to the participants to and from the center,

a hot midday meal, outreach and public information programs, and opportunities for maximum participation of senior participants and senior volunteers in the planning and operation of such centers).[9(p33)]

Title III further directs that the programs should be provided within the community in which the participants live. Accessibility is stressed. The reimbursement is primarily for social services defined in the title as follows:

1) health, continuing education, welfare, informational, recreational, homemaker, counseling or referral services;
2) transportation services where necessary to facilitate access to social services;
3) services designed to encourage and assist older Americans to use the facilities and services available to them;
4) services designed to assist older persons to obtain adequate housing;
5) services designed to assist older persons in avoiding institutionalization, including preinstitutional evaluation and screening, and home health services;
6) services designed to provide legal and other counseling services and assistance, including tax counseling and services and assistances, and financial counseling to older persons;
7) services designed to enable older persons to attain and maintain physical and mental well-being through programs of regular physical activity and exercise; or
8) any other services if such services are necessary for the general welfare of older persons.[9(pp15-16)]

During fiscal year 1974, state agencies were awarded $12,000,000 to conduct statewide model projects efforts. This was reduced in fiscal year 1975 to $5,000,000, supporting 40 projects.

$$\text{allotment} = \text{appropriation} \times \frac{\text{state population 60 and over}}{\text{national population 60 and over}}$$

An example of a Title III grant proposal for an adult day center is shown in Figure 9-2.

Title IV-B—research and demonstration projects. The Title IV research and demonstration program is designed to meet the special needs of, and to improve ways of solving the various problems of, the older adult. Congress has directed the administration to focus on better ways to help the elderly return to, or remain in, their own homes or other appropriate settings. Congress has also directed that priority be given to solutions to the mobility and transportation problems of older persons. The research and demonstration program further supports methods of improving the delivery of services to the older adult as well as encouraging the development of social gerontology in order to gain new insights into the needs, circumstances, resources, expectations, and roles of the nation's older population.

GRANT PROPOSAL

1. *Brief Background of Your Agency and Experience in Serving the Older Person, Which Indicates Your Ability to Attain the Proposed Project's Goal and Objective.*

   The Adult Day Health Center opened December 19, 1978 with one participant from Waltham attending two days weekly. On November 15, 1979 the Center had an average daily attendance of sixteen participants with two pending admission in November, and another five awaiting admission when space permits. The Center's space limits the participation in the program to eighteen participants daily at the present time.

   The participants range in age from fifty-one to eighty-six years with the average age at seventy-five. Twenty-nine of the thirty participants now participating in the program reside in communities served by Suburban Elder Services. The youngest participant is under sixty years of age. Each participant has one or more disabling physical and/or mental conditions which restrict his/her ability to utilize other community facilities serving the elderly. Eighty percent of the participants are recipients of medical assistance from the Department of Public Welfare.

   In the eleven months the Center has been operating, fifty-one older persons have been served by the Center. A total of 328 service days had been provided as of October 31, 1979. The rapid growth in participation in the Center's program, as well as the improvement observed in the participants by family members and staff, and the results of the Systematic Functional Assessment Tool, clearly indicate that the Center's program is meeting its objectives and goal.

2. *Statement of Project Goal*

   The Adult Day Health Center will provide preventive, maintenance, and therapeutic rehabilitative services to those physically and mentally disabled, low income, and minority adults sixteen years or older with particular emphasis on those sixty years and older living in the West Suburban Elder Services area.

3. *Statement of Project Objectives*

   The Adult Day Health Center program will:

   1. Prevent premature institutionalization in fifty percent of the participant population.
   2. Decrease the incidence of social isolation for one hundred percent of the participant population.
   3. Provide an environment which stimulates peer interaction for one hundred percent of the participant population.
   4. Promote health maintenance practices through an on-going health education program for one hundred percent of the participant population.
   5. Decrease the severity of physical disability in seventy percent of the participant population.
   6. Increase the participants' ability in activities of daily living in forty-five percent of the participant population.
   7. Assist families caring for a disabled participant in sixty percent of the participant population.
   8. Ease transition from community living to nursing home residence in twenty-five percent of the participant population.

Figure 9-2. Example of a Title III Grant Proposal for an Adult Day-Care Center (From Proposal submitted for a project grant under Title III of the Older Americans Act, by C O'Brien and G Dix. Newton, Mass., Nov., 1979.)

The Center's program, operating from December 1978 to November 15, 1979, has met the objectives as stated. Of the Center's present population, seventeen participants are being maintained in the community who would otherwise be in nursing homes, or be awaiting placement in a nursing home (objective 1). All participants are prevented from being socially isolated by their participation in the program and the program provides opportunities for peer interaction to all (objectives 2 + 3). Participants and their families, when applicable, are given health information by the professional nurse and licensed practical nurse through a planned educational, on-going health maintenance program (objective 4). Physical limitations have been decreased in twenty-two of the thirty persons participating in the program and twelve persons have increased their abilities to function independently (objectives 5 + 6). Nineteen participants are presently living with family members and/or relatives (objective 7). The staff provides continuous consultation and assistance to these families and relatives with referrals. Of the fifty-one participants who have participated in the program to date, twelve have been discharged to nursing home care. These twelve participants and their families were significantly helped in accepting a change in residency (objective 8).

A unit of service the Center provides is determined to be a six- to eight-hour day of participation by one participant. Therefore, at the present time, the Center provides sixteen to eighteen units of service five days weekly excluding weekends and legal holidays.

4. *Statement of Project Need*

In the eight towns served by the Suburban Elder Services, statistics show that the sixty-years-and-over population is either stabilized or on the increase. Clearly, the population of older persons is on the rise and this increase is seen in the more "at risk" frail elderly population most in need of day health services if they are to be maintained in the community.

The Adult Day Health Center was planned and implemented to reach this "at risk" group of elderly people in the community. This group includes the following:

1. The elderly infirmed and disabled person in need of a therapeutic program of social and/or physical rehabilitation, dietary services, recreation, and other restorative services.
2. Those elderly on waiting lists for admission to nursing homes.
3. Those elderly persons who no longer can be maintained solely by family members at home because of their increased need for health, psychological, and social services.

To date fifty-one persons have been served at the program. All of these persons, excluding a fifty-one year-old man, are over sixty years of age. Currently the program services eighteen to twenty persons a day. Documentation for further expansion and the evidence of unmet needs of the elderly are seen by the following:

1. An existing waiting list.
2. The receipt of one to three applications weekly.
3. The phone inquiries of ten to twenty persons a month regarding future placement possibilities.

Figure 9-2. *(continued)*

5. *How the Objectives Will Be Met*

The Adult Day Health Center will service older persons living in the Suburban Elder Services area. In providing a day health program from 8:00 A.M. to 4:00 P.M. daily, five days weekly, the center will offer all the services needed to meet the proposed objectives. In addition, the program will maintain community liaison with other organizations and agencies directly related to servicing the same target population. To date, the Adult Day Health Center has coordinated its services with the V.N.A.'s, the Community Health Center, the local hospital's Mental Health Units, the Human Services Department, and the Councils on Aging, to mention a few examples. These coordinating efforts assist the participants and their families in utilizing these agencies for meeting their financial, social, educational, and medical needs.

The objectives will be met further by a projected plan for expansion to twenty-four participants per day with a target date of February 1980 for implementation. With the expansion will be an increase in the staff to include a social worker and a program assistant.

Currently, the Center's staffing pattern includes the following:

Program Director: A registered nurse (with an M.S. in Nursing) experienced in rehabilitation and administration functions as the full-time program director. The Director has at least three years' experience in the field of gerontology and community health nursing. This individual assumes responsibility for coordination of all services offered at the Center and for supervision of staff and integration of staff activities in meeting program objectives.

The Director does all the initial interviewing with the client and his/her family. After conferring with the other team members as to appropriateness of placement in the Day Health Center, the R.N. conducts a second interview for the purpose of collecting a health history and doing an admission assessment.

The rehabilitation services for each patient are set out in writing by the patient's physician. The Director, together with the other team members, then develops the treatment plan for each participant. The Director is responsible for supervising the staff in carrying out the plan.

During the week the Director is involved with planning, public relations, inservice training and other staff and program functions. The number of hours devoted to these areas may fluctuate from week to week, but it is about six to eight hours per week.

Activities Director: An activities director develops and implements a therapeutic activity program in coordination with the occupational therapist to meet the individual needs of each participant. This full-time position requires previous experience in a social or recreation program designed for older persons.

Licensed Practical Nurse: A licensed practical nurse functions as the full-time nurse under the direction of the program director and has the ability in meeting the health needs of the elderly population.

Figure 9-2. *(continued)*

Social Worker: A social worker with a minimum Bachelor's Degree in behavioral or social sciences will be hired to function as the full-time social worker and assistant program director. The social worker will coordinate and implement individual, group, and family counseling as well as inform participants and their families of community services, make referrals, and serve as the Center's community liaison person.

Program Assistant: A program assistant with previous experience in working with the elderly will be hired to function as a full-time assistant to the professional staff. The assistant will assist with the preparation of activities, assist with individual and group projects, perform secretarial and clerical duties for the program director, accompany the participants on outings and appointments, assist with serving of the meal and snacks, and monitor the Center activities during staff meetings, family conferences, and interviews.

Consultants: Physical Therapy, Speech Therapy, and *Dietary, Social Worker:* The Center has signed a written policy agreement with the following consultants: P.T., O.T., S.T., nutritionist to provide services in accordance with the department of Public Welfare's conditions of Participation for Restorative Services. The consultants develop therapy programs appropriate to the needs and limitations of the participants in compliance with the physician's orders.

Occupational Therapist: The occupational therapist supervises the activity-socialization aspects of the treatment plan. The occupational therapist is trained and has a minimum of two years' experience in the field of geriatric rehabilitation. The occupational therapist is responsible to the Director of the Center.

The Physical Therapist: A registered physical therapist supervises the physical therapy program and gives direct services where appropriate and ordered by the physician. The physical therapist is trained and has a minimum of two years' experience in the field of geriatric rehabilitation and long-term care. The physical therapist is responsible to the Director of the Center.

The Speech Therapist: A registered speech therapist supervises the speech therapy program, and gives direct service where appropriate and ordered by the physician.

Nutritionist: An employee of the Nursing Home who is a graduate of an approved program in the field of nutrition provides consultation to the staff, participants, and their families in menu planning and nutrition.

Volunteers: Volunteers are an important part of the day health center's staffing. They are used in all facets of the program as they are available. The role of the volunteers, their tasks, and responsibilities are clearly defined; screening, training, orientation, and supervision of volunteers is provided and on-going.

Figure 9-2. *(continued)*

Citizen/Professional Advisory Council:
The Adult Day Health Center has a seven member Advisory Council. Its members represent the citizens and agencies which serve the elderly and disabled of the west suburban area. At least fifty percent of the members will be non-providers of health care. Any significant problems concerning the Center's program and operation are discussed, negotiated, and resolved in a cooperative spirit by this committee to the benefit of the community and its residents. This committee will receive a yearly report from the program director. It makes evaluative visits and reports its findings to the Director. The Director of the Center is responsible for educating the committee members.

SCHEDULE OF A PROGRAM DAY

8:00–9:30 A.M. Arrival Time
This is an unstructured social period for all participants. Reading interests, handicrafts, and social conversation are encouraged during this time.

9:30–10:00 A.M. Snack Time
This is a social time of sharing food, discussing current events, making announcements, and presenting the day's events and news about Center activities.

10:00–10:30 A.M. Exercise
This is a time when all participants sit in a circle and perform range-of-motion exercises led by the activities director or nurse and adapted to their needs.

10:30–11:30 A.M. Projects and Crafts
This is an hour of group and individual participation in specific projects (i.e. wreath making, printing, cards, games, knitting, embroidery). Nursing treatments, bathing, and therapy are done during this time.

11:30–12:00 A.M. Preparation for Lunch
During this time the participants clear off the activity tables and set them for lunch with assistance as needed from the staff.

12:00–1:00 P.M. Lunch
Lunch is served by the staff with participants helping as they are able. The meal is prepared according to each participant's physician-ordered diet and one-third of the day's nutritional requirement is met at this time.

1:00–2:00 P.M. Rest and Relaxation
Participants requiring a nap recline on lounge chairs at this time while others elevate their feet and rest while listening to music. During this time a group of confused participants are given a half-hour of reality orientation.

2:00–2:30 P.M. Group Activities
At this time group entertainment, slide shows, speakers, singing, and/or discussion groups are provided. Holiday parties and birthday celebrations are included at appropriate times throughout the year.

2:30–3:00 P.M. Afternoon Snack
This is a time for the serving and sharing of a refreshing drink and snack as well as providing a time to reflect on the day's activities before departure.

3:00–4:00 P.M. Departure
At this time the activities are put away and the Center arranged for another day. Participants are assisted in preparing for their departures and assured that they are departing in the appropriate vehicle when it arrives.

Figure 9-2. *(continued)*

6. *How the Project Will Be Monitored, Measured, and Evaluated.*

    Program evaluation was established at the Adult Day Health Center during the planning phase of the program's development. During this process many types of evaluation methods were discussed. From these discussions a decision was made to use both formative and summative methods.

    Included in the formative methods are the use of the problem-oriented record, participant and family meetings, consultation from the Department of Public Welfare's survey staff and the registered nurse consultant, weekly team meetings, and a semi-annual advisory council meeting. In addition, the Systematic Functional Assessment Tool, which is a comprehensive assessment and evaluation tool, will be used for both formative and summative evaluation at admission, six months later, yearly, and at discharge.

    Included in the summative evaluation methods are retrospective audit of the participant's records and the reasons for discharge. Moreover, the participant and family benefits are also analyzed. Yearly records will be reviewed to evaluate the number of participants attending the program, for how many days, what services they receive, and how many are participating in each activity.

    Along with looking at program effectiveness in terms of participant/family outcomes, a serious look is given to program cost effectiveness in relation to other alternatives available in the community.

7. *Plans for Project Continuation After Funding Terminates.*

    It is anticipated that after one more year of funding the Adult Day Health Center program will be self-sustaining. This will be possible through the implementation of the final phase of program development. Program growth will be completed when the daily participant census is twenty-four persons a day and five full-time staff members are employed by the Center. Changes in the project costs, which will make the program continuation without additional funding possible, are:

    1. Completion of construction with termination of construction costs.
    2. Completion of purchasing required equipment.
    3. Maintenance of a ninety percent participation rate of twenty-four persons daily, five days weekly.
    4. Maintenance or an increase in the ratio of private paying participants to participants on DFW medical assistance.
    5. Increase in the Medicaid reimbursement rate by fiscal year 1981.

Figure 9-2. *(continued)*

8. Itemizing Budget				
TITLE III BUDGET INFORMATION				
Applicant __Adult Day Health Center__		Fiscal Year __1980__		
Cost Categories	Federal Title III Cost	Non-Federal Costs		Total
^	^	Cash	In-Kind	^

Personnel:
  Program director
  Licensed practical nurse
  Activities director
  Social worker
  Program assistant
	
	 18,360
	 11,130
	 10,700
	 11,770
	 8,000			

Fringe benefits @ 20%	11,992			
Sub-Total (a)	71,952			
Staff travel	500			
Rent & utilities	10,200			
Communications	1,200			
Office expense	1,000			
Equipment purchase—per attached	4,270			

Other:
  Consultants
  Crafts supplies
  Cleaning
  Medical supplies
  Prepared foods
  Professional fees
  Other costs
	
	 960
	 1,000
	 5,000
	 200
	 23,600
	 1,000
	 5,000			

Subtotal (b)	53,930			
Total	125,882			

Total Budget	$125,882
Non-Federal Resources	$ 81,466
Prior Award	$ _____

Figure 9-2. *(continued)*

	TITLE III BUDGET INFORMATION			
Applicant _____				

Cost Categories	Federal Title III-C Cost	Other Resources Cash	Other Resources In-Kind	Total

Equipment purchase:
  Desk
  Lighting
  Telephones
  Reclining chairs (4)
  Table
  Chairs
	250
	475
	625
	475
	45
	200			

Total equipment purchase	2,070			
Other: Construction costs	2,200			
Total other	2,200			
Direct services:				
Total Direct Services				

Figure 9-2. *(continued)*

9. *Budget Narrative*

Personnel: The personnel costs as listed include a seven percent salary increase for the four full-time professional staff. The staffing pattern meets the Department of Public Welfare's regulations requiring a professional staff of: a full-time registered nurse, a full-time social worker, and a full-time activities director when twenty-four or more participants are served by the Center daily. The regulations further state a minimum staffing of one full-time person for every six participants. These regulations specify staffing for direct service. Since the Adult Day Health Center has a high percentage of handicapped and disabled persons in need of nursing services, a full-time licensed practical nurse was hired to assist the R.N. Director in fulfilling these needs. With the expansion of the program to twenty-four participants daily, a full-time position of a social worker must be filled to meet DPW regulations. In addition, a program assistant has been included in the staffing pattern to provide much-needed assistance to the staff and adequate staffing coverage when other staff members are absent (i.e., sickness, vacations, educational programs, and conferences).

Staff Travel: This category includes staff educational costs and travel costs.

Rent and Utilities: This cost includes the 1218 square feet of space being used in the Nursing Home by the Center, as well as the heat, water, and electricity usage.

Communications: This figure is an estimate based on last year's printing costs, copying, mailings, and the cost of service for one telephone by the Center.

Office Expense: This cost is based on the previous year's office supply expenses with considerations for the increase in staff and its needs.

Equipment Purchase: Due to the planned increase in participation and staffing, costs are listed here which include needed additional equipment as well as another telephone and the expenses of service for that telephone. Also listed is an estimate on construction costs for the additional space required for expansion based on estimates received to date.

Other:

Consultants: This is a minimum cost based on the consultations of four consultants required by the DPW regulations, providing service to the Center staff one hour every month at $20 per hour.

Crafts-Supplies: An estimated cost of all activity materials provided the 24 participants, five days weekly.

Cleaning: This figure is computed as a percentage of the cost of providing cleaning services to the Nursing Home. The cost is based on the service to the area now being cleaned as well as additional space to be cleaned. Cleaning services include daily cleaning of the activity-dining area, office, rest space, and two bathrooms, plus supplies of paper products and soap.

Medical Supplies: This cost includes emergency equipment, maintenance of a stock supply of non-prescription medications for administration as needed, maintenance and repair of blood pressure equipment, thermometers, and paper products for dispensation of medications.

Figure 9-2. *(continued)*

Prepared Foods: Food products, paper supplies and preparation of food for twenty-four participants receiving a noonday dinner and two nourishing snacks (including a complete breakfast when a participant arrives without eating) is calculated to be $4 per person daily.

Professional Fees: These fees take into account the need for accountants, lawyers, and other professionals at various times throughout the year when events require their services.

Other Costs: This figure is given to provide the Center with a necessary contingency fund.

Less Non-Federal Resources:

This amount of income is based on a ninety percent participation rate with one-third of the participants being private payers and two-thirds of the participants being on Medicaid, using a daily census of twenty-four for 246 days a year. The number of days of service is based on five days weekly, fifty-two weeks a year, with ten holidays, and allowing for four weather days causing the Center to be closed.

10. *Summary of the Project Proposal*

The Adult Day Health Center is designed to fill the missing link in the continuum of care available to the isolated, physically handicapped older person living in the suburban area. Considering the unique characteristics of the target population, the Center serves to meet the community's needs for health services which offer for many an alternative to institutionalization and for others a salvation from isolation.

The Center's program is planned by a professional staff to meet the physical, social and psychological needs of its participants and their families during the day. The program utilizes health maintenance, therapeutic, social, rehabilitative, nutritional, and recreational services to promote optimal physical and psychological well-being. Through these services the disabled older person is able to remain in the community and participate in family and community life to the fullest possible extent. Family and community involvement is considered essential in the planning of care for each participant.

Evaluation and continuation of services provided are essential components of the program in meeting its objectives. Through the use of several evaluation methods and plans for becoming a self-sustaining program, the Center will continue to serve the West Suburban area's older citizen's health care needs without duplicating or overlapping other services. The Center's program will maintain participation at twenty-four persons a day, five days weekly, and five full-time staff members when the program has completed its final phase of growth.

Figure 9-2. *(continued)*

Part B of Title IV provides grants for developing or demonstrating new approaches ... including the use of multipurpose centers, which hold promise of substantial contribution toward wholesome and meaningful living for older persons; ... or for achieving or improving coordination of community services for older persons.[9(pp38–39)]

Title V—multipurpose senior centers. Grants are available from the Administration on Aging for the acquisition, alteration or renovation of facilities that will be used as multipurpose senior centers. The centers must serve as focal points for the development and delivery of social services and nutritional services designed primarily for older persons and be in close proximity to the majority of users.[9(p43)]

The federal government will be responsible for not more than 75% of the costs, and the remaining portion must be guaranteed by the contractee. Additionally, the center must remain in use for at least ten years, sufficient operating funds must be demonstrated, and it may not be used for sectarian purposes. Preference is given to areas where a comprehensive and coordinated system under Title III of the Older Americans Act is being developed.[9(p44)]

Title V, Part A, provides mortgage insurance and annual interest grants, and Part B provides grants for the staffing of the center. The latter grants may not exceed 75% of the total cost of staffing the first year; 66⅔% the second year; and 50%, the third year.

Title VII—nutrition program for the elderly. In 1972, a new Title VII was created, authorizing a nutrition program for older Americans. It was extended in 1974 and is designed to provide those aged 60 and over at least one hot meal per day that assures a minimum of one-third of the daily nutritional needs of the individual. It must be provided in a congregated setting, since isolation of the elderly is part of what is being remedied. Supportive social services; health, welfare, and nutrition counseling; and educational and recreational activities must also be provided.

Those elderly who are specifically addressed by this title are those who

do not eat adequately because: 1) they cannot afford to do so; (2) they lack the skills to select and prepare nourishing and well-balanced meals; (3) they have limited mobility which may impair their capacity to shop and cook for themselves; (4) they have feelings of rejection and loneliness which obliterate the incentive necessary to prepare and eat a meal alone.[10(p5)]

Preference is further given to low-income individuals.

The Administration on Aging may make grants to cover up to 90% of the cost of the purchasing, preparation, and delivery of the meals, and individual supporting services that are found necessary and are not covered through other programs. The Administration on Aging will establish the criteria for costs deemed reasonable and necessary for the conduct of the nutrition program. Each state receives an allotment from the appropriated funds based on the formula

$$\text{allotment} = \text{appropriation} \times \frac{\text{state population 60 and over}}{\text{national population 60 and over}}$$

except that the allotment shall never be less than ½ of 1% of the appropriation.

Table 9-2 shows nutrition-program appropriations of past years at the national level. In 1975, an additional $35,000,000 was authorized in the Title III Amendments to the Older Americans Act (Section 309) for the purpose of providing "supportive transportation services in connection with nutrition projects. . . ."[10(p6)]

Table 9-2
Title VII nutrition program for the elderly appropriations table

Fiscal Year	Amount of Appropriation
1973	$100,000,000
1974	$150,000,000
1975	$150,000,000
1976	$262,500,000
1977	$250,000,000
1978	$275,000,000

From *The Social Security Act and Related Laws*, US Government Printing Office, 1978.

Community Services Act of 1974

Title II of the Community Services Act of 1974 provides for urban and rural Community Action Programs. Section 222 (a) of Title II, Part B, sets forth special programs which include "The Senior Opportunities and Services (SOS) Program." This program is designed specifically to meet the needs of *poor persons above the age of 60 and to remedy gaps and deficiencies* in the existing service system.

Community Action Agencies which sponsor the Senior Opportunities and Services Programs may themselves establish Adult Day Care Programs or may fund other programs sponsored by agencies or organizations which have a history of involvement with, and special interest in, low-income persons.[5(pII-16)]

Revenue Sharing

Revenue Sharing is available for all state, county, municipal, and town governments. It may be used for any government-approved project, including capital expenditures. Discrimination on the basis of age is explicitly forbidden. Unfortunately, funds are limited, and competition for these funds is tremendous. In addition, the program requires renewal, through congressional approval, in 1980.

National Health Insurance

As a national issue, the type and extent of health-insurance coverage has been a matter of concern for some time. The debate over the many national health-insurance proposals has focused on the extent and type of coverage to be made available under legislation. In particular, the number of uninsured persons and their characteristics have been a matter of interest and investigation. As seen in the previous section, those persons over 65 who are not eligible for Medicaid and those who have decreased incomes without private insurance are often unable to pay for and attend adult day-care programs. It is this group that have the need for the coverage of such services under national health insurance. Indeed, the Kennedy proposal provides for a comprehensive plan that would cover the entire population, but limits adult day-care services to mental health.

This restriction of the type of participant served in day-care centers is in need of change. To accomplish this change, much lobbying is needed within Congress, as well as consciousness-raising within the group that will benefit from the services of the program.

Private Funding Sources

Private Insurance

Under most forms of private insurance (including self-insurance) the participant in adult day-care services bears the ultimate responsibility for payment. Since the contract for insurance is between the participant and the carrier, the adult day-care center has no direct dealings with the carrier, except to act as the participant's collection agent. Currently, there are persons who are attending adult day-care services who are receiving payments for such services from their private insurance companies (examples in Massachusetts are Aetna, Blue Cross, Blue Shield, and Mutual of Omaha). For the most part, decisions about such coverage are being made on a case-by-case basis. Therefore, participants holding private insurance policies should contact their companies in relation to payment for adult day-care services. Table 9-3 presents information concerning the five most common types

Table 9-3
Number and percent of persons with health-care coverage under major private or public plans. United States, 1976*

Major private or public plan or program	All ages number in thousands	percent	Under 65 years number in thousands	percent	65 years and over number in thousands	percent
All plans or programs	210,643	100.0	188,844	100.0	21,799	100.00
Private hospital insurance	159,957	75.9	146,340	77.5	13,617	62.5
Medicare	19,412	9.2	420	0.2	18,992	87.7
Medicaid	16,392	7.8	13,835	7.3	2,557	11.7
Other plans or programs†	4,868	2.3	4,790	2.5	78	0.4
Private surgical insurance	156,276	74.2	143,450	76.0	12,826	58.8

*From United States Department of Welfare *"Advanced Data" from Vital and Health Statistics of the National Center for Health Statistics.* US Government Printing Office, 1978.
†Excludes private surgical coverage only.

NOTE: Types of coverage do not sum to the population total. The table reflects extent of coverage of each type and, thus, does not exclude double counting.

of health-care coverage, without eliminating those persons who have more than one type of coverage.

A person covered by both private health insurance and federal Medicaid insurance is listed in both categories. Although the table gives data from the 1976 Health Interview Survey, the primary source of data on private insurance is usually the Health Insurance Association of America. For 1976, their estimates of the number of persons protected by private insurance were 176,581,000 persons of all ages; 164,027,000 persons under 65 years of age; and 12,554,000 persons aged 65 years and over. From these numbers, it is readily seen that the percentage of the population insured under private insurance decreases with age. Statistics from the Health Insurance Association of America also state that the percentage of persons with private coverage increases directly with increasing income. Among persons who belonged to families with incomes of less than $3000, 51% of the population were insured. Among persons who belonged to families with incomes of $15,000 or more, approximately 92% were insured by private insurance. These statistics certainly document the fact that fewer persons over the age of 65, particularly those with lower income who attend adult day-care centers, are covered by private health insurance. Therefore, they must rely on private payment out of their own pockets or other public funds for reimbursing the services they receive at these programs.

Foundations

A private foundation is any nongovernmental, tax-exempt organization whose principal function is to give away money in response to a given request. There are approximately 26,000 organizations in the United States that presently satisfy this definition of a private foundation. In the course of a year, these foundations make 500,000 grants with a combined value of $2 billion. About half of these grants are for less than $1000; only 20% exceed $5000. Even though the 26,000 possibilities seem large, the number of these foundations having direct interest in adult day-care centers is much smaller: first, an overwhelming majority of these 26,000 foundations are small, family foundations whose annual benefactions reflect the personal interests of the family members; second, most foundations have strong regional or local biases; third, many private foundations have well-defined interests that may not include such programs as adult day care.

In general, the foundations are managed by professionals who are competent people seeking to fund innovative programs that will eventually be self-sustaining. Therefore, the quality of a proposal that one submits to obtain support should reflect the focus of the foundation being solicited for funds and project the program as innovative and necessary. Further, the proposal should demonstrate that the program will contribute significantly to the foundation's field of interest and that the benefit will be regional rather than local.

Foundations, as mentioned earlier, play a role in funding for some 166 adult day-care programs. Although most foundations will not support programs that have already been tried, some will support programs of social significance even when they have been developed elsewhere.

The five types of foundations that persons working in adult day care should consider are shown in Figure 9-3.

Community Organizations as a Funding Source

Seed money (a small grant to cover at least part of the cost of writing a proposal or beginning a program) can be requested from various community organizations (churches, United Way, industries), service clubs, and local banks. When request-

---

Figure 9-3. Funding Sources for Adult Day Care (From *Developing Successful Proposals in Women's Education Equity,* vol I by US Department of Health, Education and Welfare. Washington, DC 1977 p 19.)

FUNDING SOURCES FOR ADULT DAY CARE

1. *National General Purpose Foundations:* As the name implies, these foundations are interested in projects with a national scope, pilot or demonstration projects, and popular programs that will draw attention to the foundation. These large funding agencies, such as the Ford and Carnegie Foundations, award about half the money that comes from foundation grants. They seldom make awards designed to cover the operating expenses of a project another agency has funded, or grant funds for the extension of old projects.
2. *Community Foundations:* This is your best bet for getting local programs funded. Community foundations are usually glad to give out information on their granting programs. The Cleveland Foundation is the largest of these. Check the *Foundation Directory,* which is organized by state, to see if there's a community foundation near you.
3. *Special-Purpose Foundations:* The crucial question here is whether you fit into their category, because these foundations fund only programs that reflect their special interests. The Farm Foundation, for example, has the goal of improving the conditions of rural life, while the Whitely Foundation limits its program to providing a business education to needy students of Ingham County, Michigan.
4. *Corporate Foundations:* These foundations are extensions of profit-making corporations and as such, are interested in funding local impact programs that will help the parent corporation's image in the community. Examples are the Schlitz Foundation and the Bristol-Meyers Fund.
5. *Family Foundations:* These foundations are usually small and controlled by the donor or the donor's family, with their interests reflected in the foundation's granting priorities. Frequently there are specific geographical boundaries on the limited granting policies of these foundations.

If some of your potential sources are foundations, the easiest way to find out more about them is to write and ask them for a copy of their annual reports, and a list of funding priorities or plans, if one is available. The larger foundations will be glad to mail you a free copy, but some of the small foundations may request that you come to their offices and read the reports they keep available. Also, all foundations with gross assets of $5,000 or more are required by Federal law to file a Form 990-AR explaining how they distribute their money. The regional collections of the Foundation Center have microfiche copies of the 990-AR forms from all the foundations that are required to file information on their funding activities.

The kinds of information you will need to learn about a foundation include:

1. What is its full legal name and proper mailing address?
2. Is it a community foundation or a private foundation?
3. What are its current priorities and interests?
4. How much money is available?
5. How large is the typical grant?
6. What kinds of projects have been funded?
7. What limitations are specified in the guidelines?
8. What are the application procedures and deadlines?
9. Who is the contact person?
10. Who are the officers and trustees?
11. Is there a possibility for renewals?

You should be aware that foundations do not like to be used as a supplement to public funds and do not usually consider funding programs for which there is public money available.

ing seed money, one must be specific about the amount of money or the kind of support that is needed. If the community organization cannot give money it may be willing to loan equipment or offer consultant help in a given area to benefit the program participants. Your presentation for seed money should be short, informal, specific, and made to someone in a decision-making position within the organization.

Summary

The limitations imposed by government regulations have tended to distort the emphasis in adult day care so that frequently the funding available determines what need will be met. In those states in which Title XX funds are allocated, within the state plan, to adult day care, the programs are primarily social, while in those states in which Title XIX funds are so allocated, the programs are primarily health-focused.

A second distortion exists in the effect these limits have on middle-income elderly. Unless they spend down to the $2000 Medicaid limit and lose their security in the process, they don't qualify for Medicaid coverage. Medicare, for which many of them do qualify, does not yet extend sufficiently to adult day care. All of the other programs give preference to the low-income elderly. Middle-income elderly are as vulnerable to the diseases of old age as are low-income elderly and are unable to support their own care for very long. Efforts, such as the On Lok study, are being made to remedy this inequity, but for the present it exists. Although the task of planning funding sources is an arduous one, it is very necessary and can be very rewarding to the program in the end. Thorough familiarity with the process will increase the chances of funding both now and in the future.

References

1. Robins EG: *Directory of Adult Day Care Centers*. DHEW, Health Care Financing Administration, Health Standards and Quality Bureau, May 1978, pp 3–6.

2. Health Planning Council for Greater Boston, Inc: *Newsletter*. Boston, Apr 28, 1981, p 1.

3. Aldrich EB: Funding and spending for human and non-human resources in 100 adult day care centers across the U.S.A. Warwick, RI, Apr 1978, p 1.

4. *The Social Security Act and Related Laws*. United States Senate, Committee on Finance, Dec 1978, p 407.

5. Holmes D, Holmes M: *Planning Guide to Day Care Services for Older Persons*. New York, Community Research Applications, Inc, 1978.

6. Massachusetts Department of Welfare: Adult day health cost study. Boston, June 1975.

7. Conley SR: Official summaries and project reviews: Alternatives to institutionalization for the long-term care of the impaired aged. Office of Social Services and Human Development, Office of the Assistant Secretary for Planning and Evaluation, Jan 1976, pp 39–42.

8. *Assembly Bill 1611,* State of California, Sept 24, 1977.

9. *Older Americans Act as Amended.* Administration on Aging, Office of Human Development Services, DHEW, Mar 1978.

10. *Older Americans Amendments.* US House of Representatives, Report No. 94-67, Mar 14, 1975.

III

Setting Up a Day-Care Program

10

Program Development

Carole Lium O'Brien, RN, MS

Introduction

One of the most neglected areas of planning in adult day-care programs is the development and interpretation of the program philosophy. Planners many times have implemented these programs without first developing a well-thought-out program philosophy. This lack of program philosophy has caused many problems in adult day-care programs. Because philosophies are often vague and abstract, they tend to be ignored in the implementation and evaluation phases. Within this context, it is not surprising that adult day-care programs have not carved out a unified or well-established position in the present long-term-care system.

Definition of Philosophy

A philosophy is a system of motivating beliefs, concepts, principles, and values. Webster's *Third International Dictionary, Unabridged* cites two other definitions of philosophy: 1) "a critical examination of the grounds for fundamental beliefs and an analysis of the basic concepts employed in the expression of such beliefs" and 2) "the sum of an individual's ideas, and convictions; personal attitudes."

Through these definitions one is able to see that philosophy includes ideas about values, ethics, and what is worth pursuing for itself and no other reason.

Ethics

In the United States, certain ethics are prevalent. These affect the long-term-care system as well as influence program planners. Three examples of our national ethics are

1. All men are created equal.
2. All men should have equal opportunity.
3. All men have a right to health care.

In developing programs such as adult day care, one must consider national ethics, since they are the single greatest moral force affecting a program.

Values

Values must also be considered in developing philosophies. Philosophy reflects and addresses itself to the values and beliefs of its adherents. A philosophy and the values it encompasses may be hidden but they still support the visible portion of the program structure and its responses to the currents that surround it. Values may be looked upon as concepts, customs, attitudes, or ideas by which we judge ourselves, each other, or the larger world. We acquire values over time and through many experiences. In our country, values are communicated in the long-term-care system. As such, the initiation of any adult day-care program must involve a clear, logical, and emphatic investigation of values, because values and decision-making are so totally interrelated that one cannot precede the other.

Truth

Finally, a philosophy is a statement of what one believes to be truth. Truth involves all our basic assumptions of duties, rights, productivity, and what is worth pursuing. Not all persons hold the same truth. Many times truths seem obvious to the person that holds them and can be stated as aphorisms or rules of thumb. Examples of some common truths are:

1. the Protestant work ethic
2. the child labor laws
3. the just rewards theory—"you've made your bed, now sleep in it."
4. class distinctions
5. loyalty to friends
6. roles for persons holding specific jobs

Certainly those truths that are subscribed to in planning for adult day-care programs will influence the type and kinds of services provided and the designation of a specific participant group who should receive the services.

Plato has stated that "there is a notion of study in which the various special sciences are to be related together and understood as parts of one system."[1] His statement reflects back to Chapter 1 and the discussion on systems theory in Chapter 2, which suggest that long-term-care planning be viewed as a whole. In doing so, the planner recognizes that developing a philosophy is a subsystem within planning that affects the entire planning system. Clearly planners need to be aware of the fact that a philosophy must be stated in order for program outcomes to be viewed in relation to their original intent. Without an explicitly written philosophy, it becomes difficult for the adult day-care center staff to evaluate the benefits of the program.

Relationship of Various Groups in Philosophy Development

One cannot function well within an organization without having a knowledge of philosophy. In order to develop an adequate philosophy, planners must understand and recognize the broader philosophical underpinnings of the local community, as well as the state and national philosophy of long-term care in which the community is located, for these broader philosophies do have an impact on a specific program philosophy. It is during the program development phase of planning that meetings between the planners and the local community for the purposes of identifying a program philosophy become necessary. As both groups begin to work together, their values, ethics, and truths are shared. Such sharing leads to the beginning development of the program philosophy. Once initiated, the process continues with discussions with the board, staff, and consumers of the proposed service. After all have had a chance to present their views, an appropriate and accepted philosophy is developed. It becomes the foundation for the program and affects all other planning during the program-development phase. The relationship between all these groups in planning for the program's philosophy can best be illustrated by a group of concentric circles with the forces of influence moving across the circles in both directions (see Figure 10-1).

Western Civilization and the United States

The figure shows how both western civilization and the nation's philosophies affect the long-term-care delivery system within a community. Then the philosophies of both the planner and community enable their sets of values and beliefs to influence the goals and functions of the adult day-care program.

Philosophy of Western Civilization
↓ ↑
Philosophy of the United States
↓ ↑
Philosophy of the Community and Planner
↓ ↑
Philosophy of the Adult Day-Care Board
↓ ↑
Philosophy of the Team
↓ ↑

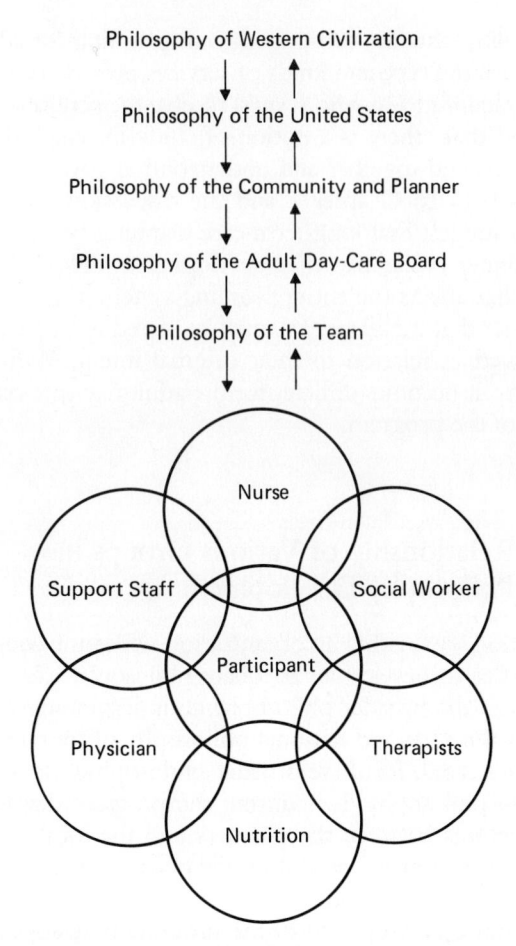

Figure 10-1. Relationship of Various Groups in Development of Philosophy

Community and Planner

The community may have varied expectations of what the program should embrace. Among these are

1. the belief that quality long-term care is given to all members of the community
2. the belief that a higher level of wellness is attained through the advancement of health knowledge by health education

3. the belief that community residents have the right to partake in decisions relating to their personal care
4. the belief that all participants deserve respect as human beings and community residents

Adult Day-Care Board

The agency's philosophy does reflect the goals of the board. For the most part, the board will express values related to the nature of the services they feel they can best provide to their participants. Since adult day-care programs offer a broad spectrum of services ranging from recreational to rehabilitative, it is important for the board to develop a philosophy explicitly stating what type of services will be offered.

Team and Participant

Within the team circle lie those philosophies of the multidisciplinary team members and participant. These may be similar by the fact that each of them responds to the values surrounding them, yet they may be different because of the nature of the service they provide and/or receive. The components of the individual team members' philosophy should express these three common elements: the nature of their participants; the nature of their profession; and the nature of the interaction between them, the participant, and other team members. Clearly, the figure exhibits the interaction between all circles. One affects the other. None exists in isolation. They are not mutually exclusive.

As philosophy is a statement of beliefs, it can be reported and written to serve as the foundation from which will rise the development of the scope and focus of the program. A unification of some philosophical elements will serve as the main foundation for any long-term-care program's sense of identity, security, and confidence. Indeed, programs with a philosophical base will have a much greater control over their future. Ultimately, it will enable them to make a much clearer identification of their purposes and goals.

An example of one adult day-center philosophy is given in Figure 10-2. Some characteristics seen in this example, which can assist the planner in developing the philosophy, include

1. the nature and degree of wellness or illness of the participants
2. the age of the target population
3. the goals of the services provided
4. the approach used in meeting the goals
5. the focus of the services

PHILOSOPHY

The Center believes that the aged have unique needs which want satisfying. In satisfying these needs, the board believes that all aged, infirmed/disabled persons should have equal access to their program. Further, the staff believes the wellness of an individual is intrinsically linked to the physical, social, and psychological aspects of that person's life. Therefore, the staff believes in a health promotion and maintenance framework. In addition, the staff is committed to the concept of Adult Day Care and to its place within the continuum of care for the physically and/or mentally handicapped aged person. Family and community involvement is considered essential in the planning of long-term care for each participant. Therefore, the staff and board believe in including community and family input at all levels of decision making. Since the goals set with each participant are aimed at obtaining the highest level of independence and wellness for that individual, the belief in individualized care is paramount.

Figure 10-2. Example of a Program Philosophy

Program Definition Stems from the Scope of the Philosophy

The scope and extent of the philosophy give support to the explanation or definition of a program. America's ambivalent feeling and confused information about adult day care are keenly illustrated in the government's inability to define the concept. This inability stems from the inadequate philosophical base, as was mentioned earlier in this chapter. Currently, adult day care is an umbrella term describing a whole host of day-care services and modalities of treatment. Consequently, the term *day care* has become a generic one describing various program definitions and models, each providing a composite of services. These services range from intensive restoration to protective services that are primarily psychosocial in nature. Several terms have evolved from the concept *day care*. Four of the most used terms are: *day care, day treatment, adult day health care,* and *day hospital*. Stemming from these four terms are several definitions of day care in current use. One of the most used definitions was developed in 1974 by the federal government.

> "Day Care" is a program of services provided under health leadership in an ambulatory care setting for adults who do not require 24-hour institutional care and yet, due to physical and/or mental impairment, are not capable of full-time independent living. Participants in the day-care program are referred to the program by their attending physician or by some other appropriate source such as an institutional discharge planning program, a welfare agency, etc. The essential elements of a day-care program are directed toward meeting the health maintenance and restoration needs of participants. However, there are socialization elements in the program

which, by overcoming the isolation so often associated with illness in the aged and disabled, are considered vital for the purposes of fostering and maintaining the maximum possible state of health and well-being.

"Impaired adult" means a chronically ill or disabled adult whose illness or disability may not require twenty-four hour inpatient care by which, in the absence of day-care services, may precipitate admission to or prolong stay in hospital, nursing home or other long-term care facility.[2]

As an active researcher in the field, William Weissert has written his version of a definition:

> Day care is essentially a program designed to serve elderly, infirmed and disabled who do not require 24-hour institutional care but who would benefit by a therapeutic program of social, physical, rehabilitation, dietary services counseling and recreation.[3]

Adult Day Care

As the spokesperson for our senior citizens, the National Council on Aging supports the following definition:

> Adult Day Care is a program of care during the day for impaired adults in a group setting away from home.[4]

Brakna Trager in September of 1976 adapted part of the 1974 federal definition:

> Adult Day Care is a program of services provided under health leadership in an ambulatory care setting for adults who do not require twenty-four hour institutional care and yet, due to physical or mental impairment are not capable of full-time independent living.[5]

Although adult day-care planners must be aware of and recognize the existence of the various definitions, they are advised by the author to initially develop their own philosophy upon which they can then proceed to define their program.

Four Models of Adult Day Care

Just as there is no one definition of adult day care, so too there is no one model. The four distinct models that are presented below were initially proposed by Edith G. Robins.[6] The author has further developed these models and elaborated the services related to each model. It should be noted that the cost figures for each model were derived in 1979 and, with the change in the inflationary rate, they could be substantially higher with time.

Table 10-1 conceptualizes four models of adult day care. This conceptualization should not lead the reader to believe that they are mutually exclusive. A blending of models and overlap of program boundaries can and do occur. For example, many social-model adult day programs in the United States offer health services. In some cases, this blending of models is favorable. The program is able to provide a broader range of services resulting in more participant individualization. Moreover, the financial base is expanded, thus providing the planner with more options for funds. On the other hand, however, the blending of models can result in negative outcomes. When several participant populations are mixed, which happens when a broader array of services is offered, these populations may be separated into groups. Program fragmentation can occur because of the different needs that each group presents. As far as staffing is concerned, program blending calls for staff with varying levels of specialized expertise. Practically speaking, it may be difficult to find such staff, and they also may be more costly to the program. Consequently, programs that attract a wide variety of participants are often the most difficult to staff, organize, and manage.

Common to all four models are recreational activities, health promotion, health maintenance, nutrition services, and transportation. There is progression from greater to lesser participant disability from Model I to IV.

Model I

The model I day-care program is for the severely disabled/acutely ill, post-hospital person who requires extensive rehabilitative and medical care. In this program, physician services are directly provided. Common reasons for referral to day hospital are for new strokes, post-surgery recovery, and acute exacerbations in arthritis. When higher levels of functioning are reached, the day-hospital participant is referred either to home or to the model II day-care program. The model I program is thus time-limited.

Model II

The model II day-care program primarily serves the mentally ill or seriously disabled population who suffer from chronic health problems. The day-treatment center offers such services as intensive restorative medical and health services (physical therapy, occupational therapy, and speech therapy) and social services. However, it does not provide physician services. There is no time limitation in this program.

Model III

Model III is primarily a health-oriented program with medical and psychiatric services being offered. It is for the "at risk population" who are in need of a long-

Table 10-1
Conceptual distinctions between the four models of day care in the United States

Facility	Clients	Services Offered	Days/wk. Offered	Estimated Cost	Time Limitation	Expected Outcome	Family Responsibility	Community Supports
Model I Hospital	severely disabled, acute post-hospital	intensive, restorative, medical, and health services (P.T., O.T., S.T.); physician services provided directly by program; activities, nutrition	5 days	$60–$70/day	yes	higher level of physical functioning	training of family members to take over on weekends and nights	usually are necessary
Model II Long-Term-Care Facility	seriously disabled (mental or physical), post-hospital, post-nursing home	intensive restorative medical and health services (P.T., O.T., S.T.); activities, nutrition	5 days	$20–$30/day	none	higher level of functioning—both mental and physical	training of family members to give care on weekends and nights	usually are necessary
Model III Long-Term-Care Facility/Community-Based	"at risk population"	long-term health-maintenance services, nursing services, activities, nutrition	5 days	$10–$25/day	none	prevention of premature institutionalization, relief to families, promotion of health	families provide health supervision in home during days not at program	offered when necessary
Model IV Community-Based	socially isolated "frail elderly," slightly disabled	psychosocial activities in a protected environment, nutrition	5 days	$5–$15/day	none	prevent mental deterioration and physical breakdown, promotion of health	families provide supervision at home if necessary	not usually necessary

Adapted from the four modules of adult day care defined by Edith Robins in "Operational Research in Geriatric Day Care in the United States," paper presented at the 10th International Gerontological Congress, Jerusalem, Israel, June 1975, with the permission of the author.

term health-maintenance program. The services included are nursing, social activities, nutritional, and health-promoting and maintaining ones. There is no time limitation on how long one can stay in this program, since it is within a long-term-care model.

Model IV

Model IV is a social program for the "frail," slightly handicapped or slightly confused older person who may need care during the day for a portion of the week. The adult day-care center does provide a safe, pleasant atmosphere, various activities, health services in some, rest periods, and one nutritious meal a day. The program is not time-limited.

In all models, some type of family and community supports are necessary. For models I and II family/community supports are not only needed but many times these supports take over the responsibility for care when the individual is not at the adult day-care program. In models III and IV, the supports are still necessary but may be of a different type, as the participant tends to need less physical care and more supervision or psychosocial stimulation. In fact, many of these participants may attend the adult day-care program for the very reason that necessary daytime supervision is lacking at home.

Psychiatric Day-Treatment Programs

Similar to some adult day-care programs are psychiatric day-treatment programs. Their services can be offered by either a mental-health department or private psychiatric hospitals. The aim of the programs is to develop and monitor a comprehensive network of community supports and to coordinate the formulation and implementation of individualized followup treatment programs.

Philosophy

Like adult day-program planning, psychiatric day-treatment programs begin with a specific philosophy. An example of such a philosophy is given in Figure 10-3.

Services

With the philosophy in place, as explained earlier in this chapter, the planner for psychiatric day-treatment programs would apply the same planning process and begin to identify the program objectives. From the objectives, the program services are decided. Usually, the services of a psychiatric day-treatment center provide a full day, Monday through Friday, of treatment and rehabilitation programming to chronically mentally ill clients. Staffing can include a director, registered nurse, rehabilitation counselor, allied health professional, administrative assistant, social worker, transitional employment work supervisor, and psychiatrist. Staffing

> **PHILOSOPHY**
>
> We believe if day treatment services are flexible and focus on maximizing individual potential without penalizing limitations, that growth and restoration are possible even within the chronically mentally ill population. Goals must be modest and reachable with built-in provisions for mobilizing resources in the face of regression in order to avoid re-hospitalization and/or shorten periods of readmission. Achievement of independent autonomy is an unrealistic goal for a sizeable percentage of our client population regardless of the sophistication of post-hospital supports. One must accept the challenge that many of the psychiatrically disabled will never be capable of coping with the demands of independent living, but they are, nonetheless, entitled to a decent standard of living and the attention and interest of skilled caregivers who will not abandon them as hopeless.

Figure 10-3. An Example of a Psychiatric Day Treatment Philosophy

patterns depend upon the number of daily clients attending the program. Funding is received from the National Institute of Mental Health as well as from several other sources.

Comparison with Adult Day-Care Programs

Certainly the concepts of adult day-care programs and psychiatric day-treatment centers are alike. The main differences result from the needs of the populations being serviced and the specialization areas of the staff. In adult day-care centers, the population usually is physically disabled or mentally handicapped, but can be cared for by a rehabilitative team of various professionals. In contrast, the psychiatric day-treatment center is for chronically mentally ill persons, who are cared for by psychiatrically trained professionals.

Although some adult day-care programs provide services for mentally disabled adults, these participants are usually in need of a much less concentrated psychiatric program and can readily take part in a program lacking the heavy psychiatric orientation. Currently, in the United States, psychiatric day-treatment centers are planned and developed separately from adult day-care programs, but many exist side by side in communities and should be considered when deciding upon a specific model to implement.

Consideration of Various Adult Day-Care Choices

It is always difficult to make decisions when choices are offered. Decision-making is particularly difficult in adult day-care planning, whether it involves selecting one model or portions of models. The author feels certain that the planner's selection of an appropriate model will be made easier by reading the last few sections of this chapter and continuing to read the remainder of the text. The author also would like to refrain from giving advice about model selection at this time, since significant evaluative studies have not been carried out specifying which model is most beneficial and cost effective. Rather, the author suggests a vigorous study of the various models as well as the population and community the program is to serve, for it is through such a process that an informed decision can be made by the planner.

Program Objectives Stem from the Focus of the Philosophy

Past trends in planning have shown that in elderly services, the focus is on illness rather than wellness. This statement is also true of the United States long-term-care system as a whole and results in our stressing acute rather than preventive care. The acute-care hospital has been well defined while health-maintenance organizations and primary health-care providers are newer, less-used options in the long-term-care system.

Levels of Prevention

It is the intent of this section to present a prevention orientation to adult day-care services. For this reason, Leavell and Clark's "Levels of Prevention" framework[7] was chosen to operationalize those services which should be included in adult day-care programs.

As seen in Table 10-2, primary prevention programs are designed to prevent illness before it begins by eliminating its causes rather than by treating its effects. Such adult day-care services as nutrition, counseling, health teaching, the provision of a safe environment, provision of adequate housing arrangements, periodic examinations, use of specific immunizations, and attention to personal hygiene fall under the category of primary prevention.

Secondary prevention is aimed at curing or arresting a disease in order to prevent the complications of that disease in causing prolonged disability. Within secondary prevention, case finding in the early state of disease is important, for this is when treatment can be most effective. Such day-care services as giving medication, treatments, and nursing care for various diseases, taking blood pressure, and various therapies are classified as secondary preventive measures.

Tertiary prevention is the prevention of complete disability after the disease process becomes more stabilized. In adult day-care programs, participants needing intensive rehabilitation and restoration to regain a higher level of functioning are receiving services that fall within tertiary prevention. Some of these include physical therapy, speech therapy, and occupational therapy, as well as nursing services.

Table 10-2
Adult day care—continuum of services

Health	Illness	Restoration
Primary	Secondary	Tertiary
Nutrition services	Blood-pressure screening	Retraining in activities of daily living
Provision of adequate housing	Diabetic screening	Therapies (physical therapy, occupational therapy, speech therapy)
Counseling	Glaucoma screening	Work therapy
Health teaching	Dental screening	Education for maximum use of remaining capacities
Provision of activities program	Medications	
Periodic exams	Treatments	
Immunizations	Therapies (physical therapy, occupational therapy, speech therapy)	
Protection against accidents with safe environment	Selective examinations for various diseases	

Utilizing a framework of levels of prevention allows the planner to place the areas of health promotion, detection, cure, and restoration on a continuum of care within a given program.

Program Objectives

With the focus on the three levels of prevention, the planner can now proceed to identify the program objectives. Although philosophy statements are broad and abstract, objectives are very specific and concrete. The program objectives are usually statements made about program outcomes. They are measurable. Clearly, they are the superstructure of the philosophy foundation.

After stipulating the broad program objectives, the planner can identify more specific program objectives for goal achievement. Stipulating objectives is in itself a complex, multifaceted process. Basically, a program objective should state the purpose of the program, its anticipated benefit, who is to be served, what services are to be provided, and a time parameter. The specific objectives make clear the broader objectives. When writing objectives it is crucial to remember that accompanying each objective is a rationale, a statement of activity that will be used to achieve the objective, a study-time period, and an assessment tool that will measure the objective and criteria affecting the objective. Each objective should be listed separately. Figure 10-4 illustrates nine program objectives and the rationale for

---

OBJECTIVES

Objective 1. Prevention of Premature Institutionalization

Rationale: An adult day-care program will give support and service to inform and elderly disabled adults living alone or with family and who wish to remain in the community. It promotes the service that the institution provides and is able to serve the day-care participants on the basis of meeting their specific needs rather than insisting that they "purchase a complete package" of institutional life. An adult day-care program is one method by which a community can extend its services to disabled men and women by utilizing existing facilities and resources.

Objective 2. Minimize the Incidence and Severity of Social and Physical Disabilities

Rationale: In addition to preventing premature institutionalization, adult day care may prevent the need for a greater degree of care. For example, an elderly disabled man living with his spouse by going to an adult day-care program may eliminate the necessity of expensive care being put into the home and may improve the relationship with his spouse by redirecting stress.

Objective 3. Strengthening of Other Programs

Rationale: Day-care programs may strengthen other programs, such as homemaker, foster-home, home-care, and nursing services, by decreasing the load on these facilities and resources.

Objective 4. Social Relief and Prevention of Family Breakdown

Rationale: Adult day-care programs can ease the burden on relatives or foster families. Those who have worked with the elderly and disabled know that where there is a question of "burden," it is rarely a one-way process. For example, the elderly or disabled person, anxious about being a nuisance and disrupting the "normal" family life, may feel that he is a burden to other members of the family or relatives. Adult day-care programs will support the disabled and infirm person's desire to be as independent as possible and can help to maintain and strengthen family ties.

Figure 10-4. Example of Program Objectives

each of them. The study-time period for each and the assessment tool most appropriate for measuring each of the criteria affecting it are not presented.

Evaluation as an Integral Part of Objective Development

In planning, one must recognize the importance of not waiting until the end of the process to employ evaluative measures. Therefore, evaluation must be considered during the planning phase of any project. It has an intrinsic relationship to the planning and implementation phase. Recognizing the importance of evaluation and recognizing the importance of the written program objectives, the planner should at this point begin to consider a number of steps vital in planning for future program evaluation.

Objective 5. Prevention of Social Isolation

Rationale: Adult day-care programs are aimed at activating and sustaining the disabled and infirm persons who are most in need of social interaction and meaningful activity.

Objective 6. To Assist in Early Detection and Assessment of Illness

Rationale: Careful history and observation by the adult day-care team will facilitate timely medical and social intervention. In view of the high threshold of tolerance of discomfort, adult day care can provide a baseline of assessment, and close and frequent observation can become a vital element in early detection of physical and social illness.

Objective 7. Promote Health Teaching and Counseling

Rationale: Through counseling and use of community resources, participants are given assistance with management of their problems—for example, nutrition, diversional activities, and social problems.

Objective 8. Easing Transition of Person from Community to Nursing Home

Rationale: An adult day-care program can help to reduce the fear of transferring from community to nursing home by providing a gradual introduction to congregate living. Experiences have shown that persons entering nursing homes are fearful of the unknown. This program would familiarize prospective participants with the nursing-home environment and residents.

Objective 9. Reduce Gaps in Service

Rationale: Elderly, infirmed, and disabled persons many times require a wide range of services in order to help them select appropriate ones to meet their needs. There are now a number of available services, such as senior centers, home care by families, homemaker, nursing services, hospital-based home-care programs, Meals-on-Wheels, foster homes, and congregate housing.

There is a need for an adult day-care program that will enhance the other services and also prevent the overuse of institutions. This service is a vital element in a balanced continuum of community health and social services.

Figure 10-4. *(continued)*

Goal-Attainment Outline

The goal-attainment outline shown in Figure 10-5 will assist the planner in making provisions for future program evaluation.[8] A further discussion and example of utilizing this model by implementation of an evaluation flow sheet can be found in Chapter 14.

Quality Assurance

An important aspect that must be considered during the planning for evaluation is the development of a quality-assurance program. There are many methods and approaches being utilized in quality assurance programs, and the literature abounds with the current emphasis on the need for evaluation and quality controls in long-term-care delivery.

```
                    GOAL ATTAINMENT
    1.  Develop a philosophy

    2.  Identify a model and define the program
                                   ⎧  Ultimate    ⎫
    3.  Formulate the objectives  ⎨                ⎬   Inputs
                                   ⎩  Intermediate ⎭

    4.  Specify activities to reach objectives    ⎫
    5.  Specify needed resources                  ⎬   Throughputs
    6.  Identify specific measurement criteria    ⎭

    7.  Determine outcomes                        }   Outputs
    8.  Recommend further activity or change      }   Feedback
```

Figure 10-5. Goal-Attainment Model as It Relates to Systems

Quality assurance in the long-term-care field can be defined as those activities that are performed to determine the extent to which a phenomenon fulfills certain values and those activities that are then performed to assure changes in practice that will fulfill the highest or a predetermined level of values.[9] Quality assurance looks at the accountability of professional personnel for the quality of care they provide. Such programs are designed to evaluate the extent to which the professionals involved achieve the specific program objectives based on the program's philosophy, which contains certain values. These values are stated in terms of standards, criteria, and norms.

Standards, Criteria, Norms

In understanding the use of standards, criteria, and norms, one must be clear about their definitions, for the difference between performance standards and criteria of evaluation is sometimes unclear. A standard is what is stated by law. Standards of performance are desired or achievable levels of performance that are compared with the criteria. There are usually general minimal standards that are established to govern the quality of care. These standards speak to the safety and experience necessary for acceptable job performance.

Criteria are descriptions of variables without any value judgment placed upon them. They are developed by experts in given areas of specialty. Criteria of evaluation enable the evaluator to determine the degree and extent to which the evaluatee is performing in relationship to the established minimal standard. When planning evaluation criteria, it is imperative to include a precise description of the expected outcome.

Norm is defined as a level or range of performance regarded as typical or normal for any individual or situation. It refers to a conclusion reached as a result of empiric study of present conditions or circumstances. Norms may present problems when there are a vast number of criteria in the assessment of care that are unknown. For example, the norm for "amount of pain" continues to remain undetermined. Not until much research is conducted in this area can reliable norms be developed to test criteria. In the interim, hypothetic norms are used.

Quality assurance and cost-benefit analysis, which is discussed next, are objectives common to most programs. Evaluation of these objectives is consuming much energy today. The tools used in these kinds of programs are discussed in Chapter 14.

Cost-Benefit Analysis

Cost implications are the final element in planning for evaluation. Many times planners tend to put monetary considerations at the bottom of their list as they begin to plan and develop a given program. They assume that everything likely to benefit a specific target group must be done, irrespective of the cost. This assumption cannot be continued, for resources are not limitless, and available funds must be put to the most valuable use. Clearly, the cost implications of maintaining a specific level of benefits are most complex. For a further discussion of this topic, see Chapter 14.

Summary

Initially, focusing on the program's philosophy is certainly a crucial task in program development. Understanding and accepting a program philosophy can create a bond between the agency, the staff, the participants, and the larger community. Only after successfully completing the philosophy statement and utilizing it as the foundation of the adult day-care program can the planner then begin to make decisions about the program model, its objectives, and evaluation tools. Developing objectives from such a philosophy will facilitate the measurement of goals at evaluation. Finally, deciding on the method to be used for evaluation and being aware of cost/benefit analysis at this stage of program development are essential for carrying out future evaluations on program objectives and their benefit to the client as well as their cost to society.

References

1. *Encyclopedia Britannica*, 1968, vol 17, p 865.

2. *Guidelines and Definitions for Day Care Services to Be Carried Out In Experiments and Demonstrations Authorized Under P.L. 92-603, Section 222*. US Government Printing Office, 1974.

3. Weissert W: *Adult Day Care in the U.S.* National Center for Health Services Research, Division of Health Services Evaluation, June 30, 1975.

4. Padula H: *Developing Day Care for Older People.* National Council on Aging, September 1972, p 1.

5. Trager B: *Adult Day Facilities for Treatment, Health Care and Related Services: A Working Paper.* United States Senate Special Committee on Aging, September 1976, p 8.

6. Robins EG: Operational research in geriatric day care in the United States. Speech given at the 10th International Gerontological Conference in Jerusalem, June 1975.

7. Leavell H, Clark GF: *Preventive Medicine for the Doctor in His Community.* New York, McGraw-Hill, 1965, p 21.

8. Davidson SV: Community nursing care evaluation. *Family and Community Health: The Journal of Health Promotion and Maintenance,* 1: 41, 1978.

9. Douglas LM, Bevis EO: *Nursing Management and Leadership in Action.* St. Louis, CV Mosby, 1979, p 198.

11

Adult Day-Care Staffing

Carole Lium O'Brien, RN, MS

Introduction

Although physicians have traditionally been the primary care givers of the disabled aged, they usually do not have the time or resources to meet all the needs of the participants in adult day-care programs. The needs of these participants are such that they require, at times, intensive management of their disabilities and, at other times, psychosocial stimulation. To this end, occupational, physical, speech, and recreational therapists, nurses, nutritionists, social workers, and physicians collaborate. The anticipated result is that no part of the holistic approach is neglected, overlooked, undertreated, or mismanaged. (see Figure 11-1).

The adult day-care planner must consider staffing patterns. Only after the type of model is determined, however, can the planner proceed to decisions regarding appropriate staffing patterns. Who will be most qualified to develop, implement, and evaluate the services to be offered within a given program model is dependent on the program's purpose, goals, and objectives. Although the use of the staff described in this chapter may be central or peripheral to the program, all professional personnel spoken of should be available for consultation when necessary.

Table 11-1 describes the four models of adult day-care services and suggests staffing personnel for each model.

INTERDISCIPLINARY PARTICIPANT APPROACH

Problem: Hypertension

Treatment Regimen: Thiazides

Needs: Potassium replacement. Physician orders participant to take a glass of orange juice or eat one banana daily to supplement potassium loss.

Constraints: Participant dislikes both, is allergic to orange juice, or is tired of eating these replacement foods after a six-month time period.

Collaboration: The nutritionist as a team member working with all participants recognizes the participant's need and supplies the participant with a long list of low-sodium, high-potassium food sources. Then, in collaboration with the nurse, social worker, and cook, the nutritionist establishes a daily meal plan, rotating foods high in potassium that are acceptable to the participant. In addition, the nutritionist guarantees their incorporation into the participant's daily lunch menu at the center. Documentation is made on the care plan and progress notes are made in the record.

Feedback: Feedback is given to the physician on the participant's compliance with the medication regimen and ability to maintain potassium intake.

Figure 11-1. Example of an Interdisciplinary Approach in a Medical-Model Adult Day-Care Program

When selecting staff for the adult day-care program, it is crucial that a close match between staff capabilities and needs of the participants be studied. As the planners attempt to plan for adequate staffing within their programs, they must be aware of the fact that the more medical and restorative a model is, the higher number of skilled professionals is needed. Therefore, when one is developing a model I or II program, one must realize the need for a larger number of, and a better qualified, professional staff.

The organizational chart in Figure 11-2 illustrates the kind of professional and nonprofessional staff that is needed for a Model I or II program.

The ratio of professional staff to participants in these programs depends on the needs of population being served. Research has shown that, at Burke in White Plains, New York (a day hospital), there exists a ratio of 1.3 participants to each professional staff member, whereas, at St. Otto's in Little Falls, Minnesota, there exists a ratio of 5 participants to each professional staff member. In Massachusetts, the state guidelines for health-oriented programs recommended 1 staff member to 6 participants.[1(p34)]

Major Staffing Categories

Administrative

Adult day-care participants need much assistance in learning about and utilizing various and appropriate community resources. The director is in an excellent

Table 11-1
Suggested staff for the four models of adult day-care services

Model	Services Offered	Staffing Personnel

I	Medical
	Nutritional
	Nursing
	Restorative
	  Physical therapy
	  Occupational therapy
	  Speech therapy
	Clerical
	Recreational
	Social service
	Transportation
		Physician
		Dietician
		Nurse
		Physical therapist
		Occupational therapist
		Speech therapist
		Recreational therapist
		Social worker
		Possible van operator
		Secretary
		Technicians/aides

II	Nutritional Nursing Restorative Physical therapy Occupational therapy Speech therapy Recreational Clerical Social service Transportation	Dietary consultant Nurse coordinator Physical therapist Occupational therapist Speech therapist Recreation therapist Technicians/aides Social worker Secretary Possible van operator
III	Nutritional Nursing Recreational Clerical Transportation Social service	Dietary consultant Nurse coordinator Recreational director Technicians/aides Secretary Social-work consultant Possible van operator
IV	Nutritional Recreational Clerical Social service Transportation	Dietary consultant Recreational director Secretary Social-service coordinator Possible van operator

position to offer this information. Another community role assumed by the director is as a designated representative to do outreach, public relations, and educational training about the program.

In the area of education, the director is primarily responsible for the in-service education of all staff members. Furthermore, the adult day-care center can be engaged in providing experiences for nursing, social work, and other students. In this instance, the director will have a key position in student training.

Since adult day-care programs are a fairly new development of long-term-care delivery in the United States, many programs are engaged in research activities. The purposes of the research are varied (see Chapter 5). However, the overall goal

254 / Part III: Setting Up a Day-Care Program

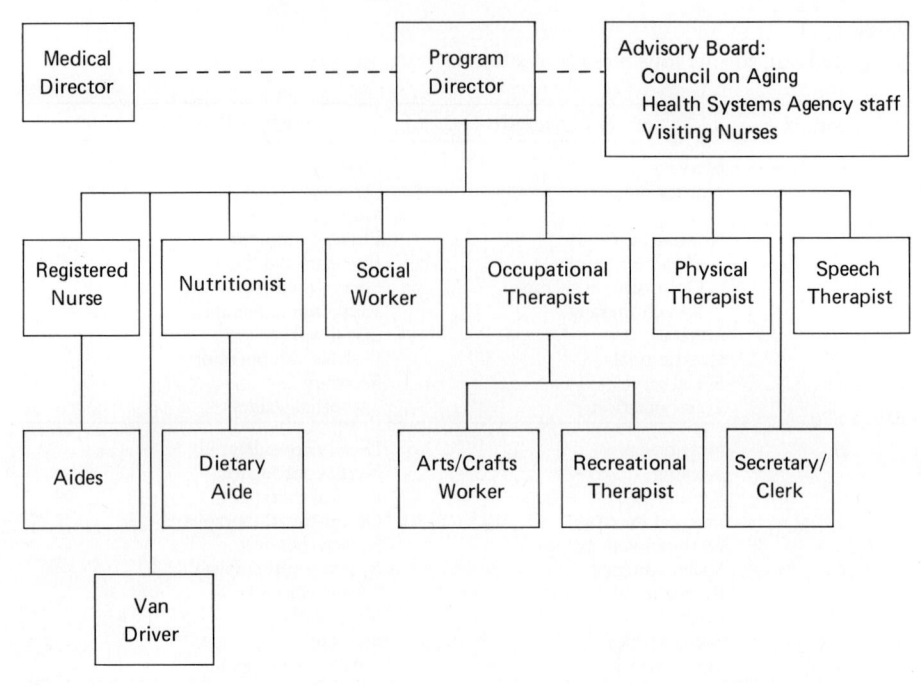

Figure 11-2. Example of a Model I or II Adult Day-Care Program Organizational Chart

for most projects is to increase the knowledge base about the concept of adult day-care services. The directors can become involved in research when their programs engage in such activities.

Recruitment, orientation, and scheduling of volunteers and the developing of an advisory board are other functions of the director. The director employs the administrative and professional staff for the program. In this capacity, the director works with staffing patterns, population mix and needs, and other community support systems that reinforce the adult day-care services when the participants are not in attendance.

Funding sources within states have a major impact on the types of models that can be reimbursed in that state. (See Chapter 9 for a further discussion of the various funding mechanisms that adult day-care centers can utilize.) Those states that offer more social adult day-care programs for the most part have larger ratios of participants to staff, whereas the states that provide health/medical programs require a smaller ratio of participants to staff. For example, programs that offer health services are in greater need of more professional staff, usually within a ratio of one staff member to five participants. Purely social programs can have a ratio of one staff member to eight or ten participants. If the models are a blend of health and social services, then the planner would consider a ratio in between those mentioned above. However, if the physical and medical needs of the participants were greater than those provided for in an adult day-care program, the participants would probably utilize a day hospital model in which each staff member works with one or two participants, as seen in the Burke example.

The program director coordinates all the functions of the interdisciplinary health-care team who share the responsibility for implementing and evaluating the program objectives. Research at the Levindale Hebrew Geriatric Center and Hospital, in Baltimore, Maryland suggests that the director plays a crucial role in coordinating communication among physician, staff, participant, and family. One effective way of keeping the channels of communication open is to obtain input from the team and have them document this valuable input in the problem-oriented record. This particular function will enable the team to provide comprehensive and well-planned care for the program participants (see Chapter 13).

Fiscal management is yet another area of the director's responsibility. The director must be acquainted with the entire budget. Direct, in kind, and indirect costs need to be considered, and available funding sources and cost-benefit and cost-effective measures need to be explored.

The directors in adult day-care programs must aspire to administrative positions and have capabilities in organization and management skills and a theoretical knowledge base of disabled, elderly persons. In addition, an understanding of the community is paramount in the director's job. Because of the way many adult day-care centers function, the director may also give direct service and should, therefore, be able to lend a hand when necessary. Caution in giving too much of a hand to the team is advised, as well as spending all his or her time in pure administration. What is needed is a director who plans and implements a well-thought-out balance between direct care and administration. Needless to say, this balance is difficult to obtain. But directors who are competent administrators as well as concerned care givers can accomplish this difficult balance.

In summary, the director in adult day care assumes a leadership role, which involves getting input from participants, conducting community education and research, coordinating all team activities, and assuming financial responsibility. The director's functions range from the simple to the complex, with more weight given to the complex.

Professional

The professional staff in adult day-care programs find themselves involved with medical and nursing services, physical, occupational, and speech therapies, psychiatric and psychological counseling, as well as grooming, feeding, supervising meals, recreation, and all social services. The range in percentage of the total amount of time spent in rehabilitation activities is from 10% to 55% of the total eight-hour day, depending on how great an emphasis is placed on restorative activities.[1(p50)]

A time survey was conducted in Massachusetts during February 1980, to study the amount of time spent in all administrative versus direct services. Over a two-week period, the staff (both professional and support personnel) in adult day-care centers documented hourly on a form the kind of activities they performed.

The partial return of data from this study showed that the directors spent 63% of their time in administrative duties. The other 37% of the time was spent assisting their staff in giving direct care. It was particularly interesting to note that the directors' service hours went up when nursing-staff members were absent. Nursing-staff members used 90% of their time in providing direct services, and activities directors spent 92% of their time in direct care. The other 8%–10% of their day was given to housekeeping or other administrative responsibilities. These results support the hypothesis that adult day-care providers spend the majority of their time giving direct services. In addition, the results document the need for adequate staffing patterns so that the director can keep up with program administration and not be pulled consistently into direct service.

Support Personnel

The number of nonprofessionals and uses to which they are put varies widely among adult day programs and depends on the extent of restorative activities versus the more social/recreational ones. The nonprofessional staff in adult day programs help the professional staff in such activities as grooming, feeding, serving meals, recreation, transportation, and clerical work. General administrative duties and some record-keeping are also carried out by the nonprofessional staff. The San Diego Senior Adult Day Program in San Diego, California relies heavily on nonprofessionals. They report that 80% of the program's health-care time is administered by their nonprofessional staff.[1(p49)] In contrast, in the Levindale Program in Maryland, 30% of the health-care services are carried out by the nonprofessional staff.[1(p40)]

Whether the program has a heavy rehabilitation emphasis or is focused more on social/recreational activities, interaction among participants and among staff is considered to be of vital importance. Team work and communication are therefore necessary at all times. The next section of this chapter discusses the various health-care team members, their roles in the program, and the services they provide.

Professional Staff Members

Nurse

Adult day-care nursing staffs should include a highly trained, geriatric and community-oriented nurse. This nurse usually assumes complete responsibility for the provision of direct nursing care. Since direct nursing care involves assessment, planning, implementing and evaluation, the nurse must be comfortable in working with the nursing process. In addition, all nursing personnel should be competent in generating plans with other team members (see Chapter 13); they must do more than passively implement physicians' orders.

Some of the various responsibilities of the professional nursing staff are as follows:

- health education
- dispensing of medications
- assisting in and carrying out good hygiene practices
- monitoring vital signs
- screening for various disease processes, such as diabetes or glaucoma
- immunizing participants
- assisting with activities of daily living
- observing all behavior
- implementing rehabilitative nursing practices
- creating, implementing, and evaluating a treatment plan

Depending on the availability of other team members to participate in the initial assessment, the nurse may find it necessary to do the complete assessment on her own. Along with the initial assessment, a complete physical and review of body systems are conducted. Once these baseline data are collected, the nurse proceeds to define the nursing problems. The nurse then collaborates with the other team members in including their problems on the problem-oriented record. Once the problems are identified, a plan is designed. Within this plan, the nurse and other team members will identify the long-term and short-term goals, thus facilitating measurement of stated outcomes. Stating participant goals in behavioral terms also facilitates measurement.

At the completion of goal development, appropriate interventions are identified through a collaborative effort among all team members. If the interventions are appropriate and effective, the results will be seen during evaluation. This process is ongoing and circular in nature; reassessment and revision are continuous.

Physical Therapist

The physical therapist—except in a Model I program focusing on intensive rehabilitation services—usually is a consultant to adult day-care programs. The physical therapist develops a plan for the restoration of physical functioning and provides direct service to many participants. In some instances, a maintenance regime of daily exercises is carried out by the nurse. Examples of services delivered by the therapist are as follows:

- active or passive exercise
- use of physical agents, such as heat, cold, water, ultrasound, and massage
- teaching the family skills to help in the care of their family member
- recommending adaptive appliances and equipment
- observing participant behavior both before and after treatment
- educating the nursing staff

The physical therapist not only works with individual participants, but also uses group experiences for participants with similar disabilities. Group therapy has been shown to be an effective mode of treatment, since group members will encourage each other during the sessions. This encouragment leads to invaluable peer support. The role of the physical therapist is truly a most important one in adult day-care programs.

Occupational Therapist

The occupational therapist provides services designed to increase range of motion, strength, and coordination and to teach adaptive techniques that will enable the participant to overcome barriers and impediments in the activities of daily living. Activities performed by the occupational therapist include

- assessment and evaluation of each participant's present capacities
- development and implementation of a treatment plan
- teaching the participant, staff, and family how to follow through with the instituted plan
- assessment and evaluation of the participant's home environment for the purpose of selecting adaptive equipment and, when possible, eliminating barriers to make the environment safer and more convenient
- improvement in the control of sensory/motor behavior and basic neurophysiological functioning

Depending on the model of adult day care, the occupational therapist may rely heavily on paraprofessionals to implement the plan of treatment. Like the physical therapist, the occupational therapist uses group work with persons of similar disabling conditions.

The occupational therapist not only is involved in direct care of the participants, but also consults with the recreational therapist to suggest appropriate activity projects for the participant. The occupational therapist is an active and valuable team member in adult day-care programs.

Recreational Therapist

The recreational therapist plans leisure-time activities for participants that will provide opportunities for enjoyment and peer support, as well as contribute to the participants' social adjustment and physical well-being. Older adults are often unprepared to cope with leisure time, and the recreational therapist must therefore be a creative, energetic, and enthusiastic person who can develop meaningful and therapeutic programs.

The recreational therapist is the newest team member to adult day-care staffs and fills a long-existing need for expert avocational guidance, particularly for those participants who live alone and are isolated and less socially oriented. One important consideration that the recreational therapist must keep in mind is that participants must be able to make choices in relation to their programs. Just as the nutritionist assesses the participants' likes and dislikes in foods, the recreational therapist must assess the participants' preference for becoming involved in specific activities. Furthermore, the therapist must be aware of the physical and mental limitations of the individual participants so that appropriate therapeutic activities can be discussed and planned with the participant.

Activities in adult day care range from very informal, spontaneous ones to more formal, structured types. One of the responsibilities of the recreational therapist is to maintain a balance between these two extremes.

In addition to giving direct services to participants, the recreational therapist also becomes involved with recruiting, training, and supervising volunteers. The recreational therapist must therefore know and be able to tap available sources for volunteers. The effective use of community volunteers helps the staff tremendously, particularly in a large, busy center with much emphasis on restorative measures.

Since religion plays a large role in many people's lives, the recreational therapist must also develop and maintain ongoing communications with several community churches. Participants should have the option of attending services of their choice, either in the community-church setting or at the center itself.

Special events, such as celebrations of national, cultural, and religious holidays and birthdays, field trips, movies, and speakers provide a stimulating and exciting change from the usual routine. The recreational therapist should plan such events adequately on a monthly basis, with input from the participants. An ad hoc participant committee can be formed to provide such input, thus allowing the participants to feel they are taking an active role in the special events.

Three newer therapeutic recreational techniques are music, art, and dance therapy. Several programs have demonstrated how these three art forms proved to be successful. The recreational therapist who is not familiar with these therapeutic techniques should consult with persons in the field about them.

It can readily be seen how versatile and skillful the recreational therapist needs to be to work with participants in adult day-care programs. Without such a person, the center would be lifeless, meaningless, and just a place to come and sit.

Speech Therapist

The speech therapist focuses on the assessment and evaluation of speech, hearing, and language disorders and designs, implements, and evaluates corrective therapies that will restore the participant's communicative processes. In addition to direct service, the speech therapist educates the other health-care professionals about the skills needed to recognize and work with speech disorders. They also teach family members how to assist participants with their treatment plan. Working within a team framework, the speech therapist offers expertise in communication problems to help develop and implement comprehensive participant-care plans.

Nutritionist

The nutritionist plays a pivotal role in adult day-care centers, in helping to provide adequate nutritional intake for the participants. Most adult day-care programs are mandated to make provision for one hot meal along with two supplemental snacks. This meal offers the participants the equivalent of one-third of their daily nutritional requirement and is planned according to their therapeutic dietary restrictions. In some adult day-care centers, breakfast and dinner are also included, but this service is the exception rather than the rule. The expected outcome of the nutrition component of the treatment plan is to provide the participant with a balanced and adequate intake of the four basic food groups in order to reach and maintain a high level of health.

In making recommendations for an adequate balanced daily intake, the nutritionist must first assess the participant's preferred food customs, for, if this assessment is not complete, the participant may not adhere to the dietary plan. Although preferred food customs should be taken into consideration, the nutritionist is constantly involved in teaching new and better ways of eating. Patience is needed because it is difficult to change old eating habits even when they are inadequate in terms of daily intake.

The nutritionist supervises participants who need assistance with cooking or food-serving skills and assesses and develops therapeutic activities in these areas in conjunction with the occupational therapist. The nutritionist also collaborates with the other interdisciplinary team members, such as the nurse, social worker, physical therapist, physician, and recreational therapist, in developing exercise programs for the participants to incorporate into their current life style and nutritional intake.

In addition, supervised individual or group shopping provides an invaluable help to those participants who live alone and have difficulty in this area. The use of the group again allows for sharing of ideas and problems relating to food purchases.

Since eating is a social behavior, the nutritionist should ensure that the environment is pleasant, that participants can choose their places at the table, and that the food is prepared and served attractively. In some instances, the participants can help with food preparation and serving, but only if such activity is therapeutic and enhancing of their independence. If the meals are prepared at the center, the nutritionist may supervise a cook. With all these responsibilities, the nutritionist serves in a pivotal role in adult day care.

Social Worker

The social worker seeks to develop a service plan that will address the participants' needs and to provide counseling, either in an individual or group setting, to help the participants overcome some of their feelings of uselessness, loneliness, and inability to deal with stress and illness. Depending on the model used, the social worker can perform administrative duties or, in fact, act as the program director.

When a social worker assumes the director's role, greater emphasis is placed on the social functioning of the participants within the program. Various health functions tend to be second in priority, with the nursing staff being responsible for most of these functions.

When not in an administrative role, the social worker is responsible for developing the social service component of the program and is an interdisciplinary team member. Services delivered by the social worker include

- conducting reality-orientation sessions, individual or group
- conducting counseling sessions and discussion groups designed to stimulate participants to develop new interests
- assessing, implementing, and evaluating the social-service plan for each participant
- counseling family members in order to help them understand the participant's needs and be supportive of these needs
- orienting and teaching the staff, family, and participant about available community resources
- coordinating adult day services and community supports for participants
- providing information about financial benefits to which the participants are entitled
- providing for the participants' psychosocial adjustment to the program
- collaborating with the interdisciplinary team members about the reaction of the participants to their treatment and therapies

- conducting staff meetings, which serve as a forum for problems and as a means of staff education
- assisting and implementing the discharge plan
- collaborating with other community agencies in preparing the participant and family for discharge to their programs

The social worker in adult day-care programs serves as an integral team member. The role includes direct service, as well as consultation with other staff and with community agencies, and is extremely important in all the phases of program planning.

Physician

The physician can have both a direct and indirect role in planning for, implementing and evaluating adult day-care programs. The direct role of the physician includes the provision of on-site medical services and directorship of the program, with major responsibility for medical-policy formulation. The indirect role of the physician includes community-based medical supervision of participants and new-client referrals. This type of indirect care reflects a minimal amount of physician involvement with the formal adult day-care program, since the community-based physician is only contacted in emergencies or for renewal of orders, yet it is the most prevalent type of medical involvement within the adult day-care movement in the United States.

The indirect physician role can present a problem for the program director when several physicians are involved in one participant's plan of care, particularly when the director must coordinate medication regimens from many physicians. Clearly, a close working relationship between the director and physicians is essential from the outset to prevent negative drug interactions.

The physician can assume a direct role within the adult day-care center as the person who continually assesses the participant's medical status and prescribes the necessary medications, treatments, or restorative therapies. In carrying out this role, the physician must discuss the participant's care plan with the participant, other interdisciplinary team members, and the family. Such an approach by the physician is helpful in providing a therapeutic milieu at the center.

Referrals to the day-care center can be both direct or indirect responsibilities of the physician, depending on his association with the program. If the physician initiates the referral, it is a direct referral; if the referral to the center is made by the participant, family member, or community agency, it is an indirect referral. Even with indirect referral, the physician is consulted because a physical exam is required for admission, and renewal orders are due periodically. Furthermore, the physician's attitude and support are crucial to whether the participant attends the program regularly. The importance of the physician's attitude is compounded further by the fact that families look to their physicians for reassurance when they have any doubts about adult day-care involvement.

One of the most vital indirect roles the physician assumes in adult day care is in the utilization-review process. Here again, the physician must consider the relevance of the interdisciplinary team approach, in which each specialized team member reports on the progress or lack of progress observed in the participant since the last review.

Finally the physician has an important role to play in maintaining good communications with the staff, participants, and family members. By ongoing medical backup, assessments, consultation, and in-service training, the physician can foster a positive attitude within the center that will facilitate staff and participant morale.

Support Personnel

Technicians/Aides

The role of the technician or aide in adult day care is to assist the professional staff members in any way possible to augment the services being given to the participants and to help with the direct service load carried by the professional team. The services of technicians and aides are designed to assist participants in a wide range of activities of daily living. Depending on the needs of the individual, these activities can and often do include assistance in toileting, grooming, feeding, dressing, and walking. The technicians and aides also assist the recreational therapist with activities, assist the physical therapist or nurse with group exercise, assist the nutritionist with food preparation and serving, assist with transporting and delivering participants to the program, run errands, and the like.

The technicians and aides are invaluable staff members. They work closely with the participants and families, can offer many good suggestions to the interdisciplinary team about the participants, and should have the opportunity to provide input into the participant's plan of care.

Clerical

The clerical/secretarial staff are involved with maintaining, organizing, and completing all the paper work that accompanies processing admission forms. Their services include

- keeping records in order
- completing billing forms
- seeking renewal of orders
- making appointments for the director

- answering the phone
- giving information to referral agencies and families
- typing correspondence
- all the other clerical duties that capable administrative assistants perform

With an organized and skillful secretarial/clerical staff, the director can be assured that the program will run more smoothly. If the staff can be relied on to complete all their duties, the director will be free to do more of the essential tasks in program planning, implementing, and evaluating.

Auxiliary

Van driver. The van driver plays a particularly crucial role in adult day-care programs. The participants depend on being transported, many in specially equipped vans. If the driver isn't available, they are unable to come to the program. The van driver needs to be a person who can effectively communicate with the elderly and disabled and who can provide for their physical comfort while they are being transported.

Adult day-care centers are only as successful as their transportation mechanism is reliable because without reliable, efficient, and convenient transporting, the program cannot exist. In programs that do not provide transportation services, coordination must be developed with other community transporting services. Transportation is a complex task at best; it is often an ongoing problem and must be considered early on in program planning.

The services of a program's van driver may include

- transporting participants from their homes to the program
- making arrangements for and bringing participants on a field trip
- providing transportation to community social and recreational agencies
- taking participants to medical and other health-related appointments

In addition to providing all the transporting services, van drivers become involved in other types of activities in the adult day-care center, such as running errands, helping with activities, and serving meals. They are important staff members and invaluable in any adult day-care program.

Summary

Included in the participant care plan are the nurse, social worker, therapists, nutritionist, and physician. It is imperative that these disciplines plan jointly to meet the needs of the adult day-care participants. This is not to say that the participants and their families should be overlooked, for they know better than anyone their goals, resources, desires, and limitations. Indeed, one cannot stress enough the importance of gaining the coorperation of the participant and family members in developing treatment plans.

The staff, whether professional or nonprofessional, must be chosen carefully. Selection of staff cannot be overemphasized because, without the appropriate staff, an interdisciplinary team approach is impossible. Indeed, without a team effort in planning, implementing, and evaluating the participant's care plans, fragmentation will occur.

References

1. Weissert W: *Adult Day Care in the U.S.: A Comparative Study*, Rockville, Md, National Center for Health Services Research, Health Resources Administration, Public Health Service, Department of Health, Education and Welfare, 1975.

2. Massachusetts Department of Public Welfare: Application to become an adult day care program provider under the Medical Assistance Program. Boston, 1978, p 7.

12

Implementation

Gretchen Dix, RN, MS

Introduction

The lack of an adult day-care center for the elderly in a given community has prompted many concerned community-agency leaders and professionals to investigate the process by which this service can be offered to the community's residents. Once the determination of need has been established and the community's supportive services have pledged their support to such a program, the components important to the development of an adult day-care-center program are ready to be addressed.

Presently, the two *most* familiar models of adult day-care centers in the United States are the psychosocial model and the medical-rehabilitative model (see Table 12-1). The primary differences between these two models are in their emphases. The psychosocial model emphasizes the importance of psychosocial well-being and the need for social interaction, while the medical-rehabilitative model focuses on physical, as well as psychosocial, well-being and the use of rehabilitative and restorative services to obtain and maintain optimal functioning level. Both models, however, are based on a holistic concept of wellness. Familiarity with both types of models helps the planner decide which type of center can best meet a given population's needs.

Table 12-1
Comparison of psychosocial and medical rehabilitative models of adult day-care centers

Psychosocial Model	Medical-Rehabilitative Model
Type of Client	*Type of Client*
Persons in a stable medical condition; may require some health supervision; in need of socialization	Persons whose mental and/or physical status requires health supervision; at risk of institutionalization
Staff	*Staff*
Staff-participant ratio varies: 1 staff to 10–15 participants Social worker(s): frequently the director Registered nurse: part- to full-time Recreational director Senior aides Volunteers	Staff-participant ratio according to state regulations: 1 staff to 6 or less participants Registered nurse(s): frequently the director Social worker Licensed practical nurse Consultants: physical, occupational and speech therapists, social workers, physicians Senior aides Volunteers
Services	*Services*
Social-work services—counseling, group dynamics: Nursing services: administer medications Recreational activities Assistance with activities of daily living Lunch and snacks	Nursing services—full time: Social-work services Recreational activities Assistance with activities of daily living Supervision of personal hygiene Lunch and snacks Health education Rehabilitative services/therapies
Site	*Site*
Architecturally barrier-free location: Space for individual and group activities Space for dining Bathrooms	Architecturally barrier-free location: Space for individual and group activities Space for dining Bathrooms for the handicapped Treatment and therapy room Bathing facilities

Medical-Rehabilitative Model of Adult Day Care

Although the outline of the medical-rehabilitative model of adult day care presented here may serve as a guide to the organization of an adult day-care program, it must be pointed out that adult day-care services characteristically differ from one another. No statement can be made regarding participant population, services, or staffing that will pertain to all centers. The most common characteristic of all adult day-care centers is their ability to adapt to the local aged and handicapped populations' needs and provide services that do not duplicate any other health-care system available in that community.

The adult day-care center's philosophy and objectives are the foundation on which the development of the adult day-care program is based. The type of program to be established is determined by the identified needs of the elderly population, their families, the agencies serving them, and the financial supporters. Once the philosophy and objectives of the program are agreed upon and established, implementation is directed at fulfilling the purpose for which the center is being created and assuring that the objectives are met. All planning of the program is therefore focused on meeting the objectives. Keeping this focus in mind while developing the program components provides the planner with the direction needed for program implementation. State regulations may predetermine the model-type if state reimbursement is to be sought.

The implementation of an actual medical-rehabilitative model within an institutional setting in Massachusetts will be discussed in this chapter. Although this model is only one approach to establishing an adult day-care center, it includes all the components necessary to the implementation of any model, whether psychosocial or medical-rehabilitative. The program components presented here are

1. budget
2. facility requirements
3. staffing patterns
4. volunteers
5. policies
6. procedures
7. community outreach
8. admission process
9. transportation
10. family involvement
11. program activities

Budget

The first step in the planning of a program is to establish a budget. The budget for the Massachusetts program was written with existing financial constraints and available funding sources in mind.

The largest single budgetary expense was staff salaries. (For some centers, another major expense may be capital expenditures.) Start-up staffing and ongoing program staffing needs were figured to be approximately 65% of the budget. The start-up staff consisted of a program director and an activities director. These two

```
                              BUDGET
Organizational Expenses              Operational Expenses
  Equipment                            light, heat, water
    furniture                          telephone
      office                           cleaning services
      activities and dining area      food and preparation
      rest area                        supplies for arts, crafts, and games
    appliances                         medical supplies
      kitchen (coffee maker, can opener,
        toaster, cooking equipment,  Miscellaneous
        refrigerator)                  new equipment
    typewriter                         equipment maintenance and repair
    record player                      traveling expenses
  Publicity                            educational expenses
    printing costs
    postage
    open house
    advertisements
  Medical supplies
    opening inventory (stethoscope,
      sphygmomanometer, thermometers,
      oxygen, emergency supplies)
  Decorations
    drapery rods and drapes
    wall hangings and bulletin boards
    seasonal decorations
```

Figure 12-1. Budgetary Items to be Considered in Program Implementation (From Weston Manor Adult Day Health Center, Weston, Mass., 1977. Form developed by C. O'Brien and G. Dix. Reprinted by permission of the authors and Weston Manor Adult Day Health Center.)

positions met the Massachusetts Medicaid requirement of a minimum of two full time staff people for each day health program. Ongoing staff salaries were planned to meet the requirement of maintaining a staff-participant ratio of one full-time staff person for each six participants as program participation increased. Professional consultants' services were also included in the salaries budgeted.

The other budget categories were organizational expenses, operational expenses, and miscellaneous. These costs were itemized as shown in Figure 12-1.

The amounts designated for each budget item were determined by inquiring about other adult day-care-center costs, by having a familiarity with salary ranges, and by being aware of the current expenses in the institution in which the center is housed. The breakdown in percents resulted in approximately 10% for organizational costs, 25% for operational costs, and 5% for miscellaneous.

Adult day-care centers that are not institutionally based may have to incorporate the cost of rent in the budget if space cannot be arranged for as a donation by the facility involved. Costs vary widely, depending on the specific area in which a center is to be located.

Building renovations may be required in establishing a center, in order to meet state regulations. In Massachusetts, all adult day-care centers must be architecturally barrier-free. This specification required another category—capital expenditures—to be added to the proposed budget.

Once the expenses are itemized and the available funding sources known, the planner is better able to set a daily rate for participant care. The estimated income from the center's operation at 90% capacity after the first year of operation, together with the known expenses and funding available, can provide the necessary information to determine the fiscal feasibility of establishing an adult day-care center (see Figure 12-2).

Facility Requirements

The design for the Massachusetts adult day-care center took into consideration the space and environmental needs of the participants and the staff. Space was needed for

1. activities—indoor and outdoor
2. dining—activity tables are used for this purpose
3. simple food preparation
4. toileting and personal care
5. treatments
6. therapy sessions
7. resting
8. private counseling and family conferences
9. interviewing
10. telephoning and record keeping

The Massachusetts adult day-care center under discussion has the advantage of having access to the nursing home's bathing facilities, beauty shop, barber shop, laundry room, greenhouse, chapel, television room, and main kitchen. The main kitchen prepares and delivers the noon meal to the center according to each participant's therapeutic dietary needs. Food for nourishments is delivered daily by this kitchen also and stored in the center's kitchen area. Community-based centers would need kitchen facilities or a system for having the nourishments and meals transported to the center. Provision of therapeutic diets and dietitian consultation are requirements for all Massachusetts adult day-care centers.

The following environmental considerations are important to the older person who may be wheelchair-confined, prone to accidents due to diminished sensory perception and physical limitations with a need for increased auditory and visual stimulation:

1. freedom from architectural barriers
2. safety
3. lighting
4. sound
5. atmosphere

Program Name		Fiscal Year	
Description of Item	*Total Cost*	*Federal/Other*	*In-Kind Services*
A. Personnel salaries Fringe benefits Travel Equipment (purchase) Equipment (rental) Space Utilities Supplies Other: specify			
Subtotal A			
B. Contractual Consultants Communications Personnel			
Subtotal B			
C. Construction			
Subtotal C			
Total (A + B + C)			

Figure 12-2. Example of an Adult Day-Care Program Budget-Planning Sheet (From Weston Manor Adult Day Health Center, Weston, Mass., 1977. Form developed by C. O'Brien and G. Dix. Reprinted by permission of the authors and Weston Manor Adult Day Health Center.)

Income Source	Amount
A. Fees for service Third-party reimbursement Cash contributions Federal money (Title XX, III, XIX) Community development Revenue sharing	
Subtotal A	
B. In-kind resources	
Subtotal B	
Total Amount of Income (A + B)	

Figure 12-2. *(continued)*

A bright, colorful, decorative atmosphere provides a cheerful environment for the participants. Special consideration should be given to reducing glare while providing increased illumination.

The physical arrangement of the center will depend in large part on the available sites and funding sources. These lists are given as suggestions to assist the planner in search of an appropriate site.

Staffing Patterns

The staff's competence is of utmost importance to the effective operation of the program (see Chapter 11). The decision was made in the Massachusetts adult day-care center to hire professionally prepared and experienced people to fill the two start-up positions—program director and activities director. The program director was hired because she was a registered nurse with a master-of-science degree in community-health nursing and previous experience in administration and gerontological nursing. The activities director was hired for her master-of-science degree in rehabilitative counseling and previous experience in group activities and group counseling with older adults.

Since this is a rehabilitative program, consultant staffing includes a physical therapist, occupational therapist, speech and hearing pathologist, dietitian, and social worker. The institution's medical director became the medical director for the center. This appointment was felt to be important in providing ongoing medical supervision for the program. Although participants have their own physicians, the medical director provides direct services to participants when needed as well as consultation (indirect) services to the staff as necessary. This service augments the staff's ability to meet each participant's health-care needs.

Additional staffing needs were anticipated to be a registered nurse or licensed practical nurse, a secretary-typist, an activities assistant, and a nurse's aide. Since transportation is provided by contracts, a driver was not needed for this center. On the infrequent occasions when the nursing home's vehicle, the back-up system, needs to be used, one of the staff becomes the driver. The position of registered nurse or licensed practical nurse provides relief for the program director in the delivery of nursing care when she is absent because of illness, has other commitments, or has too high a case load to manage without assistance. The secretary-typist gives much needed help in record keeping, correspondence, telephone answering, and clerical duties that would otherwise consume much of the professional director's time and energies. The need of an activities assistant depends in large measure on the availability and abilities of volunteers. The number of participants requiring assistance with activities of daily living, such as bathing and feeding, determines the need for a nurse's aide. A part-time driver would be required if the center's transportation services were provided by the nursing home's own vehicles. Staffing needs are determined by

1. the maximum capacity of the center
2. the program objectives
3. the type of program
4. the availability and abilities of volunteers
5. the transportation services

Volunteers

The availability and use of volunteers has a tremendous influence on the program's operation. Volunteers augment staffing and provide additional help while contributing their special talents and skills without increasing the program's costs. Working in an adult day-care center gives the volunteers an opportunity to gain experience in the care of older adults as well as providing the center with a pool of possible staff persons for future employment.

Policies

All program planning should include the establishment of volunteer policies and the recruitment of volunteers. Volunteer policies specify

1. the screening procedure
2. orientation
3. education

4. supervision
5. evaluation

Policies were written in the Massachusetts program to define the volunteer's job description, the orientation procedure, the education and supervision the staff gives to each volunteer, and the evaluation process (see Figure 12-3). Volunteers are asked to read the policies and are queried to determine their understanding of them. Each volunteer is requested to sign a statement of commitment, indi-

---

VOLUNTEER JOB DESCRIPTION

VOLUNTEER DUTIES

1. To help assist participants in adjusting to the center
2. To help participants maintain or to increase their functional abilities—both mentally and physically
3. To help participants increase their social skills and to increase their competence in recreational activities
4. To help participants build up self-esteem
5. To be willing to
   accompany participants on trips
   find activities in the community
   function as a receptionist
   help with activities (see Activities Preference list)
   help with preparation for activities
   help with preparation of snacks
   make phone calls and answer phone
   play instrument, put on plays, etc.
   type
   type and write articles for local publications or
   otherwise use talents

POLICIES

1. Days and hours for each volunteer will be arranged at their convenience in order that attendance can be depended upon by the activities coordinator/counselor.
2. Notification is expected ahead of time if the volunteer is unable to attend as scheduled.
3. A period of orientation will be provided for all volunteers before working with the participants without supervision.
4. A minimum of 1 hour per day of supervision will be provided for each volunteer. Group sessions with volunteers will be arranged on a regular basis.
5. Every effort will be made to match the volunteer's talents and desires with the job description. However, at times, the volunteer may be asked to perform overlapping functions.

INFORMATION

The name and address of this agency are:
The phone number is:
The Director is:
The Activities Coordinator/Counselor is:
The hours are: 8:00 A.M. to 4:00 P.M. M–F

Figure 12-3. Example of an Adult Day-Care Volunteer Job Description (From Weston Manor Adult Day Health Center, Weston, Mass., 1977. Form developed by C. O'Brien and G. Dix. Reprinted by permission of the authors and Weston Manor Adult Day Health Center.)

cating days and times of service available (see Figure 12-4). The volunteer's job preferences are recorded in order to match activities with interests whenever possible. A service record is kept on each volunteer.

The volunteer screening process consists of an initial interview with each pro-

---

VOLUNTEER JOB APPLICATION

Name _____ Date _____
Phone _____ M,S _____
Address _____ M,F _____

Please state briefly your educational history:
_____
_____
_____

If a member of RSVP*, please check: ☐

Have you had experience working with the elderly in nursing homes? _____

Have you had experience in any other social service agencies? _____

State day(s) _____ hours _____ you prefer to work.

State preference for type of activity that you wish to help with:

☐ accompany participants on trips
☐ find activities in the community
☐ function as a receptionist
☐ help with activities (see Activities Preference List)
☐ help with preparation for activities

☐ help with preparation of snacks
☐ make phone calls and answer phone
☐ play instrument, put on plays, etc.
☐ type
☐ type and write articles for local publications
☐ other

Do you wish a record of your hours? _____

What do you anticipate from working at the center?
_____
_____

Please read accompanying Volunteer Job Description and Policies.

    I have received and read my Job Description and Policies.
    I understand I will not receive compensation.
    I understand my responsibilities.

    Signature: _____

Figure 12-4. Example of an Adult Day-Care Center Volunteer Job Application (From Weston Manor Adult Day Health Center, Weston, Mass., 1977. Form developed by C. O'Brien and G. Dix. Reprinted by permission of the authors and Weston Manor Adult Day Health Center.)

*Retired Senior Volunteer Program

spective volunteer, thus providing an opportunity for the staff and potential volunteer to meet and for the volunteer to see the program in action. Volunteers are asked about their previous experience in working with the elderly or disabled and why they would like to volunteer. References are requested and checked by the interviewer. The interview is conducted by the activities director, with input from the program director, who is also present. Other staff members are present whenever possible. If time permits, the prospective volunteer is observed interacting with the participants. After the interview, references are checked, and a determination is made regarding the person's interest in the program, sensitivity, and capability in working with older adults.

Once the volunteer has been asked to join the program staff, a planned orientation, with supervision and education as needed, is provided each volunteer. Regular educational programs and periodic evaluations are given the volunteers by the program director and activities director.

Recruitment

Recruitment of volunteers consists of selecting appropriate resources and explaining to them the need for volunteers. The agencies and organizations contacted for the Massachusetts program were

1. Home Care Corporation/Area Agency on Aging
2. Councils on Aging
3. Retired Senior Volunteer Programs (RSVP)
4. churches and temples
5. applicants for staff positions
6. nursing-home residents
7. elderly housing-project residents
8. hospital volunteer groups
9. local mental-health units
10. student volunteer groups in colleges and universities
11. Vista volunteers

Publicity

Free publicity for volunteers was provided by some newspapers with designated sections for volunteer recruitment; other publicity was done by attaching notices to bulletin boards and by placing articles in religious newsletters and Council on Aging publications. Frequent public-speaking engagements to local groups provide an opportunity to publicize the program as well as to recruit volunteers.

Once the program has volunteers, attention must be given to keeping them. Efforts directed at maintaining the volunteers' interest in the program and providing opportunities for personal growth and job satisfaction, together with expressions of appreciation from the staff, make for happy, contributing volunteers.

Policies and Procedures

The program's policies and procedures were written in keeping with the Massachusetts Medicaid guidelines (see Appendix B). The program's philosophy and objectives were written first, as previously discussed (see Chapter 2), to establish the focus of the program as rehabilitative. Next, job descriptions were written for each potential staff position (see Figure 12-5).

Third, agreements were made for the required services (see Figure 12-6). Contracts were written to provide for the following services:

1. emergency ambulance services
2. hospital-client transfer agreements
3. medical director
4. therapies:
   a. physical
   b. occupational
   c. speech and hearing
5. dietician
6. social worker
7. planning services
8. laboratory services
9. transportation services
   a. ambulatory
   b. nonambulatory

The necessary procedures included the admission process, the emergency plan (see Figure 12-7), medications, treatments, food services, and the discharge plan. Other policies were written stating criteria for admission, program costs, the admission agreement, and the participant's rights.

Each participant and/or participant's family are asked to read and sign an admission agreement (see Chapter 13), which specifies the services offered, the program cost, the days and times of attendance, the physician responsible for the participant's medical needs, the transportation arrangement, the hospital of choice in case of emergency, and the responsibilities of the participant and/or family (such as providing clean clothing on program days). On admission, participants receive a copy of their rights and a copy of the admission policy (shown in Figure 12-10).

A diet manual was purchased to provide the staff with a handy reference on therapeutic diets. This resource provided the necessary policies and procedures for the dietary requirements as established by the state regulations.

PROGRAM DIRECTOR

QUALIFICATIONS:

Education:

M.S. in community-health nursing
Massachusetts registration in nursing

Experience:

1. Three years' experience in community-health nursing
2. Three years' experience in rehabilitative and/or gerontological nursing
3. Previous administrative experience
4. Demonstrated ability with the aged and in program administration

RESPONSIBILITIES:

Administrative:

1. Plan, coordinate, and supervise all aspects of the Center program.
2. Recruit, orient, provide in-service, educate and supervise the Center staff.
3. Monitor and evaluate program in collaboration with the Nurse Consultant.
4. Perform staff evaluations periodically.
5. Write and maintain policies and procedures.
6. Coordinate transportation services.
7. Maintain transportation records.
8. Assist in the preparation of grants with the Nurse Consultant.
9. Maintain accurate client records.
10. Assure reporting requirements of the Department of Public Welfare are fulfilled.
11. Assure fiscal requirements of the Center program are fulfilled.
12. Report to the Administrator.
13. Represent the Center at the Mass. State Assoc. of Adult Day Health Centers.

Community:

1. Serve in a public relations role within the community.
2. Hold regular meetings of the Advisory Council.
3. Provide periodic information meetings for the interested public.

Nursing:

1. Hold an initial screening interview with each potential client and his/her family.
2. Perform an admission health assessment on all clients admitted to the program.
3. Develop a problem list and maintain a problem-oriented record on each client.
4. Develop an individualized care plan for each client.
5. Implement and perform an ongoing evaluation of the care plan in relation to the client's health status.
6. Maintain contact with each client's physician and review client's health needs and physician orders as indicated.
7. Provide health care needs and health education.
8. Supervise other staff members in their delivery of health care to the participants.
9. Administer prescribed medications and perform nursing treatments.
10. Provide for laboratory work and consultant services as ordered.
11. Serve as a member of the multi-disciplinary health care team.
12. Hold periodic meetings with client's family members.
13. Make home visit assessments when appropriate.
14. Perform an assessment on each client initially, then at six months, twelve months and yearly thereafter, utilizing the Systematic Functional Assessment tool [see Appendix C].
15. Serve on a committee for reviewing the utilization of the program by the participating clients.

Figure 12-5. Example of an Adult Day-Care Center Job Description (From Weston Manor Adult Day Health Center, Weston, Mass., 1977. Form developed by C. O'Brien and G. Dix. Reprinted by permission of the authors and Weston Manor Adult Day Health Center.)

SOCIAL SERVICES

I. *PURPOSE:*

A. This agreement provides for social services and consultation for Adult Day Health Center.

B. These services will be provided by (Name)

II. *QUALIFICATIONS:*

(Name) _____ is a graduate of (Undergraduate School) holding a (Type) degree. She has an M.S. degree from (Graduate) School of Social Work.

List other pertinent information
_____
_____
_____

III. *RESPONSIBILITIES:*

A. Social Worker
 1. Consultation
  a. Provides consultation to administration regarding program planning, policy development, and priority setting regarding social services.
  b. Provides consultation to the Center staff regarding social services.
 2. Direct Service
  a. Provides direct social case work to any participant in the Center program who is referred.
  b. Instructs Center staff concerning plans for meeting psycho-social problems influencing the participant's health status.
  c. Maintains records and reports in accordance with the policies of the Center.
  d. Bills directly for services rendered to the Center's participants by direct service.

B. Center
 1. Provides suitable space and equipment.
 2. Cooperates in arranging for consultation and service.
 3. Makes available participant's records.

C. Mutual
 1. Provides periodic review of the social service program and policies and makes recommendations.

IV. *TERMS OF AGREEMENT:*

A. This agreement may be modified or amended upon mutual agreement of the two parties and such modifications or amendments will be attached to and become part of this agreement.

B. This agreement will continue in effect indefinitely except that either party may withdraw from this agreement by giving thirty days' notice in writing to the other party of its intention to withdraw. Termination of the agreement will be effective at the expiration of the notice period of thirty days.

_____   _____
Date

_____   _____
Date   Director
                           Adult Day Care Center

Figure 12-6. Example of an Adult Day-Care Center Service Contract (From Weston Manor Adult Day Health Center, Weston, Mass., 1977. Form developed by C. O'Brien and G. Dix. Reprinted by permission of the authors and Weston Manor Adult Day Health Center.)

EMERGENCY PLAN

A. EMERGENCY EQUIPMENT
   1. Fire extinguisher
   2. Oxygen tank and nasal canula
   3. Ice packs
   4. Airway
   5. In-house emergency drug kit
   6. Bandaging, bandage strips, and tape
   7. Dressings
   8. Splints
   9. Sling
   10. Antiseptic solution and alcohol swabs

B. STAFF AND PARTICIPANT EDUCATION
   1. Orientation of staff and volunteers
      a. Information on the Fire and Disaster Plan, the fire procedure, evacuation plan, the phone number of the fire station and ambulance company.
      b. Instruction in their responsibilities in the event of a fire, disaster, or emergency.
      c. Shown how to use the fire extinguishers and fire pull station.
      d. Shown the exits and how to proceed in event of fire or disaster.
      e. Information on the quick reference file on each participant and its location.
      f. Shown the location of emergency equipment.
      g. Instruction on immediate (stat) response to:
         1. Burns
         2. Lacerations
         3. Possible fractures
         4. Eye and head injuries
         5. Choking
         6. Cyanosis
         7. Unconsciousness
         8. Seizures
      h. Information on the incident/accident report form and the need to complete this form after each incident or accident.
      i. Information on seeking assistance from the Nursing Home staff by intercom when necessary.
      j. Questioning to determine knowledge of emergency plan.
   2. Orientation of participants
      a. Information on the fire procedure and evacuation plan.
      b. Information on the need to cooperate with the staff and volunteers for an orderly procedure of evacuation when indicated.
      c. Shown the location of the fire extinguishers, fire pull station, and exits.
      d. Instruction of their responsibility in reporting an incident or accident immediately to a staff member.

Figure 12-7. Example of an Adult Day-Care Center Emergency Plan (From Weston Manor Adult Day Health Center, Weston, Mass., 1977. Form developed by C. O'Brien and G. Dix. Reprinted by permission of the authors and Weston Manor Adult Day Health Center.)

e. Instruction on the need for current up-to-date information for the quick reference file.
   f. Explanation of the fire drills, their frequency, and purpose.
3. In-service programs for staff and volunteers
   a. Hold three simulated fire drills per year with a record kept on file for educational review.
   b. Attendance at periodic meetings held by the Nursing Home and/or Center on emergency care, fire prevention, and safety.
   c. Participation in weekly discussions pertaining to the safe functioning of the Center including review of the emergency plan with all staff members and volunteers.
   d. Educational review of any accidents/incidents with emphasis on assessment, evaluation of response, and prevention.
4. In-service programs for participants
   a. Hold periodic meetings for review of the emergency plan including all participants on a regular basis.
   b. Hold weekly educational programs on fire prevention, safety factors, and/or emergency procedures with instruction on methods for obtaining help in event of an emergency in a variety of locations.

   c. Review of all accidents/incidents with the emphasis on prevention.

C. EMERGENCY CARE PROCEDURE
   1. Program director or her designate will assess the situation.
   2. Appropriate stat response will be instituted.
   3. A file for quick reference on each participant will include: physician's name and phone number; specific medications and treatment; allergies; nearest family member's (or sponsor's) name, home phone number, and business phone number.
   4. After the stat response, the participant's physician will be called for orders.
   5. Notification of the ambulance service and transfer of the participant to the hospital will take place as indicated.
   6. Notification of the family/sponsor will be done by the center staff.
   7. An incident/accident report will be completed by the staff. A copy of this report will be sent to the Department of Public Welfare, a copy will be kept in the Center's file and a copy will be sent to the participant's physician if appropriate.
   8. A referral form will be completed and sent to the hospital involved in the participant transfer.

Figure 12-7. (*continued*)

Community Outreach

The purpose of an outreach plan is to inform the communities being served by the adult day-care center of its program. The Massachusetts center plan involved initial and ongoing outreach. Both are essential to the survival of the program.

Advisory Council

Prior to the implementation of the program, an advisory council was formed as the beginning of the center's outreach plan. The seven-person advisory council includes professional and consumer representation. All members live or work in the communities being served by the center. The advisory council functions as a link between the center and the communities it serves; it provides the program director with information on the communities' needs and concerns and assists in the director's policy-making decisions. The director looks to the council for advice on the center's program operation and future direction.

Referral Sources

The next step in the initial outreach plan was to list and make contact with the potential referral sources in the communities. Many had been contacted earlier in the planning phase for the indication of need and therefore were expecting to hear of the center's progress. The referral sources listed were

1. individuals
2. physicians
3. hospitals
4. social-service departments
5. continuing-care coordinators
6. Visiting Nurse Association
7. Council on Aging
8. Home Care Corporations
9. nursing homes
10. health departments
11. mental-health units
12. clergy
13. human services

Contact was made by letter, telephone, personal visits, speaking at in-service meetings, and visits to the center.

Publicity

In order to publicize the center, a brochure and flyer were designed and professionally printed for distribution to referral sources. Letterhead stationery and envelopes were also printed. The brochure, flyer, and stationery have a logo to remind people of the center. Both the brochure and the flyer contain information on the services offered, the staff, the hours and days open, the center's name, its location, and the telephone number. The brochure also contains a description of the people served by the center, a map with directions for finding its location, and a picture illustrating the center's activities program. The flyer provides a simple, eye-catching, one-page information sheet, whereas the brochure gives more detail in a folded, illustrated format. Each serves different purposes. The flyer was designed to be posted on bulletin boards and to accompany letters prepared for mass mailings. The brochure was printed for distribution as a handout at public-speaking engagements, to people visiting the center, to prospective clients by mail, and to personal contacts.

Mass mailings to physicians, clergy, and nursing homes were done. These mailings required compiling a list of people and homes providing services to the communities' residents the center intended to serve. Physicians were sent a letter, written by the program director, which explained the program, the admission process, and the physician's role in relation to the center's program. The letter to the clergy described the program and expressed an appreciation of the clergy's position in seeing a family's need for the services offered by the center. Nursing homes were sent letters to inform them of the services in the hope that appropriate referrals would be made by nursing homes that were unable to meet the needs of potential residents. The letters were professionally duplicated on letterhead stationery and mailed with a flyer.

Initial Outreach

The initial outreach plan demands much time and energy. In the Massachusetts center numerous phone calls were made, arcticles written and distributed to local newspapers, visits to the center extended to all who were contacted, speaking engagements kept, attempts to procure television coverage made, in-service programs given, and an open house planned, with invitations sent to all the communities' health-service agencies, organizations, and institutions, as well as to the advisory-council members and concerned community leaders. When the budget permitted, advertisements were written and placed in local newspapers. Every opportunity was taken to meet with groups, speak of the program, and spread the word. A series of pictures showing the space, location, and program were displayed in a pocket-sized album for individual viewing at speaking engagements.

Ongoing Outreach

As important as the initial outreach plan is to the starting of the center's program, ongoing outreach is equally as important to the continued operation of the program. The population being served is fragile. Each participant's health status is highly changeable, and the participant census is therefore never stable. Keeping the census up is imperative to the survival of the program. The community's residents need constant reminders of the program's operation and the need for continuous referrals. The aim is to establish a waiting list and maintain at least a 90% participation rate.

The plan for ongoing public relations is not as extensive or as concentrated as the initial plan. Once the program has established itself as a viable health service and the staff is 100% involved in the program's operation, less time and energy are spent on outreach. The director makes limited speaking engagements and confines visits to the center by interested persons to monthly, scheduled group visits. Deviations from the scheduled visits are by invitation and appointment only. Mailings are done by request only. Efforts are continued to procure free television and newspaper coverage. Newspaper advertisements are used when indicated by previous advertisement response and the participant census. All inquirers are asked how they heard of the center. The future plan for publicity is largely determined by the results of this information.

Admission Process

The criteria for admission to the center's program are determined by the program's model type. Since admission criteria are part of the center's program publicity (see Figure 12-8), the community residents have information regarding the kind of people the program aims to serve. If there is any question concerning the appropriateness of a particular potential participant, the referring agency or person calls the center for clarification. Additional information and application forms are sent out on request.

When a referral is received in the form of a completed application, the admission process begins. The staff reviews the application together, and a call is then made to the potential participant and/or responsible family member to verify information, obtain additional information, and arrange for a personal interview. The interview preferably includes the prospective participant, as many family members as possible, and at least two staff members, one of whom must be the nurse-director.

The interview gives the staff an opportunity to screen and make a health assessment (see Figure 12-9) prior to admission; it provides necessary information on the potential participant's health needs, psychosocial condition, and the supports available when the person is not at the center. The interview also serves as an opportunity for the prospective participant and family to meet the staff, ask questions, and gain additional information about the program.

The ideal location for the interview is the center because of the opportunity it affords the potential participant and the family to see the center. If feasible, the interview should be scheduled during operating hours to allow them to see the group and observe the program's activities.

When the interview cannot be arranged at the center, a home interview is made. The home visit has the advantage of giving the staff information about the prospective participant's physical and psychosocial environment. In order to give the prospective participant and the family some idea of the center's space and activities, the portfolio of pictures is taken along for viewing. At least two staff persons, one being the nurse-director, make the home visit. Family members are also asked to be present for the home interview.

ADMISSION CRITERIA

Goal Statement

The primary goal of the staff will be to encourage independence. The Center staff will work in conjunction with the participants to develop the best program to meet their needs.

Relatives will also be encouraged to participate in designing the program. Emphasis will be on self care activities (ADL) in order to maintain optimal level of functioning.

Eligibility

Candidates for Adult Day Care will emerge through:

a. Self-referral
b. Family referral
c. Physician referral
d. Agency or organizational referral
e. Personal-care waiting lists
f. Outreach

Admission assessments will be performed by a panel consisting of an R.N. who serves as program director; social caseworker; S.T., P.T., O.T., and Nutritionist who serve as program consultants. This panel will look at the candidate in relation to the established admission criteria which comply with guidelines of the State Department of Public Welfare.

Criteria for Long-Term Participants

To be considered for long-term maintenance in Adult Day Care, the client must:

1. Require services to maintain his current state of emotional, physical, and social health so he does not deteriorate to a point where admission to an institution is necessary.
2. Have limited social contacts.
3. Have physical limitations that prevent him from attending other community facilities where he lives.
4. Have limited access to other facilities where he lives.

Participants who meet two or more of these criteria will be considered for long-term maintenance in the Adult Day Care setting. Participants will be maintained in Adult Day Care from one to five days a week, dependent on their needs.

Figure 12-8. Example of an Adult Day-Care-Center Admission Criteria (From Weston Manor Adult Day Health Center, Weston, Mass., 1977. Form developed by C. O'Brien and G. Dix. Reprinted by permission of the authors and Weston Manor Adult Day Health Center.)

Criteria for Short-Term Clients

The participant will be considered for short term placement in Adult Day Care if he has the potential for:

1. Motivation or remotivation to attend other community facilities.
2. Resolution of emotional or physical problems to a point where he/she can function effectively in the community without assistance.

Short-term care will vary in Adult Day Care according to patient needs—maximum eight months. Each participant has a definite goal set for him and is discharged when this goal is reached.

Criteria Would

1. Benefit the individual. This benefit would be greater than the sum benefits of the individual services provided to him in the community because the catalytic effects of social-interactional opportunities benefit the other services offered in the program.
2. Influence the cost of required services. These may be more costly or less accessible delivered in the home setting or in an institutional placement.
3. Defer costlier inputs in community services through early intervention-prevention.

Priority Would be Given To

1. Those on waiting lists of personal-care homes, who have already been shown to require more care than is available in the home with provision of other available community support services.
2. High-risk groups who are anxious to maintain independence, who, without this support, would be on a waiting list or already institutionalized.
3. Those whom the program has most capacity for benefiting according to admission criteria.

Figure 12-8. (*continued*)

After the interview, the staff members present during the interview have a group discussion and come to a joint decision on the appropriateness of the prospective participant's application. If the decision is made to admit the person to the program, the person and the family are informed of the decision. The desirability of having the person participate in the program is then pursued with the prospective participant and the family. When there is mutual agreement, they are told that the admission process will proceed with the understanding that the person will participate in the program for a one-month trial period. Additionally, they are told that, at the end of this period, a group evaluation involving the participant, the family, and the staff will be done to determine if the program is

ASSESSMENT GUIDE

Initial Screening

At first the participant, his family, or a referring physician or an agency will discuss the need for service. This inquiry will be passed on to the program director who then will proceed to schedule an interview with the client and his family either jointly or separately. In this initial interview, basic information about Adult Day Health Care will be given to the participant and his family with the understanding that neither we nor they are making a commitment that the participant will enter the Adult Day Health Care. This interview is usually conducted by phone.

Initial Assessment

After the initial screening, an interview is set up for the admission assessment. This occurs only if the participant and/or his family, as well as the day-care program director decide that this service is appropriate for the person, and that his needs cannot be met by other community resources. If a family asks for services for someone not able to qualify, then the family will be made aware, and referred to other community services. However, if in the initial screening the person seems to need day-care services, the initial assessment will be carried out by the panel already discussed. Home visits will be made to assess living arrangement, family support, etc., when this seems necessary.

Information Necessary for Assessment

1. Medical Status
2. Mental Status
3. Social Status
4. Physical Status
5. Functional Status
6. Family and Client Feeling and Request of Day

While utilizing the SFA [Systematic Functional Assessment] tool [see Appendix C] in the initial assessment, the panel will be looking at the following:

1. Goals
2. Frequency of participation
3. Duration of participation
4. Plans for subsequent evaluation

The Planning Pattern Would Be:

Assessment/Contract/Evaluation/Recontract

Figure 12-9. Example of an Adult Day-Care-Center Participant Assessment Guide (From Weston Manor Adult Day Health Center, Weston, Mass., 1977. Form developed by C. O'Brien and G. Dix. Reprinted by permission of the authors and Weston Manor Adult Day Health Center.)

meeting the health needs of that individual and of the family as a whole. At this time, problems are discussed and solutions sought. A participant's continued participation in the program is determined by this evaluation, and changes are made in the attendance schedule and care plan as necessary. When a prospective participant decides the program is not appropriate or when the staff decides the candidate is inappropriate for the center program, a notation is made regarding the disposition, and the application is filed for statistical purposes. Whenever possible, referrals are made to other community agencies who might be able to offer the help being sought.

The next step in the admission process is to receive the prospective participant's physician's orders. The center's preadmission medical form is sent to the designated physician, with a note attached indicating the person's desire to participate in the center's program and a brief explanation of the center's purpose. Frequently, a phone call is made to the physician's office to expedite the process. The medical form requests past medical history and medical orders for care. No prospective participant is admitted to the program until this form is completed and returned to the center. For Medicaid participation, a Medicaid assessment form is completed at this time (see Figure 12-10).

The admission process usually takes two to three weeks from the time of receiving the application to the first day of attendance. The length of the waiting period is frequently determined by the physician's response.

Upon admission each participant or responsible person is given copies of the participant's rights and the admission policy. The rights state each participant's rights as a member in the center's program. These rights include the right to refuse treatments, to have access to information regarding care, to participate in the plan of care, to have privacy during the rendering of care, to have information on the costs of services provided, and to discontinue participation in the program at any time. The admission policy states the conditions under which a participant will be asked to discontinue participation in the program. These conditions are that the participant becomes a safety hazard to the group or to himself or herself (that is, a chronic wanderer, physically or verbally abusive, or unable to participate in any of the group activities). Since the admission process may not provide the information needed to determine that these conditions might exist, this policy informs the participant and family when the staff has a right to discharge a person from the program.

Transportation System

Careful thought and investigation of possible transportation arrangements should precede the planning of a transportation system for the proposed center. Any transportation system must include a provision for back-up services. If both non-ambulatory and ambulatory persons are to be accepted into the center's program, transportation must be available that can safely transport both kinds of participants to and from the center.

Whenever possible, the family is expected to provide the participant's transportation. The family is always asked if one or more family members can meet some, if not all, of the participant's transportation needs. However, in many instances this is not possible. Sometimes it may be possible for the family to solicit the help of friends and neighbors in helping with the needed transportation.

The most desirable system of transportation, other than the family, is one provided by the center, with designated staff persons functioning as drivers. Since most of the problems with transportation are in the areas of dependability and communications, the center-operated system can help to alleviate these problems. The center's director can assign the same driver to the same participant routes and communicate with drivers on a regular basis regarding changes in schedules and potential problems in transporting new participants. Being able to instruct the drivers how properly to transport participants is another advantage in using a center-operated and monitored system of transportation.

Since center-provided transportation is not possible for many programs,

---

MASSACHUSETTS DEPARTMENT OF PUBLIC WELFARE
ADULT DAY-CARE PROGRAM — PARTICIPANT ASSESSMENT FORM

Adult Day-Care Facility _____ Date _____

Participant Identifying Information

Participant Name _____ Participant No. _____
Admission Date _____ No. of Scheduled Days per Week _____
Address _____
    Street   Apt.   Town   State   Zip
Participant's Telephone No. _____ Marital Status: S M W D Sep
Sex: M F   Birthdate _____ Race _____
Religious Preference _____ Birthplace _____
Medicaid No. ___/___/___/___ Medicare No. _____ Plan: A B
Blue Cross No. _____ Social Security No. _____
Other Health Insurance (specify) _____
Relative/Guardian _____ Relationship _____
Address _____ Telephone No. _____
Participant Referred From _____

Medical/Social Services (on admission)

Physician _____ Address _____
Telephone No. _____ Date of Physical _____
Participant Hospital Affiliation _____
Certified Home Health Agency (VNA): Nurse ☐ Frequency _____
   Home Health Aide ☐ Frequency _____ Homemaker ☐ Frequency _____
   Other (describe) _____
Therapy at Admission (specify frequency): OT _____ PT _____
   ST _____ Inhalation Therapy _____ SS _____
   Other _____
Hospitalization in Past 2 Years (indicate dates and why) _____

Previous Long-Term Care Facility and Period of Stay:
   Chronic Hosp. _____ Rehabilitation Facility _____
   Mental Health Facility _____ Level I/II NH _____
   Level III NH _____ Rest Home _____
                                       Staff Signature _____

Figure 12-10. Example of a Participant Assessment Form (From Massachusetts Department of Public Health, Adult Day-Care Section. Boston, 1977.)

290 / Part III: Setting Up a Day-Care Program

Participant Name _____

Medical Visits (indicate the date last seen by the following medical professionals. If exact date is unknown, enter the month and year.)
1. Consultant Physician (type of specialist) _____
2. Dentist _____
3. Podiatrist _____
4. Psychiatrist/Psychologist _____
5. Audiologist _____
6. Optometrist _____
7. Other (specify) _____

What affiliation does the participant have with the Department of Mental Health?
_____
_____
_____

Why Is This Person Appropriate for Adult Day Care?
_____
_____
_____
_____
_____
_____
_____

Staff Signature _____

Impairment Items

Sight:	☐ impairment with no compensation	☐ impairment with compensation	☐ complete loss
Hearing:	☐ impairment with no compensation	☐ impairment with compensation	☐ complete loss
Speech:	☐ impairment with no compensation	☐ impairment with compensation	☐ complete loss

Staff Signature _____

Figure 12-10. *(continued)*

arrangements must be made for other systems of transportation. In the Massachusetts center, three different transportation services were contracted with—the Home Care Corporation, a private ambulance company, and a taxi company. Each agreement offers necessary but different services and varies in cost according to the services used. These three contracts offer participants alternatives and include

	Participant Name _____
Medication (Write each medication in its category of primary use. Indicate dose, frequency and route of administration.)	*Medical Diagnosis and Problems*
Analgesics/Narcotics	
Antacids	
Antibiotics/Anti-infection	
Anticoagulants	
Anticonvulsives	
Antihypertensives	Weight Height B/P
Bowel Regulators	*Therapeutic Procedures (Describe specific treatments and whether they are to be delivered by ADH staff or other.)*
Cardiac Regulators	
Diuretics/Electrolytes	
Insulin/Hypoglycemics	
Sedatives/Barbituates	
Tranquilizers/Antidepressants	
Vasodilators	
Vitamin/Iron	
Others (specify)	*Specific Diet*
Allergies	Staff Signature _____

Figure 12-10. *(continued)*

all the needed forms of transportation for both ambulatory and nonambulatory persons. Each form of transportation has its own back-up system to assure service as agreed upon.

The Home Care Corporation provides limited free transportation under federal funding of the Older Americans Act to persons 60 years of age and older. The

Participant Name _____

Functioning Status Items (Please check appropriate boxes and describe following the corresponding statement. State the number of people needed for human assistance.)

1. Mobility Level:
   ☐ Goes outside with help of equipment/device _____
   ☐ Goes outside with human help _____

2. Walking (If the participant uses a wheelchair, do not check.):
   ☐ Uses equipment/device _____
   ☐ Uses human help _____

3. Wheeling (If participant is wheelchair bound.):
   ☐ Human help needed _____
   ☐ Is wheeled (does not participate) _____
   Does the person use electric or manual chair? _____

4. Eating/Feeding:
   ☐ Uses equipment/adaptive device _____
   ☐ Uses human help _____

5. Bathing:
   ☐ Uses equipment/device _____
   ☐ Uses human help _____

6. Dressing:
   ☐ Uses equipment/device _____
   ☐ Uses human help _____

7. Toileting:
   ☐ Uses equipment/device _____
   ☐ Uses human help _____

Staff Signature _____

Figure 12-10. *(continued)*

vans used are equipped with seats and slots to accommodate wheelchairs. This form of transportation is used to provide transport for participants who have no other way of getting to and from the center.

The private ambulance company offers chair-car shuttle service as well as ambulance service. This service is best able to handle the more difficult transportation problems, but is the most costly too. The drivers are specially trained, and

Participant Name _____

Psycho-Social Characteristics
 	
Orientation:
   ☐ Disorientated intermittently   ☐ Day   ☐ Night
   ☐ Disoriented   ☐ Day   ☐ Night
 	
Follows instructions:
   ☐ Follows complex instructions
   ☐ Follows simple instructions
   ☐ Does not follow instructions
 	
Remarks on psycho-social characteristics
_____
_____
_____
_____
_____
_____
_____
_____
_____
_____
_____
_____
_____
_____
_____
_____
_____
_____
 	
Staff Signature

Figure 12-10. *(continued)*

extra personnel are used as needed to lift and transport nonambulatory participants.

The taxi service provides transportation at the lowest cost. However, it is recommended only for ambulatory, alert, well-oriented participants with no physical limitations requiring the help of another person.

Transportation has proven to be the most difficult, ongoing problem many

Participant Name _____
Education (Circle highest grade completed.) Grades 1 2 3 4 5 6 7 8 9 10 11 12   College 1 2 3 4   Masters   Ph.D.
Employment ☐ Currently employed   ☐ Retired   ☐ Sick leave   ☐ Never worked Past or present profession _____
Home and Family Does the participant live: ☐ Alone   ☐ With others (specify) _____ Housing: ☐ Apt.   ☐ Rooming house   ☐ Single family home   ☐ Congregate housing   ☐ Senior housing   ☐ Other _____ On what floor does the participant live? ____   Is it a walk-up?   ☐ Yes   ☐ No What bathing facilities are available?   ☐ Bath   ☐ Shower   ☐ Neither No. of adults in household ____   No. employed in household ____   No. of minors ____ Minors' age range _____ Who will care for the participant on evenings and weekends? Is this person employed? _____ Is this a comfortable arrangement for all? _____ Is the participant on a nursing home waiting list? _____ What services would the participant require without day care: ☐ Family Care   ☐ Friends ☐ Self   ☐ Home Health Services   ☐ Home Care   ☐ Institutionalization ☐ Other _____ Which services are currently delivered but would need to be increased? _____
Transportation How will the participant be transported to and from the Adult Day-Care Facility: ☐ Family   ☐ Community vehicle   ☐ Program van   ☐ Livery   ☐ Taxi ☐ Chair car   ☐ Other _____ If the participant is transported by chair car, why is this transportation necessary? _____   Staff Signature _____

Figure 12-10. *(continued)*

day-care centers face. This center is no exception. Even with a well-planned system and contractual arrangements to help assure the provision of service, multiple problems exist. The Home Care Corporation system of transportation requires that arrangements be made each week and ordered a week in advance. Service is limited to three times weekly for each participant. On certain days and at certain times, no transportation is available. A participant's scheduled days of attendance are therefore governed by the transportation service. The ambulance chair-car shuttle service is available when needed, dependable but expensive. It more than doubles the daily cost of program participation when a round trip is added to the program cost. Although the cost decreases by half when two or more participants ride together, the person designated as the first rider pays the full amount. The taxi service is the most inconsistent in services provided and requires daily calling to inform the service of the participants riding each morning and recalling for the return trip each afternoon. The drivers vary greatly in their willingness to assist participants in and out of their homes as well as in their ability to comprehend a participant's needs in transit.

In an effort to coordinate all the services with the center's operation, transportation is arranged for by the center's staff. The family's cooperation is essential to the smooth operation of the transportation system designed for each individual participant.

Transportation for day trips and outings is another important consideration. Since this adult day-care center has the advantage of being based in an institution where a van is available for participant use, the van is the vehicle of choice in transporting the participants for day trips. However, the van is not equipped to accommodate wheelchairs. When wheelchair-confined participants wish to be included in a trip, another form of transportation (chair-car shuttle service) is used. The cost of renting such accommodations is defrayed by fund-raising projects throughout the year.

Family Involvement

Since, in most instances, the participant is a member of a family, the participant's state of health must be viewed in terms of the family's health. The center's program emphasizes the importance of the family's involvement in the program and aims to meet their health needs as well. The staff's efforts to improve the participant's health are seen as improving the family's health.

The family's involvement is encouraged by the center's staff from the first inquiry about the program, through the admission process, to the followup plan of care upon the participant's discharge from the program. As previously discussed, the participant's family is urged to be present for the interview before admission to the program. The family as a unit makes the commitment to assure the participant attends the center as scheduled. The family assists the staff in planning the transportation and assures that the participant is ready for being transported as planned.

Communication between the staff and the family is a continuous process. Since the family provides the participant's care when he or she is not at the center, it is essential for the staff to develop a harmonious working relationship with the family. The ability of the staff to establish this relationship with the family is of utmost importance in assuring that the participant's plan of care is continued at home. In order to establish and maintain this relationship, the staff uses several methods of communication with the family: frequent telephone conversations, regularly scheduled staff-family reviews of the care plan, meetings when requested by the family with a time and place convenient for the family, family-group discussions centering on common problems, and family counseling sessions.

The family's involvement continues through the discharge of the participant from the program to the carrying out of the discharge plan of care. The family and the staff together agree on the discharge plan. The staff makes the appropriate contacts and referrals, but it is the family who must assume the responsibility for assuring the plan is carried out. In order to support the family in their efforts to follow through with the care plan, the staff maintains contact with the family up to four months or longer after discharge from the program. When possible, the staff arranges for appropriate interventions in order to assure compliance with the plan. A reevaluation of the plan may be necessary. When changes are needed, they are discussed with the family, and referrals are made as indicated. At times, readmission to the center's program may be advised.

In the absence of a family, the center and the community serve as the participant's family. When services other than the center's program are necessary to meet the participant's health-care needs, the center's staff coordinates the services to assure continuity of care for the participants away from the center.

Program Activities

Each day-care center's program is as different as its participants' interests and as innovate as its staff's creativity. Though certain activities are basic to every program, the variety of activities is largely determined by the participants' needs, abilities, and interests (see Figure 12-11). Every program day is, however, structured and purposeful. The week's plan of activities is posted at the beginning of every week, with the schedule for each day's activities, from the time of arrival to the time of departure, five days a week.

The purpose of this day-care center's program, to provide a therapeutic environment and rehabilitative activities for its participants, can be seen in the outline of a program day shown in Figure 12-12.

An awareness of the fraility of the elderly and their functional activities is important in deciding what activities are to be offered at what times during the day. The family's need for arrivals and departures in keeping with their working schedules and arrangements for continuing care before and after the day-care services are other considerations. Days of attendance may need to be adjusted according to the person's energy levels, family schedule, and center's attendance schedule.

TO FIND OUT WHERE ADULT DAY CARE PARTICIPANTS' INTERESTS LIE USE CHECK LIST

	YES	NO			YES	NO
FOOD SERVING			**BIRTHDAY RECOGNITION**			
1. Coffee, tea	☐	☐	1. Announcement and presentation of those having birthdays	☐	☐
2. Pastries	☐	☐			
3. Regular luncheon	☐	☐			
4. Regular dinner	☐	☐	2. Singing of "Happy Birthday"	☐	☐
5. Meals on special occasions	☐	☐	3. General congratulations	☐	☐
QUIET GAMES			4. Party hats	☐	☐
1. Cards	☐	☐	5. Crowning of the oldest man and woman having birthdays	☐	☐
2. Dice games	☐	☐			
3. Bingo	☐	☐	6. Refreshments	☐	☐
4. Puzzles	☐	☐	7. Special cake(s) with candle(s)	☐	☐
5. Shuffleboard	☐	☐	8. Decorations	☐	☐
6. Croquet	☐	☐	**EXCURSIONS**		
7. Horseshoes	☐	☐	1. Libraries	☐	☐
8. Checkers	☐	☐	2. Museums	☐	☐
9. Chess	☐	☐	3. Parks	☐	☐
10. Guessing games	☐	☐	4. Concerts	☐	☐
11. Writing games	☐	☐	5. Lakes	☐	☐
12. Spelling bee	☐	☐	6. Zoos	☐	☐
13. Other table games	☐	☐	7. Historical sites	☐	☐
ACTIVE GAMES			8. Churches	☐	☐
1. Volleyball	☐	☐	9. Industrial plants	☐	☐
2. Handball	☐	☐	**HOME TALENT**		
3. Badminton	☐	☐	1. Poetry	☐	☐
4. Golf	☐	☐	2. Imaginative skits	☐	☐
5. Bowling	☐	☐	3. Square dancing	☐	☐
6. Skating	☐	☐	4. Folk dancing	☐	☐
PARTIES			5. Individual singing	☐	☐
1. Birthdays	☐	☐	6. Group singing	☐	☐
2. Special Holidays	☐	☐	7. Instrumental playing	☐	☐
3. Costume parties	☐	☐	8. Rhythm band	☐	☐
4. Carnivals	☐	☐	9. Newspaper writing	☐	☐
			10. Recitations	☐	☐
			11. Local history chats	☐	☐
			12. Dramatics	☐	☐

Figure 12-11. Example of a Survey of Adult Day-Care-Center Participants' Interests (From Weston Manor Adult Day Health Center, Weston, Mass., 1977. Form developed by C. O'Brien and G. Dix. Reprinted by permission of the authors and Weston Manor Adult Day Health Center.)

	YES	NO			YES	NO
OUTSIDE ENTERTAINMENT			**ARTS AND CRAFTS**			
1. Visual aids	☐	☐	1. Clay and plastercraft	☐	☐
2. Humorists	☐	☐	2. Needlecraft	☐	☐
3. Musicians	☐	☐	3. Woodcraft	☐	☐
4. Dancers	☐	☐	4. Leathercraft	☐	☐
5. Singers	☐	☐	5. Drawings	☐	☐
GENERAL EDUCATIONAL PROGRAMS			6. Painting (all tempera)	☐	☐
1. Book reviews	☐	☐	7. Weaving	☐	☐
2. Lectures	☐	☐	8. Metal	☐	☐
3. Discussions	☐	☐	9. Mosaics	☐	☐
4. Travelogues	☐	☐	10. Flower making	☐	☐
5. Citizenship programs	☐	☐	11. Flower arranging	☐	☐
6. Current events	☐	☐	12. Jewelry	☐	☐
SPECIFIC EDUCATIONAL PROGRAMS			13. Belts	☐	☐
1. Personality courses	☐	☐	14. Quilting	☐	☐
2. Budgeting on a small income	☐	☐	15. Bookbinding	☐	☐
3. Nutrition	☐	☐	16. Printing	☐	☐
4. Housing	☐	☐	17. Repair toys	☐	☐
5. Family relations	☐	☐	18. Make toys	☐	☐
6. Decline of hearing	☐	☐	19. Fly tying	☐	☐
7. Eyesight conservation	☐	☐	20. Lapidary	☐	☐
8. Avoidance of home accidents and their treatment	☐	☐	**COMMUNITY SERVICE**			
			1. Philanthropic fund-raising	☐	☐
9. Social action (ex. better neighborhood lighting)	☐	☐	2. Civil defense activity	☐	☐
			3. Assisting youth-serving	☐	☐
			4. Service to community bodies	☐	☐
VISITS TO SHUT-IN AND/OR ILL			**OTHER**			
1. Sick committee	☐	☐	1. Bachelors' and widowers' sewing service	☐	☐
2. Home calls	☐	☐				
3. Remembrances	☐	☐	2. Ladies' night	☐	☐
4. Audio-visual aids	☐	☐	3. Corn roast	☐	☐
5. Writing letters for the ill	☐	☐	4. Business meetings	☐	☐
6. Reading to the shut-in	☐	☐	5. Visiting or reading at club gatherings	☐	☐
			6. Gardening	☐	☐
			7. Upkeep chores around home	☐	☐

Figure 12-11. *(continued)*

The prime considerations in program planning are

1. participant/staff involvement
2. equal spacing of meal and snacks

3. maximum energy activities in the morning
4. alternating activity with quiet times.

Examples of a week's programs for recreational and nursing-care activities are shown in Figures 12-13 and 12-14.

PROGRAM ACTIVITIES

8:00–10:00 A.M. *Arrival time and socialization period*—This is determined by the transportation system being used and the participant's ability to be ready for the transportation. As the participants arrive the program day is started by greetings and conversations with the staff and others. New participants are introduced. To enhance reality orientation a large printed calendar and clock inform participants of the time, day, and date. In addition events of the day and program are discussed. During this discussion snacks are available for all participants. The participants are encouraged to help themselves when this is possible. This is also a time for special announcements such as birthdays or holidays, etc. Other business items affecting the group can also be mentioned at this time, and reports from special committees within the group are made at this time.

10:00–11:30 A.M. *Individual projects*—Each participant is encouraged to use skills known and develop new skills through individual projects (i.e., painting, writing, knitting, reading) according to personal interests. At this time attention should be given to new group members or members not motivated to participate in an individual project.

8:00–3:00 P.M. *Nursing treatments and medication*—Nursing care is provided throughout the day as ordered by the participants' physicians and as determined as needed by the nurse.

Therapy—Therapy is given as ordered by the participants' physicians.

Personal care—Participants receive assistance with their bathing, dressing, and grooming needs as required.

Health teaching—Both informal and formal health education is given the participants, in groups and individually, throughout the program day and every program day.

Counseling—Group and individual counseling is offered to assist participants with any social, family, or personal problems.

Therapeutic diets and nourishments—Every participant is served at lease one-third of the recommended dietary allowance as stated by the National Research Council. Meals and snacks offered are in keeping with the participants' prescribed diets.

Figure 12-12. Example of Program-Activities Outline for an Adult Day-Care Center (From Weston Manor Adult Day Health Center, Weston, Mass., 1977. Form developed by C. O'Brien and G. Dix. Reprinted by permission of the authors and Weston Manor Adult Day Health Center.)

11:30-12:30 P.M. *Lunch period*—Lunch is served at this particular time and it is the consensus that lunch should be served at the table family style. Tables should be arranged attractively with tablecloths and flowers. Since there may be many slow eaters or disabled participants the lunch period should be for a full hour. Special occasions could be observed at this time. One-third of the participant's daily nutritional intake is received at this meal. Diets are adhered to in the preparation of the noon meal.

12:30-1:30 P.M. *Quiet hour*—Compulsory rest time for some is required. Those not needing a rest period can at this time continue with their own individual projects but should not interfere with those who need rest time.

1:30-2:30 P.M. *Group activities*—all activities are designed to meet the physical, social, emotional, spiritual, and/or educational needs of the participants. These activities include:

exercises	bowling
singing	shopping
dancing	rest
games and cards	picnics
gardening	concerts
cooking and sharing food	museums churches
discussion groups	theatres
trips	community service
sporting events	

2:30-3:00 P.M. *Afternoon snack*—This period is structured as the morning period. Again, juices, milk, a hot beverage, piece of cheese, toast, or other healthy tidbits are served.

3:00-5:00 P.M. *Departure time*—As with the arrival time, this is determined by the participant's form of transportation. Farewells are made with a reminder of the day and date the staff will be seeing the participant again. Individual projects are sent home with the participants if they so desire. When left at the Center, the projects are identified and stored for the participant until further work is to be done on them at the Center. The program day has ended. It has been between six and eight hours the participants have spent together at the day health Center. During those hours the program provided the participants socialization, reality orientation, nursing care, therapy, health care, education, counseling, nourishing foods, relaxation, recreation, and exercise.

Figure 12-12. *(continued)*

The key to any successful day-care-center program is flexibility. Thoughtful, careful interviewing must go into the hiring of the staff and into the planning of the program. Experimentation involving participant-staff input each step of the way is essential to a growing, productive, and well-balanced program. If the staff is flexible and willing to readily adapt to necessary changes, the participants will follow without much difficulty as long as changes are integrated slowly and with advanced preparation.

| ADULT DAY-CARE CENTER: _____ |
| SCHEDULE FOR WEEK OF: _____ |

MONDAY	TUESDAY	WEDNESDAY	THURSDAY	FRIDAY
8:00 Welcome	8:00 Welcome	8:00 Welcome	8:00 Welcome	8:00 Welcome
8:00–9:00 Reality orientation	8:00–9:00 Reality orientation	8:00–9:00 Reality orientation	8:00–9:00 Reality orientation	8:00–9:00 Reality orientation
9:00 Snack & news discussion	9:00 Snack & news discussion	9:00 Snack & news discussion	9:00 Snack & news discussion	9:00 Snack & news discussion
9:30 R.O.M. exercises & *outdoor activities	9:30 R.O.M. exercises & *outdoor activities	9:30 R.O.M. exercises & *outdoor activities	9:30 R.O.M. exercises & *outdoor activities	9:30 R.O.M. exercises & *outdoor activities
10:00 †Individual projects	10:00 †Individual projects	10:00 †Individual projects	10:00 †Individual projects	10:00 †Individual projects
11:30 Lunch	11:30 Lunch	11:30 Lunch	11:30 Lunch	11:30 Lunch
12:30–1:30 Quiet time	12:30–1:30 Quiet time	12:30–1:30 Quiet time	12:30–1:30 Quiet time	12:30–1:30 Quiet time
1:30–2:30 Community service work	1:30–2:30 Group project	1:30–2:30 Group project	1:30–2:30 Group project	1:30–2:30 Bingo
2:30 Snack	2:30 Snack	2:30 Snack	2:30 Snack	2:30 Snack
3:00 Departure	3:00 Departure	3:00 Departure	3:00 Departure	3:00 Departure

*Weather permitting
†Individuals are allowed optional choices.

Figure 12-13. Example of a Week's Calendar for an Adult Day-Care-Center's Recreation Program (From Weston Manor Adult Day Health Center, Weston, Mass., 1977. Form developed by C. O'Brien and G. Dix. Reprinted by permission of the authors and Weston Manor Adult Day Health Center.)

| ADULT DAY-CARE CENTER: _____ |
| SCHEDULE FOR WEEK OF: _____ |

MONDAY	TUESDAY	WEDNESDAY	THURSDAY	FRIDAY
8:30–9:30 Baths & shampoos	8:30–9:30 Baths & shampoos	8:30–9:30 Baths & shampoos	8:30–9:30 Baths & shampoos	8:30–9:30 Baths & shampoos
	9:30–3:30 Beauty & barber shop open	9:30–3:30 Beauty & barber shop open		
11:00–12:00 Treatments & therapy sessions	11:00–12:00 Therapy sessions	11:00–12:00 Treatment & therapy sessions	11:00–12:00 Therapy sessions	11:00–12:00 Treatment & therapy sessions
11:30–12:00 Stroke club		11:30–12:00 Stroke club		11:30–12:00 Stroke club
12:45–1:00 Healthy hints	12:45–1:00 Healthy hints	12:45–1:00 Healthy hints	12:45–1:00 Healthy hints	12:45–1:00 Healthy hints
1:00–1:30 Baths & shampoos	1:30–2:30 Nail care	1:00–1:30 Baths & shampoos	1:30–2:30 Shampoos & nail care	1:00–1:30 Shampoos & nail care
			Podiatry care 1 Thursday each month	
2:00–2:30 Individual instruction for home treatment as needed	2:00–2:30 Individual instruction & reminders for home treatment as needed	2:00–2:30 Individual instruction & reminders for home treatment as needed	2:00–2:30 Individual instruction & reminders for home treatment as needed	2:00–2:30 Individual instruction & reminders for home treatment as needed

Figure 12-14. Example of a Week's Calendar for an Adult Day-Care Center's Nursing-Care Activities (From Weston Manor Adult Day Health Center, Weston, Mass., 1977. Form developed by C. O'Brien and G. Dix. Reprinted by permission of the authors and Weston Manor Adult Day Health Center.)

Role of the State Association

In the fall of 1978, the Massachusetts Association of Adult Day Care Centers was formed by a small group of energetic day-care-center directors who recognized a need for an organized support group. Membership was open to all Massachusetts day-care centers, with dues set on a yearly basis. Although still in its embryonic stages, the association represents 34 of the 43 adult day-care centers in Massachusetts.

With the bylaws established and the officers elected on a yearly ballot, the association has moved in a positive direction by establishing committees on standards of practice, education, personnel policies, public relations, legislative information, and liaison relationship with state departments. The association has quarterly meetings, at which communications are shared, committee reports are given, and current issues pertinent to day-care services on the state and national levels are discussed. Recently, the association directed its efforts toward presenting its rationale for a rate increase under Medicaid to the Massachusetts Rate Setting Commission.

Another example of the evolving trend toward statewide adult day-center associations is in Michigan. The Michigan Association of Senior Day Care Centers (MASDCC) was formally founded in the fall of 1978. It began with nonprofit senior day-care-center directors and coordinators exchanging information on the operation and problems of their centers. As a result of these early meetings, the MASDCC has formulated goals based on the primary purposes of adult day care and the barriers to its accomplishments.

It has stated that senior day-care centers are established to prevent, postpone, and/or limit institutionalization of disabled persons over 60 years of age. In addition, it has identified the following goals:

1. to promote the independent living of older people to the highest degree possible
2. to provide information and education to the community regarding day-care services for older people
3. to assist in the orderly development of day-care services for the older person as an appropriate health-care and social service
4. to advocate policy that provides a continuum of appropriate health-care and social services for the older person
5. to advocate policy that identifies senior day-care centers as an essential part of the continuum of appropriate health-care and social services

The MASDCC will not only assist persons in obtaining the appropriate care, but will also be of assistance to persons wishing to develop a nonprofit senior day-care center in their community.

Associations such as these are beginning to be recognized in various states as the organizations that represent adult day-care centers, their purposes, and responsibilities to the public. Hopefully their strength and influence will continue to grow and represent the directors of adult day-care centers collectively, thereby having a positive impact on the long-term-care system for the elderly. Another important development in solidifying a national perspective for adult day care is

Resource, a newsletter published and distributed by the Massachusetts Department of Public Welfare's Adult Day Health Services Department to inform adult day-care directors of issues pertaining to adult day-care centers in the United States.

Summary

The previous discussion has been limited to those program components important to the implementation of a rehabilitative model of an adult day-care center within an institutional setting. Obviously, some considerations of primary concern to planners of community-based centers or of other model types may differ slightly or include additional components. However, all the program components discussed are essential to a well-planned, successful day-care center. Where the primary emphasis is placed in the planning of a program will depend on the program's philosophy and objectives.

It is important to remember that each step of the process toward program implementation requires information on federal and state guidelines regarding adult day-care services, knowledge of funding sources, and the services of competent health, social service, and business professionals. Whatever the model type or location of the center, the planner must be prepared to address these elements, which are critical to the successful planning and operation of a day-care center. When this process is followed, the center's program goals will be achieved.

13

Records and the Problem-Oriented Record System

Carole Lium O'Brien, RN, MS

Functions of a Record System

Over the last century, health- and human-service professionals have been using the same style of recording information on their clients. Gradually, these records evolved into specialty-oriented data collectors, seemingly focused more on who did what and when rather than on a logical, ordered plan of care clearly identified to resolve the client's problem. Moreover, data on one client problem ran throughout the entire record and made it difficult to find specific information about the problem.

In order to correct this deficit and maintain adequate records, planners must clearly understand the purpose of a record system. The well-organized and maintained recording and reporting system serves two main functions. First, it serves as a control system that assures that needed services are provided according to an identified and prescribed plan. In the process of setting goals, certain specific outcomes are enumerated, often with measurable indicators of accomplishment (see Chapter 14 for further discussion of program evaluation). Record keeping is made easier through the use of a well-defined record system, which can supply the basic data required for program evaluation.

Second, the record system provides a rich source of information for planning and evaluating the care being given. Identification of the population characteristics will determine the types of services needed. For example, older population groups usually require more extensive and time-consuming professional services than younger populations. By reviewing the records periodically, the service provider has a basis for deciding the extent to which the services provided are relevant to the particular needs of the population served. In short, the provider can judge whether or not the care approaches appear to be suitable and can then decide whether they are as effective as possible. The directors of adult day-care centers, by reviewing the composite record, also provide themselves with the information needed to decide whether or not the level of staffing is adequate to the work being performed.

Types of Record Systems

The record-keeping system in any agency includes many types of records. Each type of record is composed of numerous forms. Agencies select the type of record or record system from many different sources. When computer analysis is part of the record system, certain parts of the reporting must be on standardized forms so that they can easily be converted to the computer. For the purposes of discussion in this chapter, identification of various types of records will be made, but full discussion will be given only to the problem-oriented record system, because it is the most adaptable to adult day-care centers and uses a multidisciplinary team approach.

The various types of record-keeping systems are

1. The service record system, which provides a register of services rendered to the participants of a program.
2. The accounting record system, which helps calculate time and effort expenditures. This system may serve as a valuable system for adult day-care centers that wish to conduct a detailed time study showing how their staff is spending their time daily in certain activities.
3. The control record system, which assures the director that program goals are met through tabulating requests for service, developing a waiting list, and estimating future trends for the types of services that will be needed. In an adult day-care center, one easy way to implement such a system is to develop an index file that follows a number system. This type of information can also be stored and retrieved in a computer.
4. The problem-oriented record system, which provides a multidisciplinary team approach to care being given to the participants in a program.

Criteria for a Record System

Although the adult day-care-center directors make the ultimate decision about the record-keeping system to be used in their programs, they should include input from all the multidisciplinary team members in making their decision. In order to make this decision, it is helpful to understand the criteria that the system is expected to meet. An effective record system should meet the following criteria:

1. It should possess suitable uniformity to provide for easy recording and tabulation, which permits interunit and interservice collation.
2. It should require the minimal amount of time consistent with the record's purpose.
3. It should be quickly obtainable to the service provider.
4. It should be subject to coordination on those parameters considered important for planning and evaluation.
5. It should provide for a participant's privacy while in use.

The Computer

The use of computers in adult day-care centers is becoming increasingly common. This advancement is particularly significant in decreasing the amount of time that professionals and paraprofessionals expend in record keeping. In Massachusetts, computerized billing is a service that assists adult day-care programs in billing accuracy, as well as more immediate reimbursement from Medicaid. Furthermore, it enables quick storage and retrieval for future use. The directors involved in this system must use the forms provided by the computer company and complete them by a specific date. Ability to comply with these two requirements assures a smoother functioning of the whole process.

The Annual Report

The director who is writing an annual report should consider that it will inform the advisory board members, the agency's board of directors, and the community at large. Furthermore, it should specify problem areas needing further work. Several points should be considered by the program director in writing the annual report:

1. Develop an outline.
2. Include all areas of major accomplishment in the body of the report.
3. Illustrate with examples some of the year's highlights.
4. Organize the report so that essential information can be easily found.

5. Recognize other professionals and agencies who have been involved with and assisted in the program.

An example of an annual report is given in Figure 13-1.

Overview of the Problem-Oriented Record System

In the past ten years, frequent references to the problem-oriented record system in long-term-care settings have appeared in all types of health and other professional literature. The problem-oriented system, the core of which is the problem-solving process, provides a method for communicating, documenting, and evaluating health-care activities performed by the members of the multidisciplinary team on behalf of the program participants. This chapter addresses the use of the problem-oriented record as an evaluation tool. Long before the problem-oriented system achieved its popularity, however, problem-solving methodology had been recognized as an inherent part of providing health care. Figure 13-2 (on page 316) gives parallels between the scientific method and the problem-oriented system.

The problem-oriented record system, like every system, has parts and components and cannot function well without them. In such a system, the quality of each component determines the quality of the overall results. Furthermore, all components of the system must relate to one another. When all the parts are in place and the connecting feedback loops are functioning, the system will come alive and work very effectively.

This problem-oriented record system entails the three following parts:

1. the record itself
2. the audit of the record
3. the correction of deficiencies [1(p6)]

In 1969, Dr. Lawrence L. Weed worked on developing such a system at the University of Vermont, where, with his guidance and direction, the system of problem-oriented records became the accepted standard for all medical and surgical services.[2] Through his influence, the problem-oriented record has become an accepted practice in the health-care system. Not only health-care facilities, but also other disciplines (for example, social work), private practices, and educational institutions throughout the country have taken on this record-keeping system. It is believed that such a system can be utilized to benefit adult day-care participants. In addition to providing a logical, organized, and systematic approach to client management, it enhances all levels of education of professionals working in adult day care and, further, it contributes to research in this field.

Dear Reader:

It is with great pleasure that I report to you the success of the Weston Manor Adult Day Health Center's first year of operation. The Center opened on December 19, 1978 with one participant and is presently providing services for eighteen to twenty older people Monday through Friday. Participants attend the Center two to five days weekly with the exception of one participant who attends one day weekly due to financial limitations. At this time, there is a waiting list for admission.

The staff has seen significant positive changes in the persons attending the Center and their families continually express their appreciation and satisfaction with the program. The objectives of the program have been met and the staff's efforts will continue to be directed toward fulfilling the program objectives and meeting the Center's goals.

Sincerely,

ADVISORY COUNCIL
1978–1979

Mrs. _____, Director, _____ Council on Aging
Ms. _____, Executive Director, _____ Elder Services, Inc.
Mrs. _____, Assistant Professor, Boston College School of Nursing
Mrs. _____, Social Worker, _____ Council on Aging
Dr. _____, Physician
Mrs. _____, Director, _____ Council on Aging
Ms. _____, Assistant Director, _____ VNA
Mrs. _____, _____ Council on Aging

The Advisory Council linked the Weston Manor Adult Day Health Center to the communities it served. The Council provided the director with information on the communities' needs and concerns. Additionally the Council assisted the director in her policy-making decisions. The director sought the Council's advice on the Center's program and future direction.

Figure 13-1. Example of an Adult Day-Care Center Annual Report (From Weston Manor Adult Day Health Center, Weston, Mass., 1979–80 Annual Report, by C. O'Brien and G. Dix. Reprinted by permission of the authors and Weston Manor Adult Day Health Center.)

PROGRAM GOAL AND OBJECTIVES

Center Goal

The Weston Manor Adult Day Health Center provides preventive, maintenance, and therapeutic rehabilitative services to those physically and mentally disabled, low income, and minority adults sixteen years or older with particular emphasis on those persons sixty years and older living in the West Suburban Elder Service area of Belmont, Brookline, Needham, Newton, Waltham, Watertown, Wellesley, and Weston.

Center Objectives

1. Prevention of premature institutionalization
2. Prevention of social isolation
3. Decrease the incidence and severity of social and physical disabilities
4. Provision of social relief for families
5. Promotion of good health practices through health teaching and counseling
6. Assistance in detection and assessment of illness
7. Assistance to families caring for a disabled family member
8. Ease transition of person from community to nursing home living

STAFF, STUDENTS AND VOLUNTEERS

In October of 1978 the Weston Manor Nursing Home nurse consultant, _____ _____, and the administrator, _____ _____, hired the Center's program director, _____ _____. The program director filled the position of registered nurse and director of the program. These positions were required by the guidelines for adult day health services by the Department of Public Welfare. Since the Center desired to be a provider of services for Medicaid recipients, the DPW guidelines had to be met, an application submitted, approval obtained, and a provider number issued prior to opening the Center. The director had to hire a second staff person to meet the requirements. The decision was made to hire a person who had the ability to plan, organize, and implement an activities program as well as serve as the Center's counselor and assistant director.

The program director hired _____ in November 1978 to be the activities director and counselor. With this staffing and the administrator, the nurse consultant, a physician, a physical therapist, an occupational therapist, a speech therapist, a social worker, and a dietician as consultants, the Center opened in December, 1978.

These two full-time staff people were the direct service providers and administrative staff for the Center from December to May. Consultants provided one or more hours a month as needed with the Weston Manor administrator and the Weston Manor nurse consultant being the primary resource people for the staff.

Due to the Center's growth, the need for nursing services by the participants, and the DPW requirements for a staff-participant ratio of one to six, a third staff position was created. The decision was made to hire a

Figure 13-1. *(continued)*

licensed practical nurse who would assist the director with the nursing services as well as serve as an assistant to the activities director. In May, 1979 _____, L.P.N. joined the Center's staff.

Throughout the summer months it became increasingly evident that the activities director/counselor was having difficulty meeting her job requirements. With the increase in participation and the wide range of disabilities and handicaps, the activities program required a person with experience in adapting activities to meet each person's abilities. (Priority had to be given the activities component of this position.) Since the activities director's strengths lay in her counseling skills rather than in the area of activities, the decision was made to make a change in the staff. This change in staffing made possible the hiring of a person skilled in activities for the elderly and handicapped, and placed the responsibilities for counseling on the director since she was the best qualified to assume that role.

After interviewing many applicants, _____ was hired to fill the now revised position of activities director. She had had many years of experience in directing activities programs for nursing home residents as well as experience as a nurse's aide. She rapidly developed a varied and interesting program which provided activities and stimulation for each participant.

These three full-time staff members met the DPW requirements and the administrative and direct service needs of the program. Their time was allocated accordingly: the program director divided her time equally between administrative tasks and direct service; the licensed practical nurse spent twenty-five percent of her time administratively and seventy-five percent providing direct service; the activities director's time was ninety percent service provider and ten percent planner and recorder.

During this year the Center benefited from having several nursing students and volunteers. They augmented the Center's program while receiving an excellent educational experience. Five nursing students, three from Northeastern University and one from Boston College, spent 234 hours at the Center. They provided nursing services while having an opportunity to learn more about the aging process, the elderly, and the management of their health problems. Nine volunteers contributed their time and talents to the program. They fulfilled many and varied needs of the participants and staff. Volunteer hours for 1978–1979 totaled 354.5 hours. In addition staff members from WSES [West Suburban Elder Services] assisted the Center staff during periods of absenteeism and staff changes.

All students and volunteers were informed of their responsibilities and of the Center's procedures. They were screened for their interest in working with the elderly and handicapped, given an orientation, provided supervision, and received on-going educational information. Having them was an enriching experience for both the staff and participants.

PARTICIPATION IN THE PROGRAM

From December 19, 1978 to December 31, 1979 fifty-three persons participated in the Center's program. Twenty-three persons were discharged from the Center during this same time period. As of December 31, 1979 there were thirty persons attending the Center with the average attendance three days weekly. Of those twenty-three persons discharged from the program: ten remained living in the community being referred to

Figure 13-1. *(continued)*

other agencies and services, seven were admitted to nursing homes, and six were admitted to hospitals.

Growth in program participation was as follows:

Month	Persons Served	Number of Service Days
Dec. '78	1	2
Jan. '79	3	9
Feb. '79	9	48
Mar. '79	13	152
Apr. '79	18	288
May '79	23	466
June '79	23	695
July '79	25	946
Aug. '79	26	1247
Sept. '79	27	1519
Oct. '79	30	1847
Nov. '79	31	2206
Dec. '79	30	2524

Participants lived in all the West Suburban Elder Service areas as well as other communities. The distribution of participation by community was: Belmont—1, Brookline—3, Framingham—3, Natick—1, Needham—3, Newton—14, Sudbury—1, Waltham—16, Waterton—7, Wellesley—3, and Weston—1. Participants were admitted to the program according to need rather than location. At the present time there is no day health program serving the outer West Suburban area.

PARTICIPANT PROFILE

Fifty-three participants were admitted to the Center from December 19, 1978 to December 31, 1979. Here is some information about them:

The average age was 75 years
The age range was 51 to 87 years of age
All 53 received nursing services and staff counseling
47 had chronic physical disabilities
26 had mental disabilities
11 lived with their spouses
26 lived with relatives
16 lived alone
12 were assisted with nursing home placement
20 were referred to other services for needs in addition to the day health center program
4 were wheelchair bound
2 used a wheelchair for transport only
21 received physical therapy consultation
10 received occupational therapy consultation
1 received speech therapy
17 had gait training with walker and/or cane
13 had an individualized exercise program
28 were taught increased independence in activities of daily living and
15 were given assistance with bladder training

SERVICES

A wide range of services were provided by the nursing staff during the past year. No applicant was excluded from the program because of nursing care requirements. However some applicants were deferred for admission until the L.P.N. was hired. The following nursing services were given: Monitoring cardiac and lung sounds, blood pressures,

Figure 13-1. *(continued)*

administration of medicines, evaluation of medication effectiveness and reactions, teaching of medication regimes, evaluation of pain and its management, consultations with physicians, emergency treatment with hospital transfer, supervision and teaching of therapeutic diets, monitoring of weights and edema, health education, diabetic foot care, special foot treatments, application of splints, braces, and prostheses, individualized therapy and exercise programs, moist and dry heat treatments, decubitus dressings, removal of ear cerumen, eye treatments, bathing, grooming, shampoos, manicures, toileting, incontinence care, bladder training, bowel training, instruction in ADL, and laundrying of personal clothing. Other services included individual and family counseling, arranging for physician appointments and transportation, taking participants to the dentist, the optician, and physicians, and making home visit assessments when necessary for the implementation of the care plan.

The staff had monthly consultation with the consultants which greatly assisted the staff's ability to meet the health care needs of the participants. These consultations were held at least monthly with the social worker, physical therapist, occupational therapist, and nutritionist. The speech therapist conferred with the staff as needed. Only one participant received speech therapy and this was for a two-month period. The physician consultant was available; however in most cases the participant's personal physician was consulted rather than the physician-consultant.

Additional services were provided by a podiatrist and a laboratory technician. The podiatrist visited every four to six weeks to offer foot care to those who needed it. Lab work was done as ordered by the physician.

A program of reality orientation for the confused participants was started in September by the director. Every day five to eight participants spend one half hour in a group apart from the others receiving basic information. These sessions were originally led by the director but in late October one of the alert participants assumed responsibility for the program and has competently led the group since then under the supervision of the staff.

ACTIVITIES

A structured program of therapeutic, social, and recreational activities which offered stimulation and variety was planned and implemented throughout the year. Group and individual activities were an integral part of the program. Some of these activities included craft projects such as: creweling, greeting card making, rag dogs, book holders, planters, decorative art works, and holiday decorations. Other activities were: community service work with R.S.V.P. recognition, table games, card games, word games, cards, bowling, ball throwing, walks, cooking, story-telling, sing-a-longs, indoor and outdoor gardening, and trips.

During the fall, items such as yarn dogs, pine cone decorations, greeting-card wreaths, yarn wreaths, baby blankets, shawls, sweater/cap sets, and mittens were made. In December these items were sold at the Weston Manor holiday bazaar. The participants made ninety dollars on the sale of their hand crafted articles and decided to spend the money on a stereo system for the Center's enjoyment.

Other activities were: outings, speakers, slide shows, and special events. Trips were taken to the Arboretum, a Waltham resident's private estate and gardens, Wilson's Farms in Lexington, Ashland State Park, and

Figure 13-1. *(continued)*

Christmas shopping at the Natick Mall. Maggie Kuhn, Congressman Robert Drinan, a Boston Edison representative, and B.C. and Northeastern nursing students presented educational information to the participants. Slide and Movie presentations included: The Smithsonian, Williamsburg Gardens, Flowering Trees, Plants and Shrubs, Gardens of Italy, Scenes of Italy, Aging Process, and Rescue from Isolation. The participants were invited to the Weston Manor Nursing Home's "Nostalgia Day" in October. Holiday parties were enjoyed on Halloween, the day before Thanksgiving, and the Friday prior to Christmas. On December 18, the participants and staff welcomed people from the community to join in the celebration of the Center's first anniversary. On December 19, a holiday dinner was served and Santa Claus visited everyone.

During the spring and summer months an outside garden was prepared for planting. Tomatoes, cucumbers, eggplants, squash, and marigolds were grown and harvested. Marigolds adorned the tables throughout the late summer and fall. The vegetables were enjoyed with the noon meals. Each interested person had a hand in the planting, growing, and harvesting of "our" garden. In the winter indoor plants were grown and enjoyed as they flourished in the Center's warmth and eastern exposure to the delight of all.

Every participant entered into at least usually one or more activities which were designed to meet his or her interests and capabilities. These activities were held within a group setting which naturally lent itself to increased socialization. The activities program provided an opportunity for social interaction while meeting the person's need for therapeutic activities, a sense of worth, and a sharing experience with a peer group.

PROGRAM EVALUATION AND OUTCOME

Program evaluation was established at the Weston Manor Adult Day Health Center during the planning phase of the program's development. During this process many types of evaluation methods were discussed. From these discussions a decision was made to use both formative and summative methods.

The formative methods included use of the problem-oriented record, participant and family meetings, consultation from the DPW's consulting staff, weekly team meetings, and a semi-annual advisory council meeting. In addition, the Systematic Functional Assessment Tool, which is a comprehensive assessment and evaluation tool, was used for both formative and summative evaluation at admission, six months later, yearly, and at discharge.

The summative evaluation methods included the retrospective audit for the participant's records and the reasons for discharge. Participant and family benefits were also analyzed. Records received a monthly evaluation, including a look at the number of participants attending the program, for how many days, what services were received, and the participation in each activity.

Of the Center's participant population, seventeen persons were being maintained in the community who would otherwise be in nursing homes, or be awaiting placement in a nursing home. All participants were prevented from being socially isolated by their participation in the program and the program provided opportunities for peer interaction to all. Participants and their families, when applicable, were given health information by the professional nursing staff through a planned educational, on-going health main-

Figure 13-1. *(continued)*

tenance program. Physical limitations had been decreased in twenty-two of the fifty-three persons admitted to the program, and twelve persons increased their abilities to function independently. Forty families were helped through counseling and referral. Of the fifty-three participants who had participated in the program, twelve were discharged to nursing home care. These twelve persons and their families were significantly helped in accepting a change in residency.

FUTURE PLANS

The Weston Manor Adult Day Health Center plans to expand its space, participation, and staffing. The addition of another room in the Weston Manor Nursing Home to the Center's existing space will provide 1680 square feet for its program. With this increase in space, the Center plans to provide services for twenty-four participants daily and expand its staff to include a full-time social worker. At the present time six people await admission to the program with inquiries regarding the availability of admission to the program markedly on the increase since October 1979. The need for expansion has been determined. The social problems of participants and their families make the addition of a full-time social worker to the staff a priority for 1980. This professional person will greatly contribute to the present professional staff's ability to meet the participants' and their families' health needs.

FUNDING

After the owners of the Weston Manor Nursing and Retirement Home agreed to provide space to establish a day health center, the decision was made to apply for grant funding. Since the West Suburban Elder Services area plan included an elderly day health program and this was a service lacking in the area, the decision was made to apply to WSES for a grant. November 1978 the Weston Manor Adult Day Health Center was notified of a grant award for funding under Title III of the Older Americans Act. The amount of this award for fiscal year 1979 was $24,840. With this grant the Center was able to make necessary renovations, purchase needed equipment, and hire staff.

Additional income was provided by the reimbursement of $13 a day for Medicaid recipients through the DPW's medical assistance plan and by payment of $20 by the private paying person. Participants were admitted to the program according to their needs and not their ability to pay. Medicaid recipients represented two-thirds of the client population while non-Medicaid participants made up the remaining one-third of those admitted to the Center.

Application to WSES was made in November of 1979 for a second year of funding. The request for funding was based on the need for expansion of space and staffing as determined by the requests for admission to the program. Notification of a grant award for fiscal year 1980 of $15,000 was received on December 24, 1979. A most welcome Christmas present!

The recognition of the Center's need for funding and its support this past year by WSES made the program operational and its future growth a real possibility.

Figure 13-1. *(continued)*

The Problem-Oriented Record

The use of the problem-oriented record as a tool to document, plan, and evaluate participant care has long been advocated, but not effectively implemented. When properly organized, the problem-oriented record provides a framework within which the interdisciplinary team may more effectively care for their participants and integrate their professional skills. Most traditional records lack the qualities necessary to make them effective. Separate sections for laboratory results, physicians' progress notes, nurses' progress notes, and other team members' notes, in fact, cause fragmentation. Although the problem-oriented record essentially organizes the determination of participant status, the treatment plan, and progress notes, one should be aware that the procedure may vary somewhat from program to program.

There are four essential components to the problem-oriented record. These components must be present for the record to be both an effective and comprehensive tool. They are as follows:

1. the accumulation of the data base
2. the development of a problem
3. the development of a plan for each problem
4. the utilization of progress notes (SOAP format—see below) for followup and evaluation

SCIENTIFIC METHOD	PROBLEM-ORIENTED RECORD
Problem Finding	Data Base
1. Gathering information	
2. Examining information	
3. Interpreting information	
4. Identifying the problem	Problem List
5. Stating the problem	
Problem Solving	Plan
1. Developing alternatives	1. Gather more data
2. Making a decision/proposing a hypothesis	2. Treatment
3. Deciding a plan of action	3. Patient education
4. Executing the plan/testing the hypothesis	
5. Evaluating the results/analysing data	Progress Notes
6. Redefining change	

Figure 13-2. Relationship of the Problem-Oriented Record to Scientific Method

Data Base

The data base of the problem-oriented record consists of pertinent, predefined health-related information about the participant and his background. It should include family identification, present illness, any chief complaint, past history, subjective review of systems, and objective physical exam, as well as the fact sheet (that is, address, phone number, emergency number, physician's name, payment category, referring agency, responsible family member's name and address, and so on). Data should be specific and systematically collected. Inclusion should be made of nutritional status, socioeconomic status, physical functioning, emotional status, and any other pertinent data. Just exactly what data are needed depends on the type of program and the particular participant's needs. However, a standard minimal data base should be collected and retained in the participant's record.

Problem List

After the data base is completed, both defined and potential problems are listed. A problem is any area of concern to the health-care practitioner, participant, or family. Problems can be medical, social, psychiatric, economic, or vocational. Common types of problems are:

1. a symptom (for example, headache)
2. a risk factor (for example, smoking)
3. a social problem (for example, low income)
4. an abnormal laboratory finding (for example, hypoglycemia)
5. a specific diagnosis (for example, hypertension)
6. an allergy (for example, to grass pollen)

This list serves as an index on the participant and usually appears at the beginning of the record. Each problem is numbered and dated according to the time of its appearance. The participant's problem list is a permanent part of his record and provides it with continuity of care. Since the problem list is a dynamic list, it includes not only problems identified upon admission, but any problem that arises during the participant's stay at the adult day-care program. Resolved problems are dated when they become inactive.

Initial Plans

Following the problem list is the prescribed plan of care with a flow sheet. Flow sheets have become so common as an adjunct to the problem-oriented record that many have come to think that they are the record. This conception is not, however, correct. A flow sheet is not a progress note; it is merely a data-collecting device that facilitates a quick assessment of the participant for a period of days as well as the recording of ongoing, routine measurements.

All interdisciplinary team members make contributions to the plan of care. Once an overall plan or goal is conceived, other, more specific, plans are written. In deliberating the plan, the following three steps should be considered:

1. collection of additional data
2. procedures to be followed
3. proposed client education

Evaluation and Progress Notes

The progress notes include narrative notes (SOAP notes—see below) and a discharge summary. It has been said that if the problem list is the "heart" of the record system, then the progress notes are its "circulatory" system. Weed further states that each progress note should be preceded by the number and problem title of the appropriate problem. Consideration should be given to previous notes on the same problem.[3]

Progress notes are called "SOAP" notes in the problem-oriented record. The term *SOAP* stands for Subjective, Objective, Assessment, and Plan. *Subjective* refers to comments made by the participant. *Objective* refers to direct observations made by the team or definitive laboratory findings. *Assessment* refers to the team members' interpretation of the combined subjective and objective data. Once the assessment is complete, the team members can then move on to constructing a plan, which they hope will help the participant work toward solving the problem. Thus, the *Plan* becomes the prescribed regimen for each participant's particular problem.

The success of the problem-oriented record depends upon the number of disciplines that become actively involved in the process. Implementation of the record by only one discipline results in a narrower range of problems being identified and little change in comprehensive care. An integrated record requires the active participation of all involved and, consequently, the willingness of all team members to become involved. In the problem-oriented record, the participant is viewed from many different perspectives. Thus, comprehensive, holistic care should become a reality (see Figure 13-3).

The Problem-Oriented Record Format

It is obviously impossible in this book to reproduce a cross section of problem-oriented records from various adult day-care participants. The author will therefore give one case presentation, demonstrating a beginning data base (see Figure

Chapter 13: Records and the Problem-Oriented Record System / 319

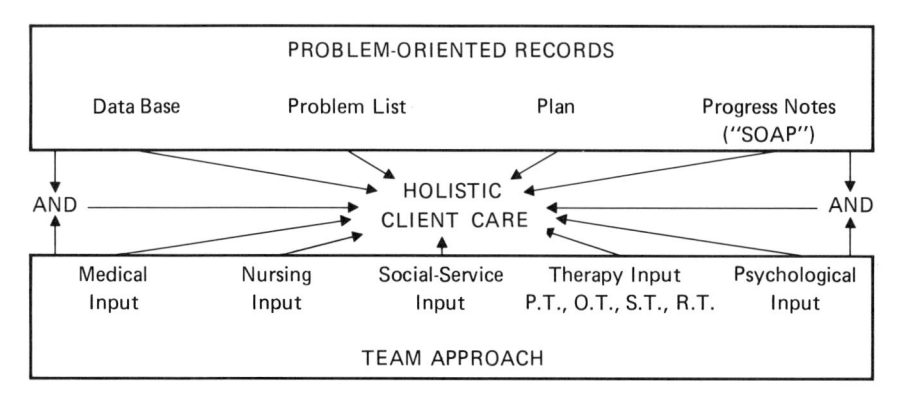

```
┌─────────────────────────────────────────────────────────────────┐
│                    PROBLEM-ORIENTED RECORDS                     │
│                                                                 │
│     Data Base        Problem List        Plan      Progress Notes│
│                                                    ("SOAP")     │
└─────────────────────────────────────────────────────────────────┘
                          ↓   HOLISTIC   ↓
   AND  ─────────────────→  CLIENT CARE  ←───────────────── AND
                          ↑              ↑
┌─────────────────────────────────────────────────────────────────┐
│   Medical      Nursing     Social-Service   Therapy Input   Psychological│
│    Input        Input         Input       P.T., O.T., S.T., R.T.  Input │
│                                                                 │
│                        TEAM APPROACH                            │
└─────────────────────────────────────────────────────────────────┘
```

Figure 13-3. Relationship of Problem-Oriented Records and Team Approach to Holistic Client Care

13-4), problem list (see Figure 13-5), plan (see Figure 13-6), and SOAP note (see Figure 13-7), to illustrate the problem-oriented record as used in one adult day-care setting. The record that follows is, by choice, that of a participant in a rehabilitation model of adult day care. Her data base was collected by utilizing the "Systematic Functional Assessment Tool" within a problem-oriented record system (see above). It is meant to be only a short, concise example of how the problem-oriented record is used.

It should be noted that there is not a single, ideal approach to the management of a participant's problems, but rather a method of recording data that permits an efficient review and audit of the problem-oriented approach to providing holistic health care.

Audit of the Record

Inherent in the record system is the goal of quality care, which is usually accomplished by allowing the day health team to identify and establish care plans for participant problems. Furthermore, the record requires that this care be audited or evaluated. To audit means to verify or examine.

Many systems have been devised to audit care, but they are usually external to the record itself. In addition, systems used in the past are extremely difficult and time consuming to audit in a meaningful way. Feedback methods that allow ongoing evaluation, change, and improvement of care while the participant is still in the day-care program are preferable to retrospective reviews done after discharge.

One must remember that formal audits, although they are facilitated by the problem-oriented record, are secondary to the continuous feedback offered by the

---

CASE PRESENTATION
BEGINNING DATA BASE

A 59-year-old woman, who lives with her husband and has had a long history of rheumatoid arthritis, generalized psoriasis, and mild diabetes, was sent to the Adult Day Health Center through the referral of a large teaching hospital. Prior to her admission to Adult Day Health Care, Mrs. S. lived at home and received services from a local home-health agency. Since their visits had to be reduced, nursing home placement became more apparent. But because of her age, desire to remain at home, and fear of nursing homes, Adult Day Health Care was suggested. The referring social worker hoped that the Adult Day Health Care placement would encourage Mrs. S. not only to receive the treatments she needed, but also to socialize more than she was able to while confined at home.

During the past 10 years, Mrs. S. was hospitalized numerous times and when at home went often to the out-patient dermatology and medical clinics. When she was admitted to the Adult Day Health Care program she had limited range of motion, many scaly, itchy, and broken areas on her body, minimal ability in activities of daily living, a poor nutritional intake, and slight depression with a lack of motivation. Once in the program, a regimen of daily tub baths with application of special ointments was begun for the scaling and broken skin areas. Physical therapy was initiated to increase her range of motion. Intensive diet teaching was started and adequate one-third of the daily nutritional intake was provided during the noon meal and snack times. Occupational therapy helped her utilize adaptive devices for increasing her functioning A.D.L. A remotivation program was instituted and participation in a planned activities program was encouraged.

Figure 13-4. Example of a Beginning Data Base

record to the interdisciplinary team offering care. Thus, the auditing shifts from an evaluation of an individual practitioner to that of holistic participant care as delivered by the entire team. This type of audit represents a major step toward evaluating the actual quality of participant care in adult day-care programs.

Once the audit is complete, deficiencies are identified and corrected. One must remember that before the problem-oriented record is used to audit or evaluate the quality of participant care, the quality of participant care that is acceptable must be defined. The audit can then determine whether the care given was carried out thoroughly, efficiently, responsibly, and with a sound knowledge base.

Two types of audit are used in adult day-care centers, general and specific.[1(p7)] In the general audit, one determines whether the adult day-care system is working (for example, whether the components of the record are consistently displayed), whereas in the specific audit, one determines the quality of care given to participants with specific problems (for example, a stroke). If the participant is discharged when the audit is done, the audit would be in retrospect (that is, the end result of the care would be evaluated).

With the audit completed, the participant's care can be identified and changes

Name	Mrs. S.		
Date of Onset	Problem List		Goals
10/59	1.	Rheumatoid arthritis	
		A. Decreased ROM	
		B. Decreased ambulation	
		C. Inability to perform ADL	
9/79	2.	Generalized psoriasis	2. Long-term goals: The participant will be relieved of itching, scaly skin in 6 months.
		A. Itching skin	
		B. Scaling skin	
		C. Broken areas	2. Short-term goals:
			A. Participant will review her current hygiene practices.
			B. Participant will identify 3 measures of hygiene practices to help her condition.
			C. Participant will demonstrate 3 methods of good hygiene practices.
8/64	3.	Diabetes Mellitus	
		A. Inadequate intake	
		B. Lack of knowledge of dietary restrictions	
10/78	4.	Slight depression	
		A. Lack of motivation	
		B. Decreased socialization	
1/79	5.	Worried about future	
		A. Fear of nursing-home placement	
4/69	6.	Frequent hospitalization	

Figure 13-5. Example of an Active Problem List

made if necessary. Changes in care require ongoing communication among those directly and indirectly involved in care and active involvement in the changes. Periodic interdisciplinary team meetings (usually once a month) will facilitate ongoing communication and enable the team to make the necessary changes in the care plan.

The degree of participant contact and scope of activity for any given team member will vary according to the participant's problems and the type of adult day-care center. In any case, it is necessary for all individuals to interact in the identification of needed changes and see that these are made.

```
Name  Mrs. S.           Participant # 23        Page 3
                        Age  59      Diet  1200 Cal Diabetics    Year 1979
Physician  Dr. S.
Date       Problem No.   Problem                 Plan of Care
3/3/79     2             Generalized psoriasis
           2A            Itchy skin              2A  Teach good skin care, types of
                                                     clothes to wear, environmental
                                                     conditions to avoid
           2B            Scaly skin              2B  Pat skin areas dry
           2C            Broken skin areas       2C  Apply prescribed ointment
                                                     daily
```

Figure 13-6. Example of a Plan of Care

```
Name  Mrs. S.
Date       Problem No.   Problem       Progress Note
3/3/79     2A            Itchy skin    Subjective—"Since I began receiving
                                       daily baths, my skin is less itchy"
                                       Objective—Mrs. S. is scratching herself less
                                       Assessment—Daily baths are relieving the
                                       itching
                                       Plan—to continue with daily baths

Nurse's signature _____
```

Figure 13-7. Example of a SOAP Progress Note

Composition of the Problem-Oriented Record

Face and Admission Referral Sheet

Each adult day-care participant should have an initial family identification (face) sheet with his/her name, address, phone number, date of birth, directions to his/her home, name and phone of responsible person to contact in an emergency (relative and/or responsible friend), previous employment, and medical coverage.

Another sheet contains a form to be completed by the referring individual; that is, the physician, family, hospital, nursing home, or community agency initiating the participant's admission to adult day care. Information such as the participant's diagnosis, treatments, medication, diet restrictions, level of ability in activities of daily living, social needs, suggested goals, physician's name, and reason for referral should be included (see Figure 13-8).

During the admission process, the participant or family should be asked to sign an admission agreement (see Figure 13-9). This agreement contracts with the participant or family for the specific services that the day-care center intends to provide and also lists the requirements that they must comply with during their participation in the program.

Medical Preadmission Sheet and Physician's Order Sheet

The medical preadmission form (see Figure 13-10 on pages 327–328) should be completed by the family physician who will be responsible for the participant in the adult day program. Included in the information should be vital signs, weight, diagnosis, significant laboratory findings, medications and dosages, special treatment, level of orientation, and communication abilities.

Since orders are required on all participants for treatments and care they are to receive, the attending physician will need to complete a physician's order sheet, which must be dated and signed by the physician (see Figure 13-11 on page 329). New orders are needed periodically, and this order sheet is therefore also used as a renewal-of-orders sheet.

Referring Social Worker's Statement Sheet

The referring social worker form should include family relationships, ethnic background, attitudes toward illness, pertinent social data, personal characteristics, language spoken, general behavior patterns, and the family members' health (see Figure 13-12 on page 329).

Participant-Profile Sheet

The participants' profile sheets are the initial collection of information taken about them and are the basis upon which problems are identified and plan of action determined. The components included in this data base are the chief-complaint client profile, 24-hour dietary recall, history of present illness, past history, family history, review of systems, laboratory data, and activity preference list (see Figures 13-13, 13-14, and 13-15, on pages 330–332). The collection of this data is the responsibility of the entire health team.

		For Office Use:			
		Date application received _____			
		Date of admission _____			

Referring agency _____ Date of application _____
Name _____ Name of spouse _____
     Last   First   Maiden
Permanent address _____ City/State _____ Phone _____
Present address _____ City/State _____ Phone _____
Birthdate _____ Birthplace _____ Marital status: S M W D Sep.
Registered voter: ☐ Yes ☐ No Languages spoken _____
Former occupation _____ Religion _____ Sex _____
Father's name _____ Mother's name _____
Citizenship _____ Alien registration no. _____
Life insurance _____ Policy no. _____
Social Security no. _____ Medex no. _____
SSI Social Security no. _____ SSI Social Security amount $ _____
Medicare no. _____ Plan: ☐ A   ☐ B   ☐ A&B

	Yes	No	Number	Office	Social Worker
Medicaid					
BC BS					
Division—blind					
Veteran's aid—city					
Veteran's aid—fed.					
Other public asst.					
Other retired income					

Family or nearest relative to be contacted in case of emergency

Name	Address	Relationship	Home Phone	Bus. Phone

Hospital affiliation _____ Date of last hospitalization _____
Attending physician _____ Phone no. _____
Clinics attended _____
Other agency services: VNA ____ Home care ____ Homemaker ____ Health aide ____
                      Visits/week _____ Hours/week _____
Planned Transportation to Day Health Program: ☐ Family/friends ☐ Taxi ☐ Other
Physician responsible for continuing care:
  Name _____ Address _____ Phone _____

Figure 13-8. Example of an Adult Day-Care-Center Face and Referral Sheet (From Weston Manor Adult Day Health Center, Weston, Mass., 1977. Form developed by C. O'Brien and G. Dix. Reprinted by permission of the authors and Weston Manor Adult Day Health Center.)

ACTIVITIES OF DAILY LIVING				Adult Day Health Care Use Only		
Name _____				Date of		
Date of application _____				assessment _____		
Activities	Ind.	Needs Assistance	Unable	Ind.	Needs Assistance	Unable
1. *Dressing*						
Shoes and stockings	☐	☐	☐	☐	☐	☐
Outer clothing	☐	☐	☐	☐	☐	☐
Under clothing	☐	☐	☐	☐	☐	☐
2. *Diet*						
Feeds self	☐	☐	☐	☐	☐	☐
3. *Personal hygiene*						
Bathing	☐	☐	☐	☐	☐	☐
Mouth care, dentures, etc.	☐	☐	☐	☐	☐	☐
Shampoo, hair grooming	☐	☐	☐	☐	☐	☐
Shaving	☐	☐	☐	☐	☐	☐
Toileting	☐	☐	☐	☐	☐	☐
Bladder functioning	— Comments —			☐	☐	☐
Continent				☐	☐	☐
Incontinent				☐	☐	☐
Catheter-drainage				☐	☐	☐
Bowel functioning	— Comments —			☐	☐	☐
Controlled				☐	☐	☐
Involuntary				☐	☐	☐
Constipation				☐	☐	☐
4. *Ambulation*						
In and out of car	☐	☐	☐	☐	☐	☐
Walk unassisted	☐	☐	☐	☐	☐	☐
Climb stairs	☐	☐	☐	☐	☐	☐
Transfer chair to toilet	☐	☐	☐	☐	☐	☐
Aids, cane, crutches, walker	☐	☐	☐	☐	☐	☐
Manage wheelchair	☐	☐	☐	☐	☐	☐
5. *Medications*						
Take as ordered	☐	☐	☐	☐	☐	☐

6. *Sleep or rest patterns*—Uses armchair, straight chair, sofa

7. *Behavior/emotional status*—Indicate if alert, confused, depressed, anxious, forgetful, etc.

8. *Special interests, hobbies, how person spends day*

Figure 13-8. *(continued)*

326 / Part III: Setting Up a Day-Care Program

Active-Problem-List Sheet

The active-problem list is the key to all the information presented in the record. It is the result of data collection and serves as the table of contents or index for the participant's record. It lists *all* the *active* problems that the participant exhibits while in the adult day-care setting, so that a required plan can be formulated while the participant attends the adult day-care program (see Figure 13-16 on page

---

ADMISSION AGREEMENT

I _____ enter into agreement with the Adult Day Health Center the following stipulations:

1. Hours to be spent at the Center to be between _____ A.M. and _____ P.M. with family or individual assuming care at night and over weekends.

2. Transportation to be provided by the family unless otherwise arranged, including any clinic appointments scheduled on days spent at the center.

3. Provide duplicate prescriptions of any medications to be taken by the person during hours spent at the center.

4. Physical examination of the person at least one month prior to admission to the program. Prior arrangement for ongoing medical supervision by the family physician or specified alternate physician.

5. Understand that ongoing involvement by the family is essential to the success of the program and that regular attendance at individual and group discussions will result in sharing the evaluation of progress and in effectively handling problems which may arise.

6. Families will contact the center in the morning or the day before if possible, if the person will not be able to attend the program on that day.

7. Participation in the program is not unlimited and is contingent on progress and needs of the person and family.

8. In case of emergency, the local hospital will be used as a back-up hospital.

The Adult Day Health Center will provide nursing care and supervision, social service with individual, group, and family counseling, and referrals to community agencies when appropriate.

One hot meal at noon, with special diets as ordered by the physician, and morning and afternoon snacks will be offered, and nutritional counseling provided.

A therapeutic program of occupational therapy, physical therapy, and social and recreational programs will be offered as needed to maximize each person's level of functioning.

_____
Program Coordinator

_____
Client or Family Member

_____
Date

Figure 13-9. Example of an Adult Day-Care-Center Admission Agreement (From Weston Manor Adult Day Health Center, Weston, Mass., 1977. Form developed by C. O'Brien and G. Dix. Reprinted by permission of the authors and Weston Manor Day Health Center.)

333). As new problems are identified or active ones become resolved, the problem list is changed. Again, all team members are responsible for adding or deleting problems on the current list.

```
                        MEDICAL PRE-ADMISSION FORM
    Name _____ Date of birth _____ Sex _____
    Permanent address _____ City/State/Zip _____ Tel. _____
    Present address _____ City/State/Zip _____ Tel. _____
    Weight _____ Blood pressure _____
    Last chest x-ray date _____ Results _____

    Diagnoses
                    Major                           Other



    Allergies
                    Foods                           Medications



    Significant Laboratory Findings



    Physician Orders
        Medications        Dosage          Frequency        Administration



    Treatments—Dressings, Lab tests, etc.



    Dietary Restrictions



    Suggested Diet
```

Figure 13-10. Example of an Adult Day-Care-Center Medical Preadmission Sheet (From Weston Manor Adult Day Health Center, Weston, Mass., 1977. Form developed by C. O'Brien and G. Dix. Reprinted by permission of the authors and Weston Manor Adult Day Health Center.)

```
┌─────────────────────────────────────────────────────────────────────────┐
│ Restorative Services                                    Plan            │
│ Physical therapy   ☐ Yes     ☐ No                                       │
│ Occupational therapy       ☐ Yes    ☐ No                                │
│ Speech therapy      ☐ Yes    ☐ No                                       │
│ Communication Abilities                                                 │
│ Vision:   Impaired ☐ Yes    ☐ No     Glasses     ☐ Yes    ☐ No          │
│ Hearing:  Impaired ☐ Yes    ☐ No     Hearing aids  ☐ Yes    ☐ No        │
│ Speech:   Aphasic  ☐ Yes    ☐ No     Language spoken _____             │
│ Functional Limitations—Please check if appropriate.                     │
│ Devices:  ☐ Dentures    ☐ Prothesis   ☐ Colostomy   ☐ Urinary drainage  │
│           ☐ Leg brace   ☐ Walker      ☐ Cane        ☐ Wheelchair   ☐ Crutches │
│ Other:                                                                  │
│                                                                         │
│ Mental Limitations—Please check if appropriate.                         │
│ Behavior:       ☐ Withdrawn     ☐ Agitated    ☐ Nervous    ☐ Wanders    │
│                 ☐ Physically abusive          ☐ Verbally abusive        │
│ Memory:         ☐ Immediate     ☐ Recent      ☐ Remote                  │
│ Orientations:   ☐ Oriented      ☐ Disoriented at times    ☐ Disoriented │
│ Purpose of Adult Day Health Center Placement—Include stability of medical status and need │
│ for health services.                                                    │
│                                                                         │
│                                                                         │
│ Contraindications to participation in ROM exercises, dance program, and/or outdoor │
│ activities:                                                             │
│                                                                         │
│                                                                         │
│ _____             │
│ Physician's Signature _____           │
│ Address _____  Tel. _____          │
│ Physician responsible for patient if other than above:                  │
│ Name _____   Address _____   Tel. _____            │
│ Physician coverage in case of emergency if other than above:            │
│ Name _____   Address _____   Tel. _____            │
│ Please include discharge summary if person has been hospitalized within the past 3 months. │
│ Date received _____                                   │
└─────────────────────────────────────────────────────────────────────────┘
```

Figure 13-10.   *(continued)*

Plan of Care and Flow Sheet

Plans for participant management follow the problem list. Each problem has plans for the implementation of care, so that all members of the health team can work together in providing thorough, nonfragmented care.

Flow sheets can be utilized for problems that elicit much data in a short period of time. If there are multiple changing parameters to be followed in a given

Chapter 13: Records and the Problem-Oriented Record System / 329

```
                        PHYSICIAN'S ORDERS
Name _____     Number _____
Vital signs _____
_____
Weight _____

Please review orders on the preceeding page and note any change in orders in space below.
If no changes are made in your orders they will be renewed as written on the care plan.




Renew current orders for 90 days except as noted above. I certify that the above-named
person is under my medical supervision and requires day health services.

Date _____   Signature _____ M.D.
Date last seen by physician _____
Please sign and return in enclosed envelope.
```

Figure 13-11. Example of an Adult Day-Care Center Physician Order Sheet (From Weston Manor Adult Day Health Center, Weston, Mass., 1977. Form developed by C. O'Brien and G. Dix. Reprinted by permission of the authors and Weston Manor Adult Day Health Center.)

```
              REFERRING SOCIAL WORKER'S STATEMENT
Include family relationships, ethnic background, attitudes toward illness, pertinent social
data, personal characteristics, language spoken, general behavior patterns, and family mem-
bers' health.




Signature _____     Date _____
Agency _____
Address _____
Telephone Number _____
```

Figure 13-12. Example of an Adult Day-Care Center Referring Social Worker's Statement Sheet (From Weston Manor Adult Day Health Center, Weston, Mass., 1977. Form developed by C. O'Brien and G. Dix. Reprinted by permission of the authors and Weston Manor Adult Day Health Center.)

PARTICIPANT PROFILE

Past Medical History

Condition	Participant	Family
Allergies		
Arthritis		
Bowel problems		
Cancer		
Heart disease		
High blood pressure		
Phlebitis		
Stroke		
Diabetes		
T.B.		
Emphysema		
Smoking		
Dental problems		
Eye problems		
Ear problems		
Operations		

Medications

At Home	Taking	Frequency	Not Taking

Diet—24-hour Recall

Breakfast	Lunch	Dinner	Snacks

Figure 13-13. Example of an Adult Day-Care Center Participant Profile Sheet (From Weston Manor Adult Day Health Center, Weston, Mass., 1977. Form developed by C. O'Brien and G. Dix. Reprinted by permission of the authors and Weston Manor Adult Day Health Center.)

situation, such a sheet would be adopted into the record. Use of the flow sheet, accompanied by appropriate instructions, will be a genuine learning experience for the team member and will present a most complete picture of the participant (see Figure 13-17 on page 334).

Chapter 13: Records and the Problem-Oriented Record System / 331

```
┌─────────────────────────────────────────────────────────────┐
│                     PAST SOCIAL HISTORY                     │
│                                                             │
│   Name _____  Participant Number _____  │
│                                                             │
│                        Date _____         │
│                                                             │
│                                                             │
│                                                             │
│                                                             │
│                                                             │
│                                                             │
│                                                             │
│                                                             │
└─────────────────────────────────────────────────────────────┘
```

Figure 13-14. Example of an Adult Day-Care Center Participant Profile Sheet (From Weston Manor Adult Day Health Center, Weston, Mass., 1977. Form developed by C. O'Brien and G. Dix. Reprinted by permission of the authors and Weston Manor Adult Day Health Center.)

Progress Sheet

After the plan is implemented, the participant's progress is evaluated through progress SOAP notes. Each problem is numbered, properly dated, and titled on the progress sheet. Then a SOAP note is written discussing the specific problem, its progress, its relation to the progress of all other problems, and its relation to previous progress of other related problems.

In this section of the record, all members of the health team record their notes, thus eliminating the physician's progress sheet, nursing and social worker notes, and the consultant's record-keeping notes. Such a progress sheet provides for a method to modify the care plan, monitor the participant's progress, and evaluate resolved problems (see Figure 13-18 on page 335).

Discharge Sheet

Each problem should be summarized on the discharge sheet at the state of resolution that exists when discharge occurs. The summary should be written in a problem-oriented format and should adhere to the principles inherent in the system—that is, the health-care or social worker must continue to identify each problem by its originally assigned number (see Figure 13-19 on page 336).

NAME _____ DATE _____

ART
- ☐ Art appreciation
- ☐ Ceramics
- ☐ Painting, drawing
- ☐ Photography

DRAMA
- ☐ Movies, slides
- ☐ Play reading (participation)
- ☐ Puppet theatre

CRAFTS
- ☐ Basket making
- ☐ Book covering
- ☐ Cooking
- ☐ Flower arranging
- ☐ Gardening ☐ indoors ☐ outdoors*
- ☐ Holiday decorations
- ☐ Jewelry making
- ☐ Knitting, crocheting
- ☐ Leatherwork
- ☐ Metal work
- ☐ Needlework
- ☐ Sewing
- ☐ Tile creations
- ☐ Toy making
- ☐ Weaving
- ☐ Woodworking

EDUCATIONAL ACTIVITIES
- ☐ Degree preparation
- ☐ Discussion groups
- ☐ Language lessons
- ☐ Health education
- ☐ Nature study

GAMES
- ☐ Ball games, bean bag, etc.
- ☐ Bingo, pokeno
- ☐ Card games (poker, bridge, etc.)
- ☐ Circle games
- ☐ Charades
- ☐ Chess, checkers
- ☐ Bowling
- ☐ Horseshoes
- ☐ Shuffleboard
- ☐ Party games
- ☐ Tournaments for games

LITERATURE
- ☐ Book reviews
- ☐ Creative writing
- ☐ Listening to readings
- ☐ Reading on own

MUSIC
- ☐ Group sing-alongs
- ☐ Music appreciation
- ☐ Music lessons
- ☐ Small band

PARTIES
- ☐ Dancing parties
- ☐ Dinner parties
- ☐ Holiday parties
- ☐ Monthly birthday parties
- ☐ Potluck parties

TRIPS
- ☐ Ball games
- ☐ Exhibitions
- ☐ Libraries
- ☐ Live TV shows
- ☐ Museums
- ☐ Parks*
- ☐ Picnics*
- ☐ Restaurants
- ☐ Zoos

WORK
- ☐ Bird feeding
- ☐ Hostessing
- ☐ Table setting, clearing, serving
- ☐ Party preparations
- ☐ RSVP
- ☐ Volunteer work

*Seasonal

Chapter 13: Records and the Problem-Oriented Record System / 333

Figure 13-15 *(at left)* Example of an Adult Day-Care Center Participant Profile Sheet (From Weston Manor Adult Day Health Center, Weston, Mass., 1977. Form developed by C. O'Brien and G. Dix. Reprinted by permission of the authors and Weston Manor Adult Day Health Center.)

		ACTIVE-PROBLEM LIST		
Name _____ Participant number _____					
Problem Number	Date of Onset	Active Problems	Long-Term Goals and Short-Term Goals	Date Resolved

Figure 13-16. Example of an Adult Day-Care Center Active-Problem-List Sheet (From Weston Manor Adult Day Health Center, Weston, Mass., 1977. Form developed by C. O'Brien and G. Dix. Reprinted by permission of the authors and Weston Manor Adult Day Health Center.)

334 / Part III: Setting Up a Day-Care Program

```
                          PLAN OF CARE
Name _____  Participant no. ____  Diagnosis _____  Page ____
Physician _____  Age ____  Diet _____  Year ____
```

Date	Prob. No.	Plan of Care/Medications	Hour	Code of Care Provided

Codes:
- C — Direct care (Vital signs & measurements enter in space)
- E — Evaluation
- N — Progress notes
- R — Referral
- S — Supervision
- T — Teaching/counseling
- A — Absent visit

Enter Date Here

Signature & Title

Figure 13-17. Example of an Adult Day-Care Center Plan of Care Sheet/Flow Sheet (From Weston Manor Adult Day Health Center, Weston, Mass., 1977. Form developed by C. O'Brien and G. Dix. Reprinted by permission of the authors and Weston Manor Adult Day Health Center.)

Authorization and Release Sheet

The authorization and release sheet serves as a contract between the adult day-center and the participant. It states that participation in the program is agreed that individual and that participation for continuation in the program

	PROGRESS SHEET	
Name __Mrs. S.__		
Problem No.	Date	Progress Notes
2A	10/79	S. "I am bathing my skin twice a day, drying it well and applying my medication." O. The broken areas seem to be healing and look less red. The skin is not as rough. A. The treatment plan seems to be working well. No additional broken areas are noted. P. To continue Mrs. S. on the same plan and recheck skin in one week. Nurse's Signature _____

Figure 13-18. Example of an Adult Day-Care Center Progress Sheet (From Weston Manor Adult Day Health Center, Weston, Mass., 1977. Form developed by C. O'Brien and G. Dix. Reprinted by permission of the authors and Weston Manor Adult Day Health Center.)

is contingent on the participant's progress and need for such services as offered by the adult day-care center. Furthermore, this sheet serves as an agreement between the center and the participant, stating that the center can release information about the participant as may be necessary (see Figure 13-20).

Participant's-Rights Sheet

The participant's-rights sheet is an important consideration for all adult day-care centers. Included in it is information that all adult day-care participants should be made aware of before they decide to become participants in such a program. It is the first form signed by the participant and should be a permanent part of the participant's record (see Figure 13-21).

Daily Attendance and Transportation Sheet

The utilization of a daily attendance sheet for each participant will facilitate evaluation of individual goal attainment. For the individual who attends the program as designated in his or her plan, attainment of goals should be realized if the program objectives are being met. In measuring individual outcomes, it is there-

```
                    MULTIDISCIPLINARY DISCHARGE PLAN
Participant's name _____ Age ____ Admission date _____
Admitting diagnosis _____
Anticipated length of stay _____
Potential discharge problems _____
Functional level _____
Goals:  Short-term _____
        Long-term _____
Nursing needs _____
_____

Social service needs _____
_____

Therapy needs _____
_____

Dietary needs _____
_____

Educational and activity needs _____
_____

Initial date _____
Dates reviewed   1. _____   Evaluation _____
                 2. _____              _____
                 3. _____              _____
                 4. _____              _____
```

Figure 13-19. Example of an Adult Day-Care Center Discharge Sheet (From Weston Manor Adult Day Health Center, Weston, Mass., 1977. Form developed by C. O'Brien and G. Dix. Reprinted by permission of the authors and Weston Manor Adult Day Health Center.)

fore important to review the attendance sheet to see the amount of exposure an individual participant has had in the program. Attendance will be recorded daily and a summary of the individual's participation in the program will be noted.

The sheet also gives information about how the participant comes to the adult day-care center. Such information is an important consideration, since transportation can affect attendance. In addition, the transportation component has many implications for the cost of day care and the numbers of individuals that can be served. The transportation record is therefore an important part of the overall record (see Figure 13-22).

Chapter 13: Records and the Problem-Oriented Record System / 337

AUTHORIZATION AND RELEASE SHEET

Name _____

I agree to be a participant in the Adult Day Health Center Program. I realize I am subject to the Center's rules and regulations of which I have been advised. I understand that participation in the program is not unlimited and is contingent on my progress and health care needs.

Date _____ Participant or Sponsor's Signature _____

I hereby authorize the release of information as may be necessary for completion of forms and/or claims which are directly related to my participation in the Center program.

Date _____ Participant or Sponsor's Signature _____

Figure 13-20. Example of an Adult Day-Care Center Authorization and Release Sheet (From Weston Manor Adult Day Health Center, Weston, Mass., 1977. Form developed by C. O'Brien and G. Dix. Reprinted by permission of the authors and Weston Manor Adult Day Health Center.)

PARTICIPANT'S RIGHTS SHEET

You may have access to information regarding your care.

You are encouraged to participate in your plan of care and may attend any team meetings concerning your care plan.

You may refuse to participate in any part of the program.

You may refuse any prescribed medication and/or treatment with the understanding you assume the responsibility for that decision.

You may discontinue participation in the program at any time.

You have the right to privacy during medical treatment and/or other rendering of care.

You have the right to know the daily cost of the program and all services included in this cost. You have the right to know all services not included in the daily rate and the cost of those services.

Participant's Signature _____ Date _____

Figure 13-21. Example of an Adult Day-Care Center Participant's-Rights Sheet (From Weston Manor Adult Day Health Center, Weston, Mass., 1977. Form developed by C. O'Brien and G. Dix. Reprinted by permission of the authors and Weston Manor Adult Day Health Center.)

ATTENDANCE AND TRANSPORTATION SHEET												
Participant Name	Mode of Trans.	1	2	3	4	5	28	29	30	31	Attend Days	Absent Days	Remarks

Absence
A = Non-medical absence
A/1 = Medical absence
S = Snow day
H = Holiday

Transportation Code   *Total Trips (One Way)*
T = Taxi
T1 = One-passenger trip
T2 = Two-passenger trip
T3 = Three-passenger trip
T4 = Four-passenger trip

C = Chair car
C1 = One-passenger trip
C2 = Two-passenger trip
C3 = Three-passenger trip
C4 = Four-passenger trip

F = Family transportation
V = Program vehicle
R = Community resource van

Figure 13-22. Example of an Adult Day-Care Attendance and Transportation Sheet (From Massachusetts Department of Public Welfare, Boston, 1977.)

Community Referral Sheet

Services to which the participant or family are referred will be documented on a community referral sheet.

Another form should be sent to the referred agency and include pertinent data about the individual. This form will have a section that is to be returned to the adult day-care program from the community agency with their recommendations for action (see Figure 13-23).

Advantages of the Problem-Oriented Record System

Participant Advantages

Since the problem-oriented record system encourages a multidisciplinary approach to care, it provides a pool of health team expertise that should improve the quality of care.[2(p17)] The quality of care can be measured through record audit, thus enabling the team to learn from their mistakes. Furthermore, the system requires that the care received by each participant be reviewed and compared to an established standard developed prior to audit.[2(p17)] In addition, data can be retrieved more quickly and in chronological sequence because this system has eliminated the need for the team to chart meaningless data such as "good day." Another advantage is that the problem list serves as a means of obtaining essential data for the assurance of continuity of care.

Finally the problem-oriented record lends itself to research pursuits because problems are organized into a meaningful whole through the team approach in caring for the participant.[2(p20)] When similarities arise in the participant's problem list, the staff can deal more intelligently with the specific participant's problems in regard to utilization of resources and response to prescribed treatment.[2(p20)]

Personnel Advantages

Since plans that are scrutinized by team efforts are likely to be superior to those made by an individual, it is evident that the problem-oriented record effects better team planning. The problem-oriented record also affords team members the opportunity to evaluate each other's performance and increases their accountability. Clearly, it enhances problem-solving logic. The team derives a great degree of satisfaction from pooling their expertise, as well as a more satisfying feeling of accomplishment regarding the participants' progress. Another advantage to personnel of the problem-oriented record is the satisfaction received from the planning and implementing of preventive care through the team's efforts in promotion of health and early detection of impending problems.[2(p25)]

Provider Advantages

Today, when emphasis is being placed on program evaluation and outcomes, one must be concerned with advantages to the provider as well as to the participant and personnel. Audit is one method of evaluating outcomes. It is an integral part

```
                    COMMUNITY REFERRAL FORM
                       (Fill Out in Duplicate)
From _____      Participant admission number _____
Address _____      Name _____
Zip _____ Tel. _____     Address _____
Admission date _____      Zip _____ Tel. _____
Today's date _____      Floor _____ Apt. No. _____
                                  Age _____ Birthdate _____
To _____      Sex: M F   Marital status: S M W D Sep.
Address _____      Religion _____
Zip _____ Tel. _____     Relative or guardian _____
                         /        Address _____
Medicare no. & letter _____ Plan: A B  Blue Cross no. _____
Social Security no. _____     Other _____
Clinic appointments _____ Date _____ Time _____

Signature Day Health Personnel _____

Instructions: Complete all the items below for transfer of participant information to Adult
              Day Health Center.

Diagnosis _____

Allergies _____

Reason for transfer _____

Return report of findings? _____

New orders _____

Recommendations _____

Signature of person returning _____

Time medications last given _____

Attending physician _____ Tel. _____
Completed by _____ Tel. _____
```

Figure 13-23. Example of an Adult Day-Care Center Community Referral Form (From Weston Manor Adult Day Health Center, Weston, Mass., 1977. Form developed by C. O'Brien and G. Dix. Reprinted by permission of the authors and Weston Manor Adult Day Health Center.)

of the problem-oriented record system, and continuous documentation and accountability are therefore important. Because of this record-keeping system, data collection and necessary treatments relate to an identified problem.[2(p27)] Unnecessary care is not given, thus reducing the cost of care to the participant and to the taxpayer.

Summary

The more comfortable service providers are with records, the less troublesome records become. If service providers adopted a positive attitude toward records and analyzed record data effectively to assisting themselves in their work, they would probably resent less the time it takes for record keeping and use the information in the record more constructively.

In concluding, one must remember the three parts of the problem-oriented system needed to reach the goal of quality participant care: (1) utilization of the problem-oriented record; (2) audit of the record for the identification of deficiencies; and (3) the correction of these deficiencies. All three parts must be implemented for the problem-oriented record system to be successful.

Adult day-care centers approaching the problem-oriented record system will certainly want to become attuned to its basis. It demands thoroughness, reliability, and sound thought because the audit is not only done on individual participants but also on the system itself.

Utilization of the problem-oriented system in adult day care will reflect the type of care being given. Indeed, the quality of care can be accurately assessed against accepted standards of care. The problem-oriented record can serve as an educational tool for all team members as they each bring their skill and knowledge to work on specific problems. All team members can work and share with the participant in a true partnership, contributing as intelligent, responsible team members.

References

1. Vaughan-Wrobel B, Henderson B: *The Problem-Oriented System in Nursing. A Workbook*. St. Louis, Mo, The CV Mosby Co, 1976.

2. Readey H, Berni R: *Problem-Oriented Medical Record Implementation*. St. Louis, Mo, the CV Mosby Company, 1974.

3. Weed, LL: *Medical Records, Medical Education and Patient Care*. Cleveland, Ohio, Case Western Reserve University, 1970.

14

Evaluation

Carole Lium O'Brien, RN, MS
Sarah J. Schiermeyer, RN

Introduction

Evaluation in the long-term-care field is an emerging social, medical, nursing, and political issue.[1] The increasing costs of these services and the growing government involvement in funding and delivering personal-care services have caused much interest in program and client evaluation.

Evaluation is inherent in all categories of adult day-care services. To decide on appropriate evaluative methods, it is essential that the planner understands the concept of evaluation. It is the purpose of this chapter to discuss those aspects of evaluation that affect the planning for suitable adult day-care outcomes.

Definition

Evaluation is a means to measure the value or amount of an outcome in relationship to a goal. These expectations, states Douglas, are either in the form of established criteria or expected outcomes specific to a health agency, care giver, or client.[2] It is both logical and necessary that plans for adult day-care services and for evaluation of their outcomes be made concurrently and that these plans be based on the achievement of objectives and compliance with criteria demonstrable at the end of the study period.

Evaluation can directly answer the following questions. Did the services provided make a difference to the clients and/or the community? Could the expected client outcomes be measured by a prescribed behavior change? Did any changes occur in the environment or community? Were more community people aware of the program? Did the original program assumptions develop into valid conclusions?

Evaluation is not an end in itself. It is a diverse process including the collection of data, not only about the measurable outcomes of a program, but also about the process itself and the facets of the environment in which the process occurs. Inherent in adult day-care evaluation is the appraisal of the worth of the program, as well as the results of the program. Evaluation can determine the extent to which program objectives, both the degree of progress and level of attainment, were met. Furthermore, it can identify the strengths and gaps within a system. When the objectives and the evaluation of them are reciprocal, the level and degree of progress are rated. If the evaluation is more comprehensive than the original objectives, absolute conclusions are invalid, but ideas for further study are illuminated. Evaluation can indicate the need for developing alternate approaches and procedures and can be used later to measure their effectiveness. Finally, evaluation is able to meet the demand for public accountability by providing justification for either continuing or discontinuing a program.

Evaluation is composed of judgments, appraisals, ratings, and interpretations. Evaluation involves judgment based on one's experiences and education. It involves appraisal based on comparison with known parameters and known cause and effect units. In addition, it involves rating based on comparison with criteria and standards. Finally, it involves interpretation of both subjective and objective conclusions and applies a value system. The criteria for each of these four areas of evaluation can be seen as either objective or subjective in nature.

Objective evaluation is that which can be definitively measured and to which statistical analysis can be applied. Objective evaluation can be performed if both the assessment and evaluation steps use the same assumptions and tools. Assessment and evaluation measurements must reflect the same variables as well as the same orientation to be considered valid comparison tools.

Subjective evaluation is used when objective evaluation cannot be applied because of the absence of data, insufficient data, or uncontrollable variables. Subjective evaluation is both necessary and desirable and, in the case of no data, it is the only possible recourse.

Evaluation of outcomes against stated criteria, guidelines, and standards is one necessary aspect of the evaluation process. Another is the separate evaluation of criteria, guidelines, and standards against new objective data. The difference between performance standards and evaluation criteria can sometimes be unclear. Standards are usually the minimal performance established to govern the quality of care given. Evaluation criteria, on the other hand, enable the person evaluating the care to establish categories for review and to determine the degree and extent to which the person evaluated is performing in relation to the minimal standard. Before a standard is tested, the method or tool used must be identified as to its validity and objectivity (see Chapter 4).

An example of an evaluation criteria tool is the California Department of Health Services (DHS) Requirements of Living Scales, used to measure functional status (see Table 14-1).[3] They were developed in 1976, included in two demonstration projects (Sacramento and San Diego) in early 1977, and then required of all adult day-care programs from July 1977 on. The tool is used as part of the intake procedure and thereafter at preset intervals. The results can therefore be compared and differences defined for a given individual and group advances or declines, or lack thereof, compared to other adult day-care programs.

In conducting objective evaluation, only methodological criticism and not opinion criticism is given. A long-term goal of any adult day-care center should be to alter the balance between objective and subjective evaluation. Only objective evaluation measures change, and only objective evaluation can prove or disprove that adult day care is effectively meeting significant health or social needs. If objective evaluation is carried out, the planner must be familiar with certain specific steps in the evaluation process, as shown in Figure 14-1.

STEPS IN THE EVALUATION PROCESS

1. Define the purpose
2. Select a model
3. Determine who evaluates
4. State the rationale
5. Describe the method
6. Develop the plan
7. A. Formulate a design
   B. Develop a work plan
8. Analyze the data
9. Make recommendations
10. Report the findings
11. Initiate changes
12. Begin again

Figure 14-1. Steps in the Evaluation of Adult Day-Care Services

Relationship of Evaluation to Objectives and Assessment

Systems theory states that nothing is seen as a lone entity. Diverse interacting and interdependent elements must also be studied. Therefore, when planning for evaluation, one cannot view it in isolation. Rather, the planner must take into consideration the whole planning process and how stating philosophy, defining program objectives, and deciding on particular assessment tools will affect evaluation both during and at the end of the study period.

Evaluation is dynamic, not static, and responds to the activities and feedback generated by the other subsystems of planning, assessment, and implementation. *Dynamic* means always moving and changing in response to stimuli. The relationship between the phases of planning is progressive as well as regressive. It is progressive when the development of the philosophy leads to assessment, to the formation of objectives, implementation, and finally to evaluation. It is regressive when evaluation is used to review the implementation phase, or when evaluation is used to determine if the objectives and philosophy are being met, or when evaluation is used to measure areas of initial assessment (see Figure 14-2).

Since steps of the long-term-care planning system may overlap or occur simultaneously, evaluation is built into every step; evaluation is, without a doubt, one

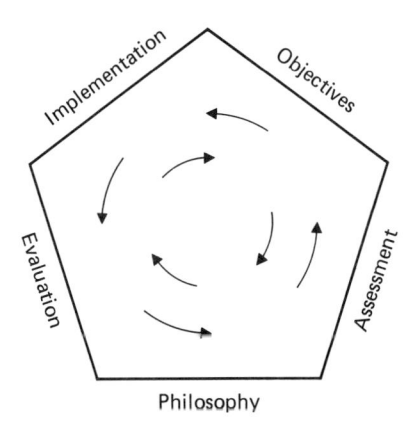

Figure 14-2. Progressive and Regressive Relationship of Evaluation to Objectives*

*The relationship of the phases of planning is progressive as well as regressive. It is progressive when the development of the philosophy leads to the assessment, the formation of the objectives, implementation and evaluation. It is regressive when evaluation is used to review the phase implementation; or evaluation is used to determine if the objectives and philosophy are being met; or evaluation is used to measure areas of initial assessment.

Table 14-1
Requirements of living scales*

Personal Care: Feeding	Personal Care: Toileting	Personal Care: Grooming/Hygiene	Home Care:	Health Care:
9 Can prepare complicated diet meals	**7 Independent in toileting need	8 Keeps self immaculately and impeccably well dressed	9 Decorates home w/ paintings, etc.	8 Can give first aid
8 Can follow directions from a nutritionist to prepare diet meals	6 Needs supervision to enable independence	**7 Independently keeps self clean and well groomed	**7 Independently maintains clean, safe home environment	**7 Seeks and follows carefully all medical directives
**7 Can independently meet own nutritional needs, including diet restrictions	5 Needs assistance in toileting	6 Bathes self w/aid of equipment	6 Capable of light housekeeping tasks	6 Could give own injections, if necessary
6 Can warm up canned or precooked food	4 Occasionally incontinent	5 Needs supervision in daily grooming	5 Needs assistance/ supervision with some tasks due to physical or mental conditions	4 Arranges with someone else to coordinate medical services
5 Can cook but not obtain proper nourishment	3 Needs assistance to schedule regular toileting	4 Needs supervision to dress appropriately	4 Arranges for others to do cleaning	3 Requires administration of oral medications
4 Can cook but forgetful (i.e., burns food, leaves stove on)	2 Incontinent, aware/not aware of need to change clothing/linen	3 Needs assistance in bathing	3 Lives in supervised environment (ex. board and care) or with relatives and others who provide home care needs	2 Requires continuous medical supervision
3 Can feed self if food is prepared	1 Totally dependent on others for toileting care	2 Needs assistance in daily grooming	2 Needs supervision in simple tasks	1 Requires intensive medical attention
2 Needs assistance in feeding		1 Needs assistance in daily dressing	1 Unable to do any housework	
1 Totally dependent on others for cooking and feeding				

Communication:	Mobility:	Service Agency Integration:	Personal Fulfillment:	Social Network Continuity:
**7 Consistently carries on intelligent conversations	8 Makes visit out of neighborhood	9 Takes active part in community affairs	8 Involved in fulfilling activities, i.e., helping others	9
6 Can seek information over telephone or by mail	**7 Moves about where he wishes to go in community	**7 Manages and budgets own finances	**7 Accepts situation, involved in pastimes and personal activities	**7 Regularly makes contacts with friends and relatives
5 Responds to questions adequately	6 Travels one or two blocks in community	6 Seeks assistance from service agencies	6	6 Would approach strangers appropriately
4 Can communicate his needs	5 Goes up and down two flights of stairs	5 Can shop in stores	5 Will engage in activities planned by others	5 Would receive visitors but would not leave his room
3 Communicates with gestures	4 Walks up 15 degree incline	4 Knows to contact social worker for needs	4 With some coercion and assistance will engage in some pastimes or activity	4
2 Communicates incoherently	3 Moves about with equipment and assistance	3 Cannot handle money properly	3 Entertains self to some degree, yet gripes about situation	3
1 Does not respond	2 Moves about in own room	2	2 Unhappy about situation, has given up trying to improve it	2 Responds inappropriately to visitors
	1 Completely dependent on others to move about	1 Completely dependent on others for all agency services	1 Unaware of his situation	1 Would sit alone for a week with no contact from outside

*From: A Review of Adult Day Health Care Pilot Projects. California Department of Finance, Report No D. 79-6. Prepared by the California Department of Health Services, May 1979.

**Indicates independent living in community.

of the most important parts of planning—it is performed after the plans are set in motion, during the implementation phase, and provides a measure of how and to what extent program activities obtained desired end results.

The development of a program structure is critical to effective evaluation. Measurement of outcomes occurs during evaluation. Feedback is defined as the return of a portion of the outcome of any process or system to the input. In addition, feedback is the information that results from a process; it is deciding what message is conveyed so that the information can be used in a constructive way. Feedback is the most important factor in assessing behavioral change. With feedback from outcomes, the program director can make necessary changes in present plans and make appropriate adaptations for future plans. Once this framework is totally understood, the planner will have little difficulty in defining program objectives that are to be evaluated later in the planning process.

California provides an example of how systematic planning for evaluation provides the feedback necessary for the systematic development and implementation of the adult day-care concept on a statewide basis. The initial program developed was On Lok Senior Health Services, which serves a homogeneous population. A data-reporting system, intake and assessment procedures, and evaluation methodology were developed for this demonstration program. Subsequently, in February 1976, the California Department of Health Services (DHS), pleased with the success of the On Lok Senior Health Services project, wished to develop additional adult day-care centers.[4(pp88-90)]

In order to expand its data base, the DHS required that the additional adult day-care demonstration projects be located in different environments (that is, geographic, demographic) and vary from the On Lok model in at least one of the following ways: organization, administration, staffing patterns, range and provision of services, payment method, or level of care provided.[4(p3)] So that the data to be acquired could be evaluated in conjunction with the On Lok data and a more precise picture of the effects of adult day care seen, the DHS required that the same data reporting system, intake and assessment procedures, and evaluation methodology be used as were used at On Lok. The two providers chosen were Sacramento Senior Day Care Center and Adult Protective Services in San Diego. Gradual accumulation of data from multiple programs using identical tools will provide data for short-term evaluation of adult day-care design and long-term evaluation of adult day-care impact. This kind of information is severely limited at present and hampers the selling of adult day care to government bodies. The California experience resulted in the passage of Assembly Bill 1611 (see Chapter 9).

Uses of Evaluation

If the philosophy is to be measured, it must first be translated into measurable outcomes (objectives). When evaluation of these objectives is completed, it can be determined if they truly reflect the stated philosophy. At that point, the planner needs to decide how the evaluation is to be used.

Areas for inclusion under the evaluative process depend on the original program objectives. These objectives are viewed over periods of time. Therefore, when objectives are written, both short-term goals and the broader long-term goals must be determined, enabling the planner to anticipate over time what should be occurring internally and externally to the proposed program. Evaluations have several uses. Among these are to examine how community needs are being met, whether the resources in the community are being utilized appropriately, if the program is beneficial in terms of participant outcomes and cost to society, and whether the staff members are functioning effectively in reaching program outcome.

It is only when the use for evaluation is determined that the planner can begin to decide on appropriate assessment tools and approaches in completing future evaluations. Also, the times when these assessments are to be carried out need to be considered. Evaluative assessments can be done during the program at different stages; that is, initially, intermediately, on discharge, or during retrospective audit (see Figure 14-3).

Adult Protective Services of San Diego, California has attempted to evaluate participant outcomes through the development and use of Effectiveness Performance Objectives. This tool attempts to measure specific improvements and the time period required to attain them. The objectives are listed below:

Objective 1: Retrain all incontinent clients with 90 percent becoming continent within 6 weeks.

Objective 2: Retrain all clients who are aphasic as a result of a stroke with the result that within 6 months, 50 percent can speak well enough to make their needs known and control short sentences.

```
Philosophy  ←————————→  Objectives

Objectives  ←————————→  Evaluation
                 ↕
            Assessment
            Initial
            Intermediate
            Discharge
            Audit
```

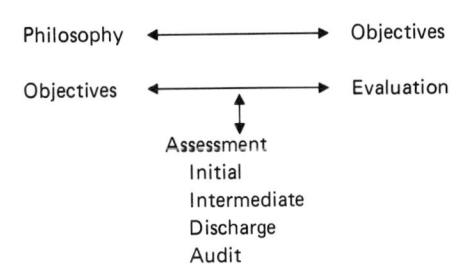

Figure 14-3. Times for Evaluative Assessments*

*Evaluation assessments can be done during the program at different stages; that is, initially, intermediately, on discharge, or during retrospective audit.

350 / Part III: Setting Up a Day-Care Program

Objective 3: Twenty-four persons transferred from nursing home back to their own homes.

Objective 4: Provide family counseling so that 75 percent of the caretakers experience sufficient decreased stress to show measurable gains, such as improved health, etc., as measured by a self-administered questionnaire.

Objective 5: Clients suffering from diabetes of age will receive counseling on self-management, such that 80 percent will be controlled cases within 4 months of enrollment.

Objective 6: 75 percent of those clients who cannot dress themselves at the time of admission will dress themselves within 60 days of admission to the program.

Objective 7: 75 percent of those clients suffering sleep disturbances such that they wander, weep, or disturb family members at night will be sleeping normally within 30 days of admission to the program.

Objective 8: Of those clients so regressed and so brain damaged as to be unaware of their own name, where they are, or what the date is 50 percent will be oriented in these matters within 90 days of admission to the program.

Objective 9: Of those admitted to the program with a diagnosis of depression, 75 percent will be symptom free within 90 days of admission.

Objective 10: Of those clients who have been told by their physicians that their only alternative to day care is nursing home or mental hygiene home care, 75 percent will be maintained at home for at least 3 months.*[4(pp88-90)]

Data collection for the program began in August 1977 and ran through March 31, 1978. After determination that a client qualified for an objective, monthly reports were made on Effectiveness Performance Update forms (see Figure 14-4). The evaluation of the results, limited as it was by the small size of the group and the fact that progress was determined by professional judgment, was encouraging enough that the California Department of Health Services feels it indicates that "improvement in performing specific functional tasks can be accomplished in persons with chronic disabilities, and gains towards independence can be made."[4(p87)]

The San Diego project illustrates the use of evaluation to measure client outcomes, as well as to challenge a health assumption, and, further, to provide a stronger health focus to the adult day-care concept.

As such projects are carried out, there will be developed a pool of definitive, objective, and concrete data relating to the original program intent and its success or failure.

*From *Adult Day Health Services*, by R. Von Behren. California Department of Health Services, 1979. This and all other quotations from this source are reprinted by permission.

EFFECTIVENESS PERFORMANCE UPDATE

According to our records _____ has begun training
for objective number _____ on _____
at _____ .

Please provide us with the following information

1. *Current Status* (check one)
   - ☐ active (in Adult Day Health Care)
   - ☐ inactive (has not attended for at least one month)
   - ☐ discharged—is independent and no longer needs ADHC
   - ☐ discharged/to skilled nursing facility
   - ☐ discharged/to intermediate care facility
   - ☐ discharged/to residential facility of board and care
   - ☐ discharged/to acute hospital
   - ☐ discharged/death

2. *For Active Participants* (circle one)
   Attendance is usually   1   2   3   4   5   days of the week

3. *Check the Appropriate Number*
   0 ☐ Discharged or discontinued before objective reached
   1 ☐ Meets the objective about 25 percent of time
   2 ☐ Meets objective about 50 percent of time
   3 ☐ Meets objective 75 percent of time
   4 ☐ Meets objective 100 percent of time.
       If 4 is checked, how long did it take? _____ months

4. *Is person still receiving training for this objective?*   ☐ Yes   ☐ No

5. *Comments: State here any of the following.*
   a. Problems that have prevented achievement, i.e., illness, hospitalization, irregular attendance, family or environmental problems.
   b. Positive examples of progress toward objective.
   c. Any significant item that should be stated to give us a better understanding.

Figure 14.4 Evaluation of Participant Progress in Meeting Effectiveness Performance Objectives (From *Adult Day Health Services*, by R. Von Behren. California Department of Health Services, 1979.)

Planning for Evaluation

Evaluation is carried out for many purposes and reasons. Inherent in these are the categories of evaluation that one must consider in planning for evaluation. As shown in Table 14-2, several questions are asked during the planning phase of evaluation.

During this planning phase, the planner must also consider the proposed areas

Table 14-2
Planning for evaluation

WHAT	is to be evaluated?	Objectives: activities, products.
HOW	will it be evaluated?	Identify alternative ways to evaluate (look at cost-benefits).
		Talk about what instruments you will use.
		Describe how data will be analyzed.
WHEN	will evaluation be conducted?	Include timetable for conducting evaluation activities.
WHO	will conduct evaluation?	Internal or external.
HOW	will results be used?	Discuss orientation of evaluation.
		How will formative and summative results be communicated to staff, people served by the program?
HOW	much will it cost?	Printing of forms, personnel to administer test instruments, computer and key punch fees, salary for people to code by hand, etc.

of evaluation and be prepared to define those areas that are to be included. Figure 14-5 gives some of the most common areas included in evaluation and their definitions.

Some questions that relate to these defined terms and that should coincide with the program's original objectives are as follows:

1. *Effort*: How much was desired? What was attained?
2. *Performance*: What was desired? What measurement tool was prescribed by the objective? What assessment tool was used? What was attained? And did it make a difference?
3. *Adequacy*: Were the objectives adequately met? What are the identified needs?

Evaluative Tools

When deciding on a category and/or categories that will be evaluated, planners must identify an appropriate tool to use, realizing that various independent tools may focus on different categories for evaluation. When planners eventually evaluate the outcome of their program against another adult day-care program, they

EVALUATIVE TERMS

Appropriateness The degree to which the program impacts on the proposed target population.

Adequacy The degree to which effective performance is adequate to the total amount of need.[5(p147)]

Benefits An economic measure of dollars saved from what would otherwise be the direct or indirect economic costs of illness.

Cost Benefits The relationship or ratio of the economic costs (direct and indirect) of a given type of illness to the benefits (defined as above in economic terms; that is, dollars served) as a result of a given disease-prevention intervention (treatment, program component, environmental strategy, and the like).

Cost-Effectiveness The relationship of the costs of a given intervention (for example, treatment) compared with the costs of a second alternative intervention in producing a desired effect (for example, relative costs of fluoridated water and of dental application of fluoride in achieving a 40% decrease in tooth decay in a given population); usually includes costs per unit (for example, dollars per decayed teeth avoided).

Economic Costs of Illness The *direct* expenditures for prevention, detection, diagnosis, treatment, and rehabilitation, plus the *indirect* costs of earnings lost by ill persons (sick days of employees, the value of housewives' services, and of those too ill—at home or in institutions—to work at all) and by those who die prematurely.

Effect The consequences, outcomes, results of an action or decision, direct or indirect regardless of intention (by individual or organization).

Effort The output, quantity, or activity of a program; that is, the number of consultations, interviews, home visits, examinations, and telephone calls. It is a strictly numerical output measure and reveals nothing about the quality of effects of program activities.

Performance outcome A measure of outcome that shows whether the effort described above made a difference.[5(p147)]

Process The procedures, methods, or arrangements by which a given effort was expended and effect(s) achieved.

Structure The human resources, knowledge, technology, organization, facilities, equipment, and finances that assist or contain the expenditure of effort and the achievement of effects or end results.[5(p3)]

Figure 14-5. Definitions of Evaluative Terms

need to be aware of the evaluative tool used by the other program. If it was a different tool and focused on categories other than their program's tool, it would definitely interfere with using crossover data.

There are several approaches to the development of an evaluation tool. In the following section, four of these approaches will be discussed. No mention is made of which one is the most valuable for adult day care because this criterion has yet to be established. After familiarizing themselves with these and other approaches, planners should be able to decide on an appropriate one for their program and, at that time, select or develop the tool that can be used with the specific approach.

The usual components of tools are as follows:

1. needs, concerns
2. questions
3. design
4. data
5. sources of data
6. analysis of data
7. workplan

Because of the complexity and individual program characteristics that are involved in the development or selection of tools, individual tools will not be discussed in this chapter.

The author, however, refers the reader to Chapter 5, which does discuss one specific assessment/evaluation tool.

One of the more frequently used evaluation approaches was developed by Suchman.[7] The five categories of criteria according to which the success or failure of a program may be evaluated are *effort, performance, adequacy, process,* and *efficiency*. Each of these categories is described in Figure 14-6, along with examples of questions answered by each criterion. The categories define the type of measure to be used in judging an activity.

Denniston and his associates, list four categories into which evaluative questions can be grouped.[8]

1. Appropriateness: Questions focus on the relative impact of the program.
2. Adequacy: Questions focus on the degree to which programs eliminate certain health problems.
3. Effectiveness: Questions focus on the extent to which programs achieve their goal, or attain preestablished objectives.
4. Efficiency: Defined as the ratio between input (resources expended) and output (net attainment of program objectives).

An application of an efficient approach can be seen in Figure 14-7.

George James also lists four categories for evaluation similar to those of Denniston and his associates.[9] However, the terms, though similar, differ in measurement used. These categories are:

1. Effort: Compare practices of program under study with local or national standards. Participant-staff ratios provides a simple, but limited, assessment of program produced.

CATEGORIES OF EVALUATION	
CATEGORY	QUESTIONS ANSWERED
Effort: the criterion of success; the quantity and quality of activity that takes place; it is an assessment of input without regard to output.	What did you do? How well did you do it?
Performance: the criterion measuring the results of effort rather than effort itself; it requires a clear statement of objectives.	How much is accomplished relative to an immediate goal? Did any change occur? Was the change the one intended?
Adequacy: the criterion of success measuring the degree to which effective performance is adequate to the total amount of need.	What portion of the target was achieved? How much progress toward an objective/goal was recorded?
Process: an analysis of the process whereby a program produces the results it does; it is descriptive and looks at the population exposed to the program, the situational context within which the program takes place, and the different kinds of effects produced by the program.	What social changes were sought? What health behavior changes were sought? What are the communication channels? Which people were most affected by the program? How much of the effect was due to locale, timing, auspices? How much of the effect was due to transportation services?
Efficiency: the criterion concerned with the evaluation of alternative methods in terms of costs—in money, time, personnel, and public convenience; it represents a rational between effort and impact.	Does it work? Is there a better way to attain the same results?

Figure 14-6. Program-Evaluation Criteria (From *Evaluative Research: Principles and Practice in Public Service and Social Action Programs,* by E. Suchman, © 1967 by the Russell Sage Foundation, New York. Reprinted by permission.)

2. Performance: What outcomes has the program produced?
3. Adequacy: To what extent has the problem been solved by this program?
4. Efficiency: Could the same result be achieved at a lower cost?

PROPOSED EVALUATION PROCESS

Initial Contact: The initial contact is generally an interview either by telephone or by mail. The interviewer should limit himself to general information but interest should be sustained pending a home visit.

Home Visit: Ideally this home visit should be made in divisions or steps: (1) contact with the family, (2) contact with the prospective guest, and (3) contact with family physician. Questions should be aimed at various levels—first at superficial and then at deeper motivations. An attempt should be made to gain insight at this time into the degree and quality of the potential guest's relationship with the family, into his general level of social and physical adjustments, and into his special interests and capabilities.

Subsequent Evaluations:

After 3rd Month
1. Family
2. Guest
3. Day-Care Staff

After 6th Month
Same as third month

12th Month (Final)
Same as 3rd month but should include contact with family physician

An evaluation should be made if guest terminates before the end of the year to determine guest and family satisfactions, dissatisfactions, suggestions, and significant changes.

INITIAL CONTACT (Appropriateness)

Family

1. How did you learn about the day-care program?
2. What about the day-care idea caused you to contact the center? (List general reasons. Ask for clarification if too ambiguous or vague. Summarize the general themes.)
3. What are some of the specific things you hope it will accomplish? (This is intended to gain a further elaboration of the general reasons and to reveal some of the more specific motivations. Summarize the specific themes as you identify them and provide the elaborating details.) For example:

    Family reasons: Seeking services for older persons not available (or not accepted) at home. Need help in supervising difficult persons. Make it possible for other member of family to continue (or start) work. Provide time for relaxation for family during day. Provide time for relaxation for older person (away from children, noise, etc.) during day.
    Other reasons:

4. Do you anticipate any problems or adverse feelings on your part or on the part of the older relative? Examples: Cost; Transportation; Reaction of the guest against it. (Feeling of being rejected, guest will be homesick or lonesome, guest is too confused to benefit); Negative reactions of neighbors; Personal feelings of your own. (Guilt over shirking family responsibilities, concern over quality of care to be given)
5. Have you talked the plan over with your older relative?
6. Special interest or background of the prospective guest which may be useful to the day care staff.
7. Obtain family evaluation of present status of guest's
    a. intellectual alertness
    b. social alertness
    c. physical alertness

Contact with Prospective Guest (Adequacy)

1. Evaluate the extent to which the prospective guest has taken part in the plan to enroll him in the day-care program?

Figure 14-7. Prospectus for Day-Care Program (From *Prospectus for Day Care Programs*. County of Los Angeles, California, Department of Senior Citizens Affairs, 1975).

2. What is his
   a. mental picture of what day-care programs are like
   b. feelings about joining the group (positive, negative, neutral; elaborate)
   c. specific feelings (positive or negative; elaborate)
3. Intellectual alertness
   a. read papers (ask what two or three recent news items were of particular interest—evaluate as to grasp, accuracy, etc.)
   b. watches television or listens to radio? What programs? Evaluate as in "a"
   c. interviewer's general impression of intellectual alertness (with brief explanation of basis)
4. Social alertness
   a. belongs to any groups (church, social, etc.) and participates (how, to what extent?)
   b. how many close friends in immediate area? What kinds of contacts? How often?
   c. maintain mail correspondence with friends elsewhere? How many? How regular? What do you correspond about?
   d. feelings toward family (general)
5. Physical alertness: General impression of interviewer with brief explanation of basis.

Family Physician (Effectiveness)

1. Evaluation of intellectual, social, physical alertness.
2. Special problems which can be anticipated.
3. Special interest or background which may be useful to the day-care staff.
4. Physician's view of what purpose day care might serve for the prospective guest and for the family.

SEQUENT EVALUATIONS (Efficiency)

Family

1. Has the day-care program served a useful purpose: If so, what? To the guest—To the family—
If not, what seemed to be the reason or deficiency? For the guest—For the family—
2. Refer to original general reasons. Ask to what extent and in what way each has been satisfied or not. Do the same for specific reasons if not already covered.
3. Refer to original listing of problems or adverse feelings. Were they resolved or did they actually present continuing and real difficulties? Specify how resolved or how they were difficulties.
4. Obtain criticism or constructive comment on the program in general.

Contact with Guest

1. What is guest's
   a. mental picture of what day-care programs are like.
   b. feelings about the group, staff, program, etc.
2. Repeat questions and evaluation of
   a. intellectual alertness
   b. social alertness
   c. physical alertness

Contact with Day-Care Staff

1. Evaluation of each guest.
   a. reactions to program
   b. special accomplishment
   c. special problems
   d. intellectual, social, and physical alertness
   e. future plans
      (1) continue
      (2) discontinue
      (3) anticipate problems
      (4) short- or long-term goals

Physician (at 12 months or on withdrawals)

1. Evaluation of present intellectual, social, and physical alertness. (What changes?)
2. Comments about value or lack of value day care has been to family and to guest.

Figure 14-7. *(continued)*

Table 14-3
Example of an evaluation flow sheet*

Participant's Name	Reason for Admission	Referral Source	Program Objectives Related to Admission†	Medical Status Functional Status Social Status
Mr. Smith 73 years old	stroke/depression/ wife recovering from surgery	hospital social worker	1,2,4,5,6,7	medical: residual damage from stroke/arthritis/diabetes
				functional: alert/ambulates with care
				social: withdrawn and depressed
Mr. Jones 65 years old	stroke/lack of socialization	community outreach worker	5,6,7	medical: right hemiplegia functional: right leg brace/alert/uses cane
				social: little social stimulation—lives alone past history of alcoholism
Mrs. White 76 years old	mental illness	family	1,2,4,5,6	medical: frequent hospitalization for mental illness
				functional: alert/ambulatory
				social: depressed/has difficulty with family

*When planners are identifying program objectives in the planning stage of the long-term-care planning process, they can create an evaluation flow sheet that includes all of the above steps.
†See Chapter 10, Figure 10-4 for exact program objectives.

Finally, Andrew Selig, in his dicussion of evaluation in the human-service delivery system, utilizes a conceptual framework including the four categories of functions, strategies, management, and operational areas.[5(p146)] The author refers the reader to Selig's article for an in-depth presentation of this model.

Evaluation Flow Sheet

A number of steps are considered vital in developing an evaluation flow sheet. These steps include:

1. identification of the objectives to be evaluated
2. specification of measures of performance
3. description of the activity

Anticipated Outcome	Program Attendance	Activities	Nutrition and Health Teaching	Medical and Nursing Care
socialization with peers maintenance of medical status balance in ambulation with cane	3 days/week 56 days to date	crafts/wood working partakes in group activities, such as singing, bingo, current events discussions	diabetic diet diabetic tool care	medical: periodic exam nursing: blood pressure once daily/hot pack 3× wk
socialization with peers improve housing arrangement/ arrange for foster home placement	3 days/week 48 days to date	little group participation prefers painting and leather-making projects	safety in current home/daily nutritional requirements with protein supplements	medical: periodic exam nursing: weights monthly/daily vitamin supplement/ protein snack
socialization with peers relationship with family/prevent further hospitalization	5 days/week 34 days to date	craft activities of various types/ beginning to participate in group discussion	—	medical: periodic exam nursing: daily antidepressant medications

(continued)

4. measurement of the degree of change that takes place
5. determination of whether the observed change is due to the activity or some other cause
6. recommendation for appropriate action in view or the variance or nonvariance between the actual results and the predetermined objectives

At the time when planners are identifying program objectives in the planning stage of the long-term-care planning process, they can create an evaluation flow sheet that includes all of the above steps. Table 14-3 gives an example of such a flow sheet.

Choice of Method

Within the context of program objectives, the need for collaboration between the planner, community, program director, interdisciplinary team, and participant

Table 14-3 *(continued)*

Participant's Name	Physical Therapy	Occupational Therapy	Speech Therapy	Social Services
Mr. Smith	group exercises 3 × wk	—	—	Encourage interaction with other participants and staff
				Encourage interaction with other day-care center participants
Mr. Jones	group exercises 3 × wk	—	—	Processing housing change to foster care
Mrs. White	—	teaching cooking skills	—	Improve feelings about family
				Encourage group socialization

should be apparent. Program directors contribute their understanding of methodologies to the identification of long-term-care service needs and their knowledge of the relationship between program objectives and overall community objectives. The interdisciplinary team is best suited to articulate strengths, areas of probable success, constraints that limit certain participant performance, and the types and amounts of necessary resources. Finally, the participants can sensitize the planner to community perceptions of the role of the program, the specific services it should provide, and how these services should be organized to maximize accessibility, acceptability and utilization. (See Chapter 3 for discussion of this material.)

At planned intervals, all objectives, outcomes processes, and inputs should be evaluated. The choice of method used for these evaluations depends entirely upon the breadth and scope of that which is to be evaluated, the original program objectives, and the initial approach used. It is important for the evaluator to remember that whatever methodology is chosen, it requires strict compliance if

Program Objectives Met	Outcomes	Future Plans
—	1. satisfied with social interactions 2. skill in wood working 3. family relationships improved 4. continues to live at home	
—	1. helping with and satisfied in new housing plans 2. more interaction noted with other participants	
—	1. no change noted in family 2. participating a little in group activities	

it is to be taken seriously. In addition to deciding on a method for evaluating these areas, the evaluator must consider the cost of program inputs as they relate to outcomes. It is much more meaningful to say that a participant in an adult day-care program has gone successfully through a prescribed treatment plan for a certain cost than to say each day in the program is costed out at a specific amount of money, with no discussion of the program's impact on the participant's well-being. Cost must therefore be evaluated to gain a picture of the balance between cost of the program and goal attainment. Various conclusions can then be drawn. These conclusions include alteration of the process, which is common to cost-effectiveness studies, and alteration of the goal, which is common to cost-containment studies.

Since evaluation of objectives common to most adult day-care programs include quality assurance, cost benefits, and cost effectiveness, some discussion of these methodologies as well as of summative/formative, structure, process, outcome methodologies will be given in this chapter.

Methodology

In designing studies for program evaluation, the planner can include both summative and/or formative evaluation procedures. Summative evaluation is an assessment of the program as a whole. The summative evaluation design should use

1. instruments that are valid and reliable
2. an adequate sample size
3. appropriate statistical methods to analyze the data collected

The summative evaluation will tell you whether you have reached your objectives on the completion of the program. It often gives little or no information about the daily operation of the program. Daily operation is assessed through a formative evaluation. Formative evaluation uses information about how things are progressing while the process is being carried out. It helps to see whether the program is doing what was intended. The planner should keep in mind that both formative and summative procedures should be included in the methodology of the evaluation design.

Structure/Process/Outcome

Another methodology used in evaluating programs includes structure, process, and outcome (see Figure 14-8).

Structure appraisal involves the evaluation of facilities and equipment used for the provision of care, administrative organization, and qualifications of professionals. If structural evaluation is used, it is assumed that using qualified staff, improved physical facilities, and an effective management system will result in the delivery of high-quality long-term care.

Process appraisal is the evaluation of the long-term-care professional's activity as related to the management of the participant's care. Process, as it applies to evaluation, refers to the sequence of events and nature of services provided. During these evaluations, management of participant care should conform to the standards and criteria set down for the performance of the involved long-term-care professionals.

Outcome appraisal is the viewing of program outcomes. Outcome evaluation assumes that beneficial results are attained by quality care. Therefore, outcome standards, criteria, and norms relate to the end point of care that is given. Actually, they are the results of the program. Although there are limitations to this approach, in that the participant may not improve even with the best care, it is these observable, behavioral outcomes that most often demonstrate quality of care. Figure 14-9 shows how the structure/process/outcome model can be used within a quality assurance model for adult day-care systems.

A quality-assurance evaluation program, as described in Chapter 10, is the best

STRUCTURE

facilities

organization
patterns

staffing patterns

personnel
qualifications

standards

funding

(resources)

PROCESS

procedures

technical aspects
of health care

health practices

provider/participant
interactions

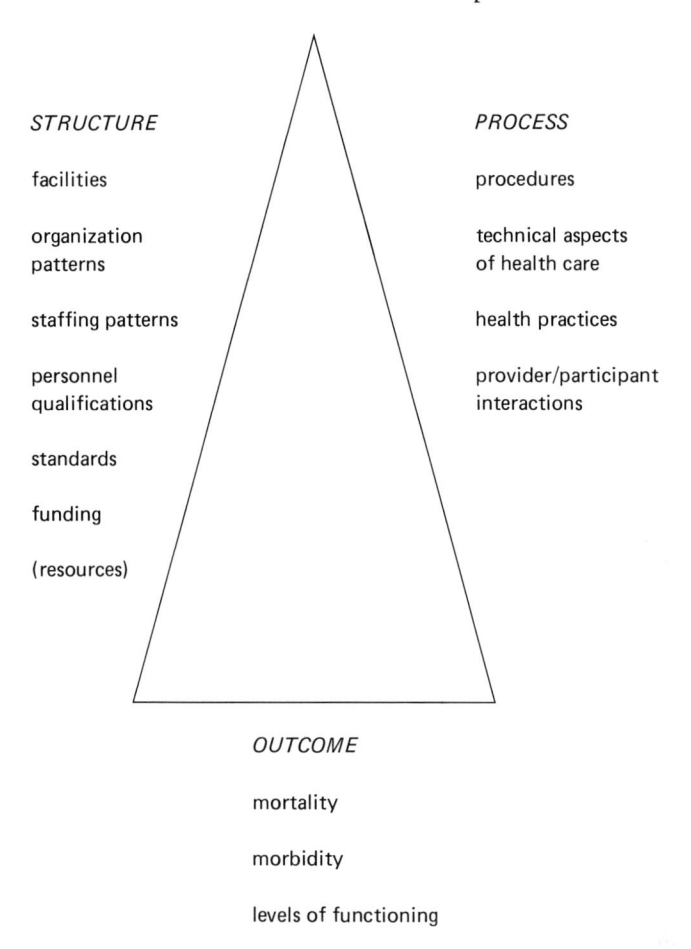

OUTCOME

mortality

morbidity

levels of functioning

Figure 14-8. Components of Structure, Process, and Outcome

overall evaluation methodology currently used by program planners. Since it cannot be covered in depth in this text, the author would encourage the planner to refer to the suggested reading list on quality assurance (see Suggested Reading) as it is important to understand for the development of an effective evaluation plan.

Cost-Benefit Analysis

As costs escalate in long-term-care delivery, providers of adult day-care services are concerned that these programs be both effective in achieving desired outcomes

364 / Part III: Setting Up a Day-Care Program

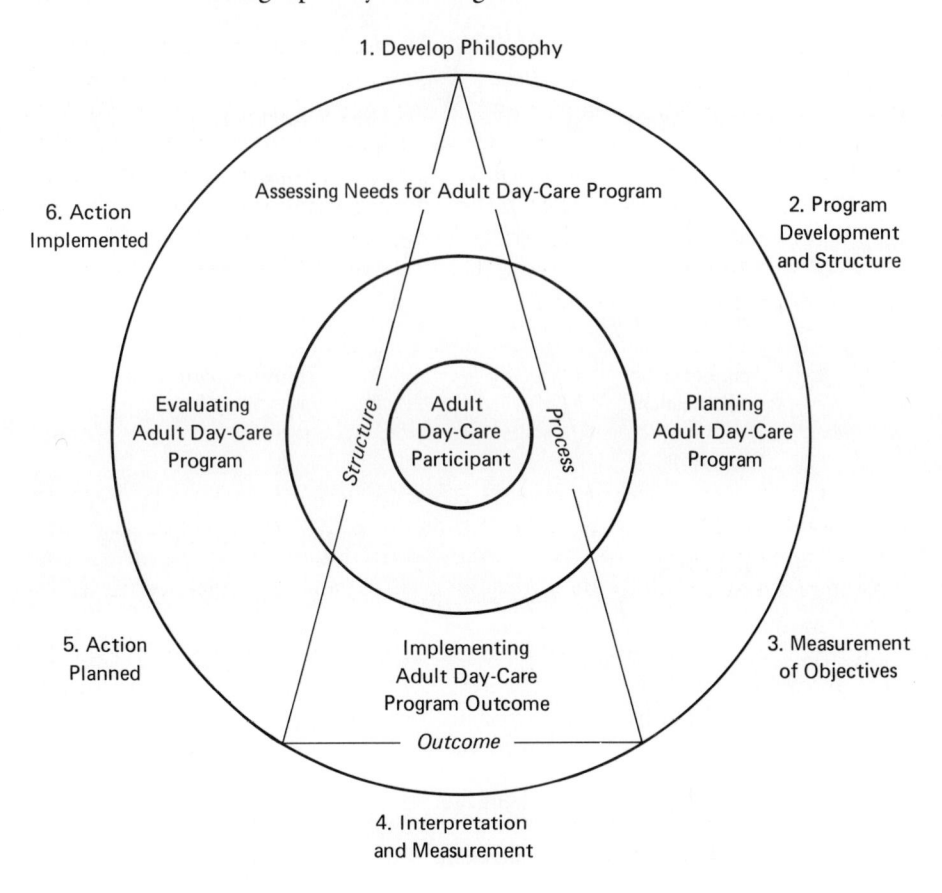

```
                    1. Develop Philosophy

                Assessing Needs for Adult Day-Care Program
6. Action                                                    2. Program
Implemented                                                  Development
                                                             and Structure

        Evaluating              Adult              Planning
        Adult Day-Care          Day-Care           Adult Day-Care
        Program                 Participant        Program

5. Action              Implementing              3. Measurement
Planned                Adult Day-Care             of Objectives
                       Program Outcome
                           Outcome

                    4. Interpretation
                    and Measurement
```

ALL AFFECT ADULT DAY-CARE PARTICIPANT

Figure 14-9. Structure/Process/Outcome Evaluation Model and Its Relationship to a Quality Assurance Model in Adult Day-Care Systems (Derived from the American Nurses' Association Quality Assurance Model as it appears in *A Plan for Implementation of the Standards of Nursing Practice*, © 1979 by the American Nurses' Association, Kansas City, Mo. Reprinted by permission of the American Nurses' Association.)

(cost-benefit analysis) and efficient in resource utilization (cost-effectiveness analysis). Not only do planners need to look at result outcomes, but they must also relate these outcomes to cost. In addition, they need to relate program costs to other alternative programs for the purpose of identifying the program's cost effectiveness.

Cost benefits are the relationship or ratio of the economic costs (direct and indirect) of a given type of illness to the benefits derived from a given program.

In order to measure the cost to society for the care of an aged, infirm participant, it is necessary to identify and measure resources used, as well as the price per unit of service. These resources (direct costs), as discussed in Chapter 3, can be supplied by state and local governments, private foundations, the family of the participant, and the participant. All resources should be evaluated to determine cost benefits, since society is foregoing an opportunity to use them in other ways in the production of goods and services for the older person.

There are many ways to do a cost-benefit analysis. The three most common areas of evaluation are the cost of

1. each client per hour of care
2. the total group intervention
3. the total year's program

In a cost-benefit analysis, an attempt is made to quantify everything. There are no established ways to complete such an analysis, and problems can arise when certain areas or items are not quantifiable. The outline shown in Figure 14-10 is recommended as a guide in identifying areas that need to be considered in a cost-benefit analysis.

Some of the resources supplied to the long-term-care participant in adult day care are indirect costs and do not involve monetary transactions—for example, a relative or friend can help the participant with shopping or errands or provide

---

STEPS IN COSTING AN ADULT DAY-CARE PROGRAM

1. Decide alternative interventions
2. Determine input* structure
3. Measure and project costs of inputs* in three ranges
   a. best estimate
   b. worst estimate
   c. possible estimate
4. Compare costs with alternatives
5. Make cost-benefits comparisons with data obtained

Inputs: time/space/equipment/supplies
Categories of Cost: Fixed—salaries/overhead/supplies/equipment
Sunk—what already put into program once
Recurring—operational items
Hidden—indirect costs

Figure 14-10. Outline of Steps in Conducting a Cost-Benefit Analysis

nursing assistance without a charge. If a price were assigned to these services, they would be considered direct costs. One technique used to determine a direct price for the indirect cost is to include the price charged for a similar service in the market as well as the value of the care giver's time, based on the wages given for a similarly educated person. In addition to such tangible items as goods and services that are the more easily measured cost benefits, indirect costs—including intangible values sacrificed, such as family feeling, control over oneself, and the unpleasantness that can be associated with having an aged parent to take care of 24 hours a day—should be taken into consideration. Qualitative, nonmonetary results (indirect benefits), such as improved family relationships or feelings of self-worth are neither easily nor objectively expressed in quantitative terms when doing a cost-benefit analysis. Figure 14-11 lists various types of cost.

It is not always clear whether certain items should be included as costs or negative benefits when the resultant outcome differs from the prescribed one. Suppose one objective of an adult day-care program is to assist older infirmed persons in maintaining their independence. In the program's attempt to meet this objective, some participants may be harmed, whereas others are helped. The issue arises as to whether the harm is counted as a cost of the program or as a negative benefit. Fisher, in *Cost Consideration in Systems Analysis*, states that "the important thing is not how we label costs and benefits, nor even which side of the equation they are on; the important thing is that all the significant consequences of our decision appear somewhere in our cost benefit analysis and that they are neither forgotten nor doubled-counted."[10]

When the evaluation is in the final step of comparing and analyzing the cost of a program in relation to the benefits produced, the evaluator must be sure to look at

1. the total program cost—that is, compare one method versus another in relation to the observed benefit
2. the average program cost—that is, the cost per participant for the benefits received
3. the marginal program cost—that is, the cost incurred by adding or removing specific services

---

LONG-TERM-CARE COSTS

1. Dollar expenditures: salaries/fringe/travel/supplies
2. Indirect costs: space/depreciation
3. Other quantifiable costs: student time/volunteer time
4. Nonquantifiable costs: effects on morale/feeling of self-worth/family relationships

---

Figure 14-11. Direct and Indirect Costs to Be Considered in a Cost-Benefit Analysis

Cost-Effectiveness Analysis

Cost effectiveness is defined by Sorenson as the comparison of all cost outcomes to identify those that are most beneficial and most economical for the type of program modality or treatment program.[11] The cost-effective analysis method developed by Sorenson explains how the costs of outcomes for a new program are seen in relation to the outcomes present, with no new program intervention (see Table 14-4). In short, do the resources utilized result in better outcomes and at what cost?

Current Evaluation Reports

The California Medi-Cal Study

The California Department of Health Services has conducted a number of cost-analysis studies of adult day-care programs as part of cost-benefit and cost-effectiveness evaluations. These studies are available upon request. Tables 14-5, 14-6, 14-7, and 14-8 show adult day-care cost figures derived from these reports. They are all Medi-Cal (California Medicaid) costs and do not include costs paid for by other payment sources or costs for services provided by families and friends. The applicability of these figures is restricted by sample size, demographics, length of study, and age of the adult day-care programs studied. Nevertheless, these figures

Table 14-4
Sequential steps in cost-outcome/cost-effectiveness analysis

Time Frame	Tasks to be Performed
One	Identifying the objective or treatment goals to be achieved (for example, increased mobility of patients, decreased length of hospital stay)
	Specifying treatment programs to be used (for example, primary versus team nursing)
Two	Determining the costs of each program cost per unit of service, and amounts of service rendered (for example, use of accounting methods, operating statistics, cost-funding, and rate-setting)
Three	Assessing the effect or outcome of the program intervention on the target group (for example, preintervention mobility versus postintervention mobility)
	Combining cost and outcome information to present cost-outcome and cost-effectiveness analyses (for example, use of cost-outcome matrices and statistical analyses to determine if program differences are greater than would be expected on the basis of chance)

From Cost outcome and cost-effectiveness analysis; emerging non-profit performance evaluation techniques, by JC Sorenson and HD Grove, *Accounting Review* 52:658–675, 1977.

Table 14-5
Cost-analysis study of adult day-care programs, at Garden Hospital* and Mount Zion Hospital and Medical Center,† November 14, 1977–June 30, 1978‡

	Garden Sullivan ADHC project		Mount Zion ADHC project		Skilled Nursing Facility (SNF)
	ADHC from Community	SNF Transfer	ADHC from Community	SNF Transfers	
Medi-Cal dollars per month per person	$153.80	$255.32	$141.89	$258.00	
Average Medi-Cal persons per month	39.12		45.25		
Average days per person per month	8.08	11.88	7.70	12.00	
Projected Medi-Cal SNF costs per month					680.00
Medi-Cal dollars per person per day	$19.03	$21.50	$19.03	$21.50	

*Garden Hospital Jerd Sullivan Rehabilitation Center of San Francisco, Calif.
†Mount Zion Hospital and Medical Center, San Francisco, Calif.
‡From *Adult Day Health Care, Nursing Home Alternative,* by R Von Behren. California Department of Health Services, 1979, p 21.

Notes: Average stay in program = 7.5 months
13% of Garden Sullivan participants were SNF transfers
2.4% of Mount Zion participants were SNF transfers

provide valuable insights into the costs of maintaining "at risk" elderly in the community.

Costs are always looked at in terms of client outcomes. Following is a summary of the California Department of Health Services' findings on client outcomes in adult day-care programs.

The effectiveness, performance update was originally conceived as a method of measuring a participant's progress in relation to a standard established for selected goals assigned to him. After a specified amount of time, each was rated on a scale from one to four in order to determine progress. The four-point scale was as follows:

1. Meets the goal 25 percent of the time
2. Meets the goal 40 percent of the time
3. Meets the goal 75 percent of the time
4. Meets the goal 100 percent of the time

Table 14-6
Cost-analysis study of adult day-care programs at Garden Hospital*and Mount Zion Hospital and Medical Center,† November 14, 1977–June 30, 1978‡

	Skilled Nursing *Facility Transfers in Adult Day-Care*	Adult Day-Care participants *Drawn from Community*	Skilled Nursing Facility (SNF)
Average Medi-Cal adult day-care costs per month	$256.66	$147.84	
Average overall Medi-Cal costs per month other than adult day care	73.97	227.77§	
Average Medi-Cal costs per month other than adult day care without hospitalizations	65.03	68.55	
Projected SNF costs per month			680.00

*Garden Hospital Jerd Sullivan Rehabilitation Center, San Francisco, Calif.
†Mount Zion Hospital and Medical Center, San Francisco, Calif.
§Major difference is caused by hospitalization of 4 participants combined sample from Mt. Zion adult day-care program and Garden Sullivan adult day-care program

Notes: Sample Size: 16 SNF Transfers, 2/Other, 14
‡From *Adult Day Health Care, Nursing Home Alternative,* by R Von Behren. California Department of Health Services, 1979, pp 23, 34, 38.

The results of the ten objectives and the ratings are as follows:

Objective 1: Retrain all incontinent clients with 90 percent becoming continent within 6 weeks.

Twenty-one clients were assigned this goal with 15 being actual active participants. Nine participants, 60 percent, received a 4 rating. Four participants, 27 percent, received a 3 rating. One participant, 7 percent, received a 2 rating and 1, also, received a 1 rating.

Ninety percent did receive a 3 or a 4 rating; though it did not occur within the time period of the standard, it was met within a median time of 8 weeks.

Objective 2: Retrain all clients who are aphasic as a result of a stroke with the result that within 6 months, 50 percent can speak well enough to make their needs known and control short sentences.

Twelve clients were assigned to the objective #2 with 7 being actual active participants. While none of the 7 participants received a 4 rating, 72 percent received

Table 14-7
Cost-analysis study of adult day-care programs at Sacramento Senior Health Day-Care Center and San Diego Adult Protective Services (19-month study period)

Average	San Diego Adult Day-Care Participants	San Diego Control	Sacramento Adult Day-Care Participants	Sacramento Control	Skilled Nursing Facility (SNF)
Costs per person other than adult day care	$784.18	$6,390.36	$635.80	$1,864.88	
Costs per person per month	41.27	336.39	33.46	98.15	$510.00
Units used per person	49.39	177.08	38.03	94.10	
Cost per unit	15.87	36.09	16.72	19.82	
Costs per person per month with ADHC dollars	226.96		226.23		
Costs per person per month with adult day care, homemaker/chore, SSI and SSP dollars*	396.51		396.51		

Source: Adult Day Health Services, by R. Von Behren. California Department of Health Services, 1979.
*Supplemental Security Income/State Supplemental Payment

Notes: Total Study group: 119 persons—55 from adult day care, 64 controls. Control group members are all Medi-Cal recipients with type and number of health problems similar to those of the adult day-care group.
Unit: 15-minute time period of Medi-Cal utilization.
75% of San Diego and 65% of Sacramento costs attributable to inpatient hospitalization and long-term-care services.
14.29% of San Diego adult day-care participants and 33% of Sacramento adult day-care participants utilized homemaker/chore services and SSI/SSP.

Table 14-8
Cost analysis of adult day-care

	Sacramento Senior Health Day-Care Center (17 months)	Adult Protective Services, San Diego (18 months)
Total days billed	10,976.18	8,862.00
Total dollars paid	$165,880.83	$137,778.76
Total number of participants	861.00	741.98
Average		
Days billed	645.65	492.33
Dollars paid	$9,763.57	$7,654.37
Number of participants	50.64	40.61
Days per person per month	12.74	11.94
Cost per person per month	$192.77	$185.69

Source: Adult Day Health Services, by R. Von Behren. California Department of Health Services, 1979 p. 9

a 3 rating within a range from 2.5 months to 12 months of training, the median being 6 months. One participant received a 2 rating with a time of 5 months and was followed by a single score of 1 which was reached within 36 months of training.

While the outcome of this goal objective didn't occur as in the standard, 50 percent did receive a 3 rating within the standard time limit of 6 months.

Objective 3: Twenty-four persons transferred from nursing home back to their own homes.

The objective of 24 persons transferred from nursing home back to their own homes was not met. Two persons were transferred home, 1 for 6 months before returning to an ICF [intermediate care facility], the other for 7 months before hospitalization.

Objective 4: Provide family counseling so that 75 percent of the caretakers experience sufficient decreased stress to show measurable gains, such as improved health, etc., as measured by a self-administered questionnaire.

Twenty-four caretakers were originally [assigned to this objective] with 17 being actual active participants. Four, or 24 percent, received a 4 rating with a range of time from less than 1 month to 1 year, the median being 10 months. Seven, or 41 percent, received a 3 rating, with a median of 4.5 months. Four, or 24 percent, received a 2 rating with an average of approximately 5 months of training. Two, or 12 percent, received a 1 with an average time of 3 months. Seventy-five percent did meet the standard within 8 months.

Objective 5: Clients suffering from diabetes of age will receive counseling on self-management, such that 80 percent will be controlled cases within 4 months of enrollment.

Of the 16 clients assigned this goal, 12 were actual active participants with 58 percent receiving a 4 rating with a range from 1 to 26 months. The median was 3 months.

Three participants received a 3 rating, all with a time of 5 months. Two participants received a 2 rating with a median of 79 weeks.

When compared to the standard for this objective, 10 participants were successful in obtaining a 3 or 4 rating within the specified time limit.

Objective 6: Seventy-five percent of those clients who cannot dress themselves at the time of admission will dress themselves within 60 days of admission to the program.

Twenty clients were originally assigned this objective with 15 actually being active participants. There were no 4 ratings. Six participants, 40 percent, received a 3 rating with a median training time of 13 months. Six participants, 40 percent, also received a 2 rating with an average time of 24 months. Three received a 1 rating with an average time of 11 months.

None of the participants were able to reach the goal within 60 days of admission to the program. All of the participants were able to reach the objective within 19 months with 75 percent achieving within 13 months.

Objective 7: Seventy-five percent of those clients suffering sleep disturbances such that they wander, weep, or disturb family members at night will be sleeping normally within 30 days of admission to the program.

Of the 15 clients assigned this goal, 11 were actual active participants. Four participants, or 36.4 percent, received a 4 rating within 1.5 months. Five participants, or 45.5 percent, received a 3 rating within 12 months. With the 3 and 4 ratings together, the median time was 4 months. There were not any 2 ratings and there was one 1 rating with 19 months. The time limit of the standard appears to be inappropriate and should probably be extended a fairly large amount.

Objective 8: Of those clients so regressed or so brain damaged as to be unaware of their own name, where they are, or what the date is, 50 percent will be oriented in these matters within 90 days of admission to the program.

Of the 60 clients originally assigned this goal, 34 were actual active participants. Eight participants, or 23.4 percent, were able to obtain a 4 rating in 5 months. Nine participants, or 26.5 percent, were able to obtain a 3 rating within 10 months of time. Eight participants, or 23.4 percent, received a 2 rating within 10.5 months. Nine participants, or 26.4 percent, obtained a 1 rating within 12 weeks. Fifty percent did receive a 4 or a 3 rating; however, it was within 6 months of time rather than the 3 months as stated in the standard.

Objective 9: Of those admitted to the program with a diagnosis of depression, 75 percent will be symptom free within 90 days of admission.

Of the 22 persons assigned this goal, 12 were actual active participants. Seven participants, or 58.3 percent, received a 3 rating with the range of from 3 months to over 36 months. The median was approximately 13.5 months. There were not any 4 ratings. Seven percent were able to reach the standard but only with a 1, 2, or 3 rating and within a median time of 13 months.

Objective 10: Of those clients who have been told by their physicians that their only alternative to day care is nursing home or mental hygiene home care, 75 percent will be maintained at home for at least 3 months.

Of the 11 actual participants for this objective, all, or 100 percent, obtained a 4 rating with the range being from 1 month to over 1 year with a median time of 14 months.[4(pp88–90)]

Functional Status

Eighty-six point one percent of the ADHC participants showed improvements in one or more Requirements of Living (ROL) scales.
Thirty-six percent did not deteriorate in any of the ROL scales.
Eighteen point one percent deteriorated in only one ROL scales.
Ninety-four point four percent were maintained at the same functional level in one or more ROL scales.
Twenty-nine point two percent improved in five or more ROL scales.
Fifty-eight point three percent were maintained at the same level in five or more ROL scales.
Nine point seven percent deteriorated in five or more ROL scales.[4(p2)]

Weissert Study

Another cost-effectiveness evaluation was carried out by the National Center for Health Services Research in 1977–78. It sought to test the effects of homemaker services and adult day-care on a Medicare-eligible population. The study used six nonrandomly selected adult day-care sites. Client selection was random within confines that required the referrers to already be aware of adult day care. After selection into the study, participants were randomly placed in control groups, the adult day-care group, the homemaker group, or the adult day-care/homemaker group. The original sample included 1871 persons, but this number was reduced to 1153 because some of the participants had an inadequate data base, some did not use the assigned service, some used additional services for which they were eligible, and some died. Subsequently, many of the persons dropped from the sample were followed for comparison.

The authors concluded that adult day care was not cost-effective in terms of reducing overall Medicare expenditures. This conclusion has been discussed and challenged by many. In question are the constraints imposed by an insufficient data base (not enough adult day-care centers have been developed and evaluated) on which to develop the study, the nonrandom selection of the sites, the construed population sample, and the use of one day hospital as a study site. The larger ratio of professional staff to participants at a day hospital significantly increases the daily rate to as much two times that of a medical-model adult day-care center. The inclusion of these costs in the total gives a medical-model adult day-care center the appearance of being costlier than it actually is (refer to Anne Klapfish's testimony in Chapter 6 for more discussion of this point).

Additional factors were considered in determining benefits. Significantly, institutionalization and mortality rates were reduced, and physical functioning, levels of contentment, mental functioning, and social activity improved in the experimental group on the average over the control group. Variables of age, sex, race, and the like were examined for patterns and impacts.

Adult day care is a long-term-care option, and the determination of who will benefit most from this option needs continual investigation. Variables such as these will have to be examined for optimal targeting for adult day-care services.

Implications for Research

Adult day care is still very young and largely experimental. Much research is required to substantiate its many hypotheses, to provide hard data for adequate funding support, and to guide us in developing adult day care as it grows. To date, too few programs have ever attempted to document carefully their development and growth. Some studies, such as those already mentioned, have tried to research a particular aspect of adult day care. Unfortunately, they have all had design inadequacies that have rendered the conclusions unsuitable for generalization. However, they have provided a large body of information to use in the designing of a new generation of research projects as the benefits of adult day care. The design of future research must include a complete accounting of the essential components of a research project. These components are as follows:

Scope

Scope includes definition of each part of the project, time parameters (six months, two years), geographic parameters (one city, one county, 240 square miles), political parameters (Indian reservation, urban, citizenship), legal parameters (AB1611, Title XX, Title XIX), complexity of parts, degree of detail or superficiality in study, interrelatedness of parts, complete description of activity and services, as well as definition of purpose.

Variables

Variables can be human (age, sex, disability), demographic (white, urban, class), monetary (funding sources, outside expenditures), geopolitical (inner city, suburb, transportation), and administrative (multipurpose senior-center staff, nursing-home site). They can be as elusive as the social histories of the participants and as concrete as incomes. They must be identified, monitored, and compensated for to establish causative relationships.

Population

The population must reflect a national body of potential adult day-care users. A heterogeneous population lends itself to generalization to large groups but introduces more variables. Sample size needs to be large enough to have results be statistically significant. In small groups, variables become more important as determinants of the outcomes.

Environment

Environmental considerations include physical layout within center, decorating of center, physical environment surrounding center, location of center, type of center, transportation modes of participants, distance and travel time of participants, housing sites of participants, noise level within and without center, special noise considerations (such as flight path of airport), temperature variations and weather patterns, and description of services at center.

Control group

The control group needs to be well matched, including variables. A control group who are more or less frail or impaired or otherwise differ markedly in kind or need cannot be validly compared to the study group. The control group must be as closely followed as the study group, to be assessed at the same points in time and to be monitored for new variables.

Tools

All the tools to be used—intake, assessment, analysis, evaluation, and so forth—should be specified and coordinated in the research design to ensure sufficient data collection, data reducibility, and utility to the purpose of the research. It must be determined in advance that the tools are actually capable of measuring what is sought. Early research on adult day care was conducted with tools designed for other care settings. Tools specific to adult day care are now being designed, but they are as much in transition as adult day care because each is building on the other. A variety of approaches to a single focus will provide the most accurate measurement. The tools should be known and understood by all the researchers and center staff since the skill of the user affects the results.

Reproducibility

The ability of another researcher to duplicate a given research project and arrive at the same results validates the results of the original project, which then become hard data. Hard data are what is needed to determine whether adult day care is a necessary long-term-care option. The research design must be analyzed to ensure reproducibility.

Summary

Finally, a complete statement of adequacy of each component to the stated purpose of the study should enable researchers to see if the research design is complete or if it needs further development before it is implemented.

Inclusion of a simple outline of the research design in the summary document of any study would allow other researchers to analyze the results with more comprehension and greater ease. Thorough and meticulous documentation of all aspects of research and retention of all records are essential to valid research.

The questions that have been researched so far are:

1. What is adult day care?
2. What could adult day care be?
3. Does adult day care improve quality of life?
4. How much does adult day care cost?
5. Is adult day care a cost-effective alternative to SNF-ICF placement?
6. Is adult day care a cost-effective means of preventing premature institutionalization?
7. Are homemaker/chore services a cost-effective means, alone or with adult day care, of preventing premature institutionalization?

A number of other questions still require study. They are:

1. What should the long-term-care continuum include?
2. Who should be served in adult day care?
3. Can various populations be effectively treated in the same program?
4. What size should a program be?
5. How many centers should be developed?
6. Who will determine where the client will be served in the noninstitutional-care complex?
7. Should homemaker services be paired with adult day care?
8. Are these services rehabilitative or maintenance? Can they be both?
9. Can social costs be measured? Should they?
10. Who will finance these services?
11. Is adult day care a form of geriatric care or should it be for all ages?
12. What determines need for institutionalization?
13. Should all existing models of adult day care be called adult day care or are they separate care modalities on the long-term-care continuum?

Both those questions that are already being researched and those that still need to be studied require much more thought and research before they are answered. Another area for research is the claim that the existing long-term-care system is fragmented, ineffective, lacks alternatives, and so forth. Although all these claims are presumed to be true, and there is a plenitude of first-hand experience attesting to them, there is insufficient documentation to claim them as a justification for adult day care development.

Adult day care needs research, and this research requires the cooperation of all who are involved in adult day care. Research will focus and direct the development of adult day care as one important option on the long-term-care continuum.

References

1. Davidson SV: Community nursing care evaluation. *Family and Community Health: The Journal of Health Promotion and Maintenance* 1: 41–45, 1978.

2. Douglas LM, Bevis EO. *Nursing Management and Leadership in Action.* St. Louis, Mo, The CV Mosby Co, 1979, p 198.

3. California Department of Health Services (DHS): *Response to: "A Review of Adult Day Health Care Pilot Projects," California Department of Finance December 1978, Report No. D79-6*, May 1979, p 30.

4. Von Behren R: *Adult Day Health Services*, Final Report, Section 1115, Project No 11-P-903549/01, California DHS, 1979.

5. Selig A: A conceptual framework for evaluating human service delivery systems. *Orthopsychiatry* 46: 140–146, 1976.

6. Rice D, Cooper B: Cost of illness. *Social Security Bulletin,* February 1976, p 8.

7. Suchman E: *Evaluation Research.* New York, Russel Sage Foundation, 1967, pp 61–71.

8. Denniston OL: Evaluation of program efficiency. *Public Health Reports* 85: 835, 1979.

9. James G: Evaluation in public health practice. *Public Health Reports* 52: 1145–1154, 1962.

10. Fisher G: *Cost Considerations in Systems Analysis.* New York, American Elsevier Publishers, Inc, 1975, p 78.

11. Sorenson J, Grone H: Cost outcome and cost effective analysis: Emerging nonprofit performance evaluation techniques. *Accounting Review* 52: 659, 1977.

12. Weissert W: *Geriatric Day Care and Homemaker Services: An Experimental Study.* National Center for Health Services Research, Department of Health, Education and Welfare, 1979.

Readings

General

Abel NE: Daytime care lets elderly people stay home at night. *Mod Health Care* **6:** 23–28, 1976.

Arie T: Day care in geriatric psychiatry. *Gerontol Clin* (Basel) **17:** 31–39, 1975.

Aronson R: Programs, I; The role of an occupational therapist in a geriatric day hospital setting—Maimonides Day Hospital. *Am J Occup Ther* **30:** 290–292, 1976.

Bagnall MK: Day care and social needs. *Gerontol Clin* (Basel) **16:** 253–257, 1974.

Barker C: Psychogeriatric day patient assessment—1. Making a visual aid book. *Nurs Times* **71:** 1292–1298, 1975.

Bendall MJ: Changing work pattern in a geriatric unit and the effect of a day hospital. *Age Aging* **7:** 229–232, 1978.

Blume RM, Kalin M, Sacks J: A collaborative day treatment program for chronic patients in adult homes. *Hosp Community Psychiatry* **30(1):** 40–42, 1979.

Brocklehurst JC: The day hospital. *Physiotherapy* **62:** 148–150, 1976.

Burke AW: Physical disorder among day hospital patients. *Br J Psychiatry* **133:** 22–27, 1978.

Cohen, MG, Cohen BS: Rehabilitation and day care—another alternative. *Md State Med J* **24:** 71–73, 1975.

Dal JL: Helping old people to continue living at home. The contribution of the day hospital. *R Soc Health J* **98:** 10–11, 1978.

Davidson SM, Nicholas M: Day treatment for the elderly mentally infirm letter. *Br Med J* **1:** 1030, 1977.

Doherty NJ, Hicks BC: The use of cost-effectiveness analysis in geriatric day care. *Gerontologist* **15:** 412–417, 1975.

Ellis LJ: Designing day hospitals. *Gerontol Clin* (Basel) **16:** 294–299, 1974.

Fairclough F: Community and day hospital care. *Nurs Mirror* **143:** 67–68, 1976.

Goldstone H: Planning a day hospital. *Gerontol Clin* (Basel) **16:** 289–293, 1974.

Gooch LA, Luxton DE: A new geriatric day hospital. *Nurs Mirror* **145:** 36–38, 1977.

Green JG, Timbury GC: A geriatric psychiatry day hospital service: A five-year review. *Age Aging* **8:** 49–53, 1979.

Greenfield PR: Day hospitals: A departmental view. *Gerontol Clin* (Basel) **16:** 307–314, 1974.

Grimaldi PL: The costs of adult day care and nursing home care: A dissenting view. *Inquiry* **16:** 162–166, 1979.

Guillette W, Crowley B, Savitz SA, et al: Day hospitalization as a cost-effective alternative to inpatient care: A pilot study. *Hosp Community Psychiatry* **29:** 525–527, 1978.

Gustafson E: Day care for the elderly. *Gerontologist* **14:** 46–49, 1974.

Hall MR: Day care and society. *Gerontol Clin* (Basel) **16:** 300–306, 1974.

Heinemann SH, Yudin LM, Perlmutter F: A follow-up study of clients discharged from a day hospital aftercare program. *Hosp Community Psychiatry* **26:** 752–754, 1975.

Hildick-Smith M: Day hospitals letter. *Br Med J* **2:** 1433, 1978.

Hildick-Smith M: A typical journey to and from the day hospital. *Gerontol Clin* (Basel) **16:** 263–269, 1974.

Isdale IC, Ridings KW: A geriatric day hospital: The first year. *NZ Med J* **85:** 177–179.

Kiernat JM: Geriatric day hospitals: A golden opportunity for therapists. *Am J Occup Ther* **30:** 285–289, 1976.

Lamden RS, Greenstein LN: Partnership in outpatient day care. *Hospitals* **49:** 87–89, 1975.

Marston PD: Day hospitals: A physiotherapist's view. *Physiotherapy* **62:** 151–152, 1976.

Mehta CM: Day care services: An alternative to institutional care. *J Am Geriatr Soc* **23:** 280–283, 1975.

Memorial hospital day house for inpatients. *Nurs Mirror* **141:** 75–76, 1975.

Minor K, Thompson P: Development and evaluation of a training program for volunteers working in day treatment. *Hosp Community Psychiatry* **26:** 154–156, 1975.

Mitchell RG: Psychiatric day centres—A sound investment. *Nurs Times* **72:** 634, 1976.

Morgan D: Gaining independence at a geriatric day hospital. *Dimens Health Serv* **56:** 23–25, 1979.

Morgan DM: Day care as an alternative to nursing homes. *Dimens Health Serv* **55:** 38–39, 1978.

O'Brien CL: Exploring geriatric day care: An alternative to institutionalization? *J Gerontol Nurs* **3**: 26–28, 1977.

Peach H, Pathy MS: Evaluation of patients' assessment of day hospital care. *Br J Prev Soc Med* **31**: 209–210, 1977.

Peach H, Pathy MS: Social support of patients attending a geriatric day hospital. *J Epidemiol Community Health* **32**: 215–218, 1978.

Pierotte DL: Day health care for the elderly. *Nurs Outlook* **25**: 519–523, 1977.

Porter KR: Day hospitals: A regional view. *Gerontol Clin* (Basel) **16**: 315–317, 1974.

Ransome HE: Physiotherapy in the geriatric day hospital. *Gerontol Clin* (Basel) **16**: 274–280, 1974.

Rathbone-McCuan E, Elliott MW: Geriatric day care in theory and practice. *Soc Work Health Care* **2**: 153–170, 1976.

Rathbone-McCuan E, Levenson J: Geriatric day care: A community approach to geriatric health care. *J Gerontol Nurs* **3**: 43–46, 48, 1977.

Ratkowski E, Liebermann R, Hochman A: Day care for cancer patients. *JAMA* **230**: 430–431, 1974.

Ridinbs KW, Indale IC: The day hospital: Efficacy and cost effectiveness. *NZ Med J* **87**: 129–133, 1978.

Russell IT, Devlin HB, Fell M, et al: Day-case surgery for hernias and haemorrhoids. A clinical, social, and economic evaluation. *Lancet* **1**: 844–847, 1977.

Saunders BM: Nurse's role in day care. *Gerontol Clin* (Basel) **16**: 248–252, 1974.

Schwartz RM: Know your community resources. Multipurpose day centers: A needed alternative. *J Gerontol Nurs* **5**: 48–52, 1979.

Shaw J: Nursing at home. *Hosp Equip Supplies* **22**: 6, 1976.

Strouthidis TM: Medical requirements of the day hospital. *Gerontol Clin* (Basel) **16**: 241–247, 1974.

Symonds PC: Social services and day care. *Gerontol Clin* (Basel) **16**: 270–273, 1974.

Thompson K: A general practitioner looks at day care. *Gerontol Clin* (Basel) **16**: 258–262, 1974.

Turbow SR: Geriatric group day care and its effect on independent living. A thirty-six-month assessment. *Gerontologist* **15**: 508–510, 1975.

Weiler PG, Kim P, Pickard LS: Health care for elderly Americans: Evaluation of an adult day health care model. *Med Care* **14**: 700–708, 1976.

Weissert WG: Adult day care programs in the United States: Current research projects and a survey of 10 centers. *Public Health Rep* **92**: 49–56, 1977.

Weissert WG: Costs of adult day care: A comparison to nursing homes. *Inquiry* **15**: 10–19, 1978.

Weissert WG: Two models of geriatric day care: Findings from a comparative study. *Gerontologist* **16**: 420–427, 1976.

Wilkes E, Crowther AG, Greaves CW: A different kind of day hospital—for patients with preterminal cancer and chronic disease. *Br Med J* **2**: 1053–1056, 1978.

Williamson F: A day hospital within the divisions of a troubled community. *Int J Soc Psychiatry* **24**: 95–103, 1978.

Wood SM, Harris WP: Adult day care: A new modality. *J Long Term Care Adm* **4**: 18–28, 1976.

Planning

General

Benedict RC: Making the health care system responsive to the needs of the elderly. *Aging*, May–June 1979, pp 25–27.

Butler RN: Questions on health care for the aged, in *Papers on the National Health Guidelines: Conditions for Change in the Health Care System*. US Dept of HEW, Public Health Service, Health Resources Administration. Publication No. (HRA) 78-642. Sept 1977, pp 98–106.

Crawford CO, Leadley SM: Interagency collaboration for planning and delivery of health care. *FCH/Community Assessment* Nov 20, 1977, pp 35–44.

Congregate Housing

Commonwealth of Massachusetts, the Congregate Housing Guidelines Committee (Department of Community Affairs, Department of Elder Affairs, Department of Public Welfare, Medical Division): *Guidelines for the Planning and Management of Public Congregate Housing for Elders*. Publication No. 11158-20-300-1-79, Sept 1978.

US Dept of HEW, Office of Human Development, Administration on Aging: Congregate housing for older people: An urgent need, a growing demand, in Donahue WT, Thompson MM, Curren, DJ (eds): *Selected Papers from the First National Conference on Congregate Housing for Older People, Conducted by the International Center for Social Gerontology*. Publication No. (OHD) 77-20284, 1977.

Williams C: *Congregate Housing for Older People in Massachusetts*. A staff report from Citizens Housing and Planning Association, Inc., 7 Marshall Street, Boston, Mass, August 1978.

Coordinated Projects

Clark AM: Adult day health services: An appropriate alternative for Malden? Masters thesis, Boston University, 1978.

Paul J: Holyoke's geriatric village. *Aging*, July–Aug 1978, pp 12–17.

Proposal for Supportive Service and Housing Program for the Elderly, Central Avenue Housing, Chicopee, Massachusetts. Massachusetts Government Land Bank, 1 Ashburton Place, Room 2109, Boston, Mass 02108, January 5, 1979.

Quinn JL: Triage: Coordinated home care for the elderly. *Nursing Outlook* 23: 570–573, 1975.

———: Lecture at Boston College on Triage Project, Sept 28, 1977.

Trebony ES: Project Find: Seeking out the isolated elderly. *Aging,* Jan–Feb 1979, pp 12–17.

Tyson T, Sytske O: The JSPOA friendship center. *Aging,* Mar–April 1979, pp 12–14.

Home Care

Massachusetts Department of Elder Affairs: *Programs and Services for Elders, 1978.* Publication No. PHL/9734-41-500-5-77/MD.

National Council on Aging: Summary of the Older Americans Act (P.L. 95-478). Aging Program Factsheet, Nov 1978.

Home Health

Assembly of Ambulatory and Home Care Services, American Hospital Association, Homemaker-Home Health Aide Services, Inc., Council of Home Health Services of the National League for Nursing: *A Prospectus for a National Home Care Policy.* New York, 1978.

Association of Massachusetts Homes for the Aging: *Statement Encouraging Parallel Services.* 5 New England Executive Park. Burlington, Mass, 1979.

National League for Nursing: Statement of the Council of Home Health Agencies and Community Health Services before DHEW Office of Policy Planning and Research, Health Care Financing Administration, Sept 15, 1978. (P.L. 95-142 Section 18. Report on Home Health and Other "In Home" Services.)

US Dept of HEW: *Home Health Care Report on the Regional Public Hearings.* Sept 20–Oct 1, 1976, Publication No. 76-135.

Hospice

Rezendes D, Abbott J: Hospice movement: Way stations for the terminally ill, *Perspective on Aging* 8: 6–10, 1979.

Neighborhood Health Centers

Massachusetts League of Neighborhood Health Centers: *Take Care of Yourself: A Directory of Massachusetts Neighborhood Health Centers.* Milford, Mass, Charlescraft Press, Inc., 1976.

Nursing Homes

Commonwealth of Massachusetts, Executive Office of Human Services, Office of Comprehensive Health Planning: *Consumer's Guide to Nursing Homes*. Boston, 1975.

Implementation

Boston, Massachusetts Department of Public Welfare: *Application to Become an Adult Day Care Program Provider under the Medical Assistance Program of the Massachusetts Department of Public Welfare,* 1978.

Commonwealth of Massachusetts, Department of Public Safety: *Rules and Regulations of the Architectural Barriers Board*. Boston, Architectural Barriers Board, 1978, pp 27–29.

Diet Manual for Long Term Care Facilities, rev ed. Prepared by a committee of consulting dietitians involved in long term care facilities, with the approval of the Massachusetts Dietetic Association, Inc. Boston, 1978.

Kinlein ML: Point of view on the front: Nursing and family and community health. *Family and Community Health: The Journal of Health Promotion and Maintenance* 1: 57–68, 1978.

Northman JE: Human service program design and the family. *Family and Community Health: The Journal of Health Promotion and Maintenance* 1: 17–25, 1978.

Special Committee on Aging: *Adult Day Facilities for Treatment, Health Care and Related Services, A Working Paper*. US Government Printing Office, 1976.

Weiler P, Rathbone-McCuan E: *Adult Day Care, Community Work with the Elderly*. New York, Springer Publishing Company, 1978.

Records and the Problem-Oriented Record System

Bjarn JC, Cross H: *Problem Oriented Practice*. Chicago, Modern Healthcare Press, 1970.

Cross HD, Burger CS, Bjorn JC: The problem oriented medical record. *Ann Int Med* 79: 46–53, 1973.

Department of Home Health Agencies: *Problem Oriented Systems of Patient Care*. New York, National League for Nursing, 1974.

Ellis GJ, Neelson, FA: *A Syllabus of Problem Oriented Patient Care*. Boston, Little, Brown & Company, 1974.

Herman H, McKay ME: *Community Health Services*. Washington, DC, International City Managers' Association, 1968.

Readey H, Berni R: *Problem-Oriented Medical Record Implementation*. St. Louis, Missouri, The CV Mosby Company, 1976.

Vaughan-Wroble BC, Henderson B: *The Problem-Oriented System in Nursing, A Workbook*. St. Louis, Missouri, The CV Mosby Company, 1976.

Walter J, Pardee GP, Mobbo DM: *Dynamics of Problem-Oriented Approaches: Patient Care and Documentation.* Philadelphia, JB Lippincott Company, 1978.

Evaluation

Blum, H: Evaluating health care. *Medical Care* **12:** 999–1011, 1978.

Conly S: *Critical Review of Research on Long-Term Care Alternatives Sponsored by the Department of Health, Education and Welfare.* Office of Social Services and Human Development, Office of the Assistant Secretary for Planning and Evaluation, Dec 1976.

Denniston O, Rosenstock I: Evaluating health programs. *Public Health Reports* **85:** 835–840, 1970.

DeGeyndt W: Five Approaches for assessing the quality of care. *Hospital Administration* **15:** 21–42, 1970.

Donabedian A: Evaluating the quality of medical care. *Milbank Memorial Fund Quarterly* **64:** 166–206, 1966.

————: Promoting quality through evaluating the process of patient care. *Medical Care* **6:** 181–202, 1968.

————: Evaluation of care: Potentials and pitfalls, in Walker JE (ed): *Evaluation of Care in the University and Community Hospitals,* New Haven, Connecticut Health Services Research Series, 1970.

————: Patient care evaluation. *Hospitals* **44:** 131–136, 1970.

————: Models for organizing the delivery of personal health services and criteria for evaluating them. Proceedings of the Sun Valley Forum on National Health, Inc., Sun Valley, Idaho, June 25–July 1, 1972. *Milbank Memorial Fund Quarterly* **2:** 103–154, 1973.

————: A perspective on concepts of health care quality. Paper read before the Fall Meeting of the Institute of Medicine at the National Academy of Sciences, November 6 and 7, 1974.

Douglas LM, Bevis E: *Nursing Management and Leadership in Action.* St. Louis, Missouri, The CV Mosby Company, 1978.

Hartman M: *Pathways to Quality Care.* New York, National League for Nursing, Publication No. 20-1636, 1976.

Levin HM: Cost-effectiveness analysis in evaluation research, in Guttengag M, Struening EL (eds): *Handbook of Evaluation Research, Vol 2.* Beverly Hills, Calif, Sage Publications, Inc., pp 89–122, 1975.

Lynch EA: *Evaluation, Principles and Processes.* New York, National League for Nursing, Publication No. 23-1721, 1978.

National League of Nursing, Department of Baccalaureate and Higher Degree Programs: *Quality Assurance.* New York, National League for Nursing Publication No. 15-1595, 1975.

Passos J: From performance measures to utilization review to quality assurance, in *Quality Assurance of Medical Care.* DHEW Regional Medical Programs Service, 1973.

Payne BC: From performance measures to utilization review to quality assurance, in *Quality Assurance of Medical Care*. Washington, DC, HEW Regional Medical Programs Service, 1973.

Popham WJ: Cost analysis considerations, in *Educational Evaluation*. Englewood Cliffs, NJ, Prentice-Hall Inc., 1975.

Rothenberg J: Cost-benefit analysis: A methodological exposition, in Guttentag M, Struening FL (eds): *Handbook of Evaluation Research*. Beverly Hills, Calif, Sage Publications Inc., 1975, vol 2, pp 55–88.

Selig A: A conceptual framework for evaluating human service delivery systems. *Am J Orthopsychiatry* **46**: 140–153, 1976.

APPENDIX A

Medicaid Community Care Act* (HR 6194)

A bill to amend Title XIX of the Social Security Act to provide for comprehensive assessments and community-based services under Medicaid.

Be it enacted by the Senate and House of Representatives of the United States of America in Congress assembled, That this Act may be cited as the "Medicaid Community Care Act of 1980."

Sec. 2. (a) Section 1905 (b) of the Social Security Act is amended—

(1) by striking out "(b) The term" and inserting in lieu thereof "(b) (1) Except as provided in paragraph (2), the term"; and

(2) by adding at the end the following new paragraph:

"(2) In the case of a State which has a community care plan approved under section 1913, the term 'Federal medical assistance percentage' means, with respect to comprehensive assessments and services listed in section 1913(a) (2) furnished to individuals determined (pursuant to an assessment) under section 1913(a) (1) to be in need of long-term skilled nursing facility or intermediate care facility services, the lesser of—

"(A) the Federal medical assistance percentage otherwise determined under paragraph (1) plus 25 percentage points, or

*From *Congressional Record*, Dec 19, 1979 p 12.

"(B) 90 per centum".

(b) (1) Title XIX of such Act is amended by adding at the end the following new section:

State Community Care Plan

"Sec. 1913. (a) A State with a plan approved under this title may apply to the Secretary to have Federal payments made with respect to home health care services and certain other services described in paragraph (2), furnished to certain individuals, at a higher rate (as provided in section 1905(b) (2) than the rate for other care and services with respect to which medical assistance is provided under the State plan. The Secretary may not approve such an application unless it is accompanied by a plan for community care assessments and for the provision of medical assistance under this title with respect to care and services described in paragraph (2) and unless such plan provides as follows:

"(1) (A) The State will provide for a comprehensive assessment of each individual eligible or applying for assistance under the State plan (including any individual who, under the State's plan pursuant to section 1902(b), would be eligible for such assistance based on such an assessment) who is likely to be in need of long-term skilled nursing facility or intermediate care facility services under the plan.

"(B) Except in the case of individuals residing in medically underserved areas (as designated under section 1302(7) of the Public Health Service Act) and under such other special circumstances as the Secretary may establish, such an assessment may not be made by an entity which, directly or indirectly, provides or benefits from the provision of home health care, skilled nursing facility, or intermediate care facility services under this title.

"(C) Such assessment shall consist of a direct, personal assessment, by trained individuals, of all factors (which may include, among others, financial resources, medical, psychological, and social needs, architectural barriers and other environmental factors, family and community support, and ability to live independently with appropriate in-home services) relating to the likelihood of the individual's requiring long-term skilled nursing facility or intermediate care facility services, and such assessment shall determine whether or not the individual is in need of such services.

"(D) The individual shall be informed of such determination and, if determined to be in need of such long-term facility services, shall be informed of the feasible alternatives, available at the choice of the individual, to the provision of such services.

"(2) With respect to individuals determined pursuant to a comprehensive assessment under paragraph (1) to be in need of long-term facility services and for whom the furnishing of medical assistance with respect to the services described in this paragraph is a feasible alternative to such assistance with respect to long-term facility services, the State plan will provide for making medical assistance available with respect to—

"(A) nursing services on a part-time or intermittent basis,
"(B) home health aide services,
"(C) medical supplies, equipment, and appliances suitable for use in the home,
"(D) physical therapy, occupational therapy, and speech pathology and audiology services,
"(E) adult day health services,
"(F) respite care,
"(G) short-term full-time nursing care,
"(H) homemaker services, and
"(I) nutrition counseling,

furnished by providers who meet such standards (including State licensure, where applicable and appropriate) and enter into such participation agreement with the State as the State established (in accordance with regulations of the Secretary), without limitation as to amount, duration, or scope, except (at the option of the State) to the extent Federal payment for such medical assistance may not be provided because of section 1903(1) (5); and, the State plan established (in accordance with regulations of the Secretary) minimum and maximum reimbursement levels with respect to each of the types of care and services described in this paragraph.

"(3) (A) The State will provide for a plan for coordinating the provision of medical assistance under the State plan with respect to services described in paragraph (2) with furnishing of such and similar services under title XVIII, under the State's plan under title XX, under the Older Americans Act of 1965, and under other similar programs operating in the State.

"(B) The State will provide to the Secretary annually, in conjunction with reports provided under section 1902(a) (6), information on assistance provided under the community care plan under this section and on the plan's impact on the amount and type of medical assistance provided under the State plan with respect to skilled nursing facility and intermediate care facility services.

"(b) The Secretary shall annually report to the Congress, in conjunction with any other annual reports required to be made to the Congress with respect to the program under this title, on the plans approved under this section and on States which have elected the option provided under section 1902(h)".

(2) Section 1902(a) (10) of such Act is amended—

(A) by striking out "and" before "(III)", and

(B) by inserting before the semicolon at the end the following: ", and (IV) the making available of services described in section 1913(a) (2) to individuals pursuant to a State community care plan approved under such section shall not, by reason of this paragraph (10), require the making available of any such services, or the making available of such services of the same amount, duration, and scope, to any other individuals".

(3) Section 1903(i) of such Act is amended—

(A) by striking out the period at the end of paragraph (4) and inserting in lieu thereof ";, or", and

(B) by adding after paragraph (4) the following new paragraph:

"(5) with respect to amounts expended for care and services described in section 1913(a) (2) for an individual during a period to the extent that such amounts exceed a reasonable proportion, promulgated by the Secretary, of the amounts which would have been expended on skilled nursing facility services for such an individual during the period had the individual been institutionalized in such a facility during the period.".

(c) Section 1902 of such Act is amended by adding at the end the following new sub-section:

(h) (1) For purposes of this title, notwithstanding any other provision of this Act, in the case of a State plan which makes medical assistance available to Medicaid institutionally eligible individuals (as defined in paragraph (2)) (A), the State may elect to have treated as such an individual any section 1913 eligible individual (as defined in paragraph (2)) (B) who meets the income and resource standards applicable to a Medicaid institutionally eligible individual.

"(2) For purposes of this subsection:

"(A) The term 'Medicaid institutionally eligible individual' means an individual who—

"(i) is in a skilled nursing facility or intermediate care facility,

"(ii) is deemed under the State plan, if the individual was not in such an institution or facility, to be eligible to have paid with respect to the individual a State supplementary payment, and

"(iii) is eligible for medical assistance under the plan in an amount, duration, and scope equal to that provided to individuals under section 1902 (a) (10) (A).

"(B) The term 'section 1913 eligible individual' means an individual who—

"(i) has been determined (pursuant to a comprehensive assessment under section 1913 (a)) (1) to be in need of long-term skilled nursing facility or intermediate care facility services.

"(ii) would be institutionalized in a 'skilled nursing facility or intermediate care facility but for the availability of medical assistance to the individual for services described in section 1913(a) (2), and

"(iii) if in such a facility, would be a Medicaid institutionally eligible individual (as defined in subparagraph (A)" . . .)

Sec. 3. The amendments made by this Act shall apply to medical assistance provided, under a State plan approved under title XIX of the Social Security Act, on or after October 1, 1980.

APPENDIX B

State Agencies Giving Population Estimates*

The following is a list of those official state agencies who work with the Bureau of the Census under the auspices of the Federal-State Cooperative Program. Further information concerning individual states and updated listings of participants can be obtained from the Federal-State Cooperative Program for Local Estimates, Population Division, Bureau of the Census, Washington, D.C. 20233. Information directed to individual states can be obtained by addressing: Federal-State Cooperative Program for Local Population Estimates, care of the agency of interest.

Federal-State Cooperative Program For Local Population Estimates

State	Agency
Alabama	Alabama Development Office 508 State Office Building Montgomery, Ala. 36104
Alaska	Division of Planning and Research Office of the Governor Pouch AD Juneau, Alaska 99801

*From *Guide to Data for Health System Planners: Health Planning Information Series,* Wash, DC: US Govt Printing Office, 1976, pp 338–344.

State	Agency
Alaska *(con't.)*	Research and Analysis Section Alaska Department of Labor Box 3-7000 Juneau, Alaska 99801
Arizona	Department of Economic Security Bureau of Planning Post Office Box 6123 Phoenix, Ariz. 85005
Arkansas	Industrial Research and Extension Center University of Arkansas Post Office Box 3017 Little Rock, Ark. 72203
California	Population Research Unit State Department of Finance 1025 P Street Sacramento, Calif. 95814
Colorado	Colorado Division of Planning Room 524 State Social Services Building 1575 Sherman Street Denver, Colo. 80203
Connecticut	Vital Statistics Section State Health Department 79 Elm Street Hartford, Conn. 06115
Delaware	State Planning Office Thomas Collins Building 530 South Dupont Highway Dover, Del. 19901
Florida	Bureau of Economic and Business Research College of Business Administration University of Florida Gainesville, Fla. 32601
Georgia	Office of Planning and Budget 270 Washington Street, S.W. Atlanta, Ga. 30334
Hawaii	Department of Planning and Economic Development Post Office Box 2359 Honolulu, Hawaii 96801
Idaho	Bureau of Vital Statistics Idaho Department of Health and Welfare State House Boise, Idaho 83720
Illinois	Illinois Department of Public Health 535 West Jefferson Street Springfield, Ill. 62706
Indiana	Indiana State Board of Health 1330 West Michigan Street Indianapolis, Ind. 46207

State Agencies Giving Population Estimates

State	Agency
Iowa	Office of State Planning and Programming State Capitol Des Moines, Iowa 50319
	Records and Statistics Division Iowa State Health Department State Office Building Des Moines, Iowa 50319
Kansas	Division of State Planning and Research 1258-W State Office Building Topeka, Kan. 66612
Kentucky	Kentucky Department of Commerce 23rd Floor Capitol Plaza Frankfort, Ky. 40601
Louisiana	Research Division College of Administration and Business Louisiana Tech University Ruston, La. 71270
Maine	Research and Vital Records State Department of Health and Welfare Augusta, Maine 04330
Maryland	Maryland Center for Health Statistics State Department of Health and Mental Hygiene 610 North Howard Street Baltimore, Md. 21201
Massachusetts	Bureau of Research and Statistics State Department of Commerce and Development State Office Building 100 Cambridge Street Boston, Mass. 02202
Michigan	Planning Analysis Unit, Budget Division State Bureau of the Budget Lewis Cass Building Lansing, Mich. 48913
Minnesota	Minnesota State Planning 101 Capitol Square 550 Cedar Street St. Paul, Minn. 55101
Mississippi	Department of Sociology and Anthropology Mississippi State University Post Office Drawer C State College, Miss. 39762
Missouri	Office of Administration State Planning and Analysis Division State Capitol Post Office Box 809 Jefferson City, Mo. 65101
Montana	Bureau of Business and Economic Research University of Montana Missoula, Mont. 59801

State	Agency
Nebraska	Nebraska Department of Economic Development Post Office Box 94666 State Capitol Lincoln, Neb. 68505
	Bureau of Business Research The University of Nebraska Lincoln, Neb. 68508
Nevada	Bureau of Business Research University of Nevada Reno, Nev. 89507
New Hampshire	Office of Comprehensive Planning Executive Department State House Annex Concord, N.H. 03301
New Jersey	Office of Business Economics Division of Economic Development Department of Labor and Industry Post Office Box 845 Trenton, N.J. 08625
New Mexico	Bureau of Business Research The University of New Mexico Albuquerque, N.M. 87106
New York	Office of Biostatistics New York State Department of Health 84 Holland Avenue Albany, N.Y. 12237
	Office of State Planning 488 Broadway Albany, N.Y. 12204
North Carolina	State Planning Division Department of Administration State of North Carolina 116 West Jones Street Raleigh, N.C. 27603
North Dakota	Department of Sociology and Anthropology The University of North Dakota Grand Forks, N.Dak. 58201
Ohio	Human Resources Development Division Bureau of Research and Analysis Department of Economic and Community Development 30 E. Broad Street, State Office Tower Columbus, Ohio 43215
Oklahoma	Research and Planning Division Oklahoma Employment Security Commission Will Rogers Memorial Building Oklahoma City, Okla. 73101
Oregon	Center for Population Research and Census Portland State College, Box 751 Portland, Oreg. 97207

State	Agency
Pennsylvania	Office of State Planning and Development Post Office Box 1323 Harrisburg, Penn. 17120
Puerto Rico	Puerto Rico Planning Board Minillas Government Center North Building, De Diego Avenue Santurce, P.R. 00908
Rhode Island	Statewide Planning Program Room 201 265 Melrose Street Providence, R.I. 02907
South Carolina	Division of Research and Statistical Services South Carolina Budget and Control Board Post Office Box 11038 Columbia, S.C. 29211
South Dakota	Public Health Statistics State Department of Health Pierre, S.Dak. 57501
Tennessee	Tennessee State Planning Office Division of State Planning 660 Capitol Hill Building 301 Seventh Avenue, North Nashville, Tenn. 37219
Texas	Office of Information Services Office of the Governor Box 13224 Austin, Tex. 78705
Utah	Utah Department of Employment Security 174 Social Hall Avenue Salt Lake City, Utah 84111
Vermont	Division of Public Health Statistics State Department of Health 115 Colchester Avenue Burlington, Vt. 05401
Virginia	Taylor Murphy Institute Graduate School of Business Administration University of Virginia Post Office Box 3430 Charlottesville, Va. 22903
Washington	Population Studies Division Office of Program Planning and Fiscal Management Insurance Building Olympia, Wash. 98501
West Virginia	Office of Research and Development Appalachian Center West Virginia University Morgantown, W. Va. 26506
	Federal State Relations Office of the Governor Charleston, W. Va. 25305

State	Agency
Wisconsin	Bureau of Health Statistics State Division of Health State Office Building Madison, Wis. 53701
Wyoming	Division of Business and Economic Research College of Commerce and Industry University of Wyoming University Station, Box 3925 Laramie, Wyo. 82070
	Administrator of Research and Statistics Division Department of Administration and Fiscal Control Room 312, Capitol Building Cheyenne, Wyo. 82001

APPENDIX C

Systematic Functional Assessment Tool

CRITERIA FOR ESCROW FUNCTIONAL SCALE*†
(Not for Persons Living in Institutions)

E—ENVIRONMENT

1. Lives in quarters that are adequate for size of the family, without major architectural barriers, accessible to convenient forms of transportation and other necessary facilities, in a safe neighborhood and free of significant or major problems.
2. Lives in quarters that are either inadequate for size of the family, with minor architectural barriers, inaccessible to convenient forms of transportation or necessary facilities, in a marginal neighborhood, or else has minor problems.

*The ESCROW profile incorporates six factors, each independently assessed and scored from 1 (most independent, or best) to 4 (most dependent, or worst).
†Reprinted with permission of Carl V Granger, MD, Professor, Family Medicine and Community Health, Brown University; Director, Physical Medicine and Rehabilitation, The Memorial Hospital, Nantuckett, RI.

3. Lives in housing with major problems but does not desire to move because of them.
4. Lives in housing with major problems and desires to move because of them.

S—SOCIAL SUPPORTS

1. Maintains a balance of social contacts by way of visiting, telephone calls, hobbies and interests, etc. Able to solve problems without undue reliance on others outside the family unit. Has one or more close or dependable friendships.
2. Social contacts are restrictive. May frequently rely on others outside the family unit to solve problems. May not readily identify a close or dependable friendship.
3. The patient or someone in the family unit occasionally requires assistance at home from a person or agency from the outside such as the visiting nurse association, home care, counselling services, etc.
4. The patient or someone in the family unit is consistently dependent upon assistance at home from a community agency at least weekly.

C—CLUSTER OF FAMILY MEMBERS
(Do Not Answer If Patient Lives Alone—A score of 4 is assigned)

1. The family unit consists of at least one member besides the patient related by marriage, kinship, or else a close personal companion; as a unit the family is sufficiently competent physically and mentally to provide adequate support to the patient at home at this time and under forseeable circumstances.
2. The family unit is as above but under particular conditions of stress they may not be able to support the patient either physically or mentally, or else particular circumstances such as a job require a crucial family member to be away from the home part of the day.
3. The impact of the disability has been such as to change either the work effort, pattern of socialization, interests and hobbies, or other important activities of some family member.
4. The impact of the disability has been such as to produce severe strain or disruptions of relationships between family members.

R—RESOURCES

1. The family is able to absorb the costs of the disability without increased indebtedness.
2. The family is required to incur debts to handle costs of the disability.

3. The family requires some form of public assistance to cover medically related costs (Medicaid).
4. The family requires public assistance to cover medical and subsistence costs (Welfare or SSI).

O—OUTLOOK

1. The individual functions independently without impairment in the following areas: problem-solving, regard for others, perceptual motor ability, judgment, reliability, and self-esteem. The individual feels *able to make decisions* easily.
2. The individual functions independently with mild impairment in some area(s) mentioned above or else has *moderate difficulty making decisions*.
3. The individual is observed to function appreciably better with assistance, supervision, cuing, coaxing or structured environment due to one or more of the problems mentioned above or else *has great difficulty making decisions*.
4. The individual is not particularly benefited by assistance with problems mentioned above or else actually *makes very few, if any, decisions*.

W—WORK/SCHOOL/RETIREMENT STATUS
FOR COMPETITIVE EMPLOYMENT, HOMEMAKER STUDENT:

1. There are no work or educational or homemaking restrictions. Essentially devotes full time to major activity(ies). Time lost does not exceed one day per month on the average.
2. The individual may have a work or educational or homemaking restriction or require some modification such as part-time, light work, etc. Time lost does not exceed more than 2 to 5 days per month on the average.
3. Work or education is attended in a special facility adapted for the handicapped *or else* time lost may exceed one week per month on the average. If a homemaker, assistance is needed from outside the home to perform household tasks.

FOR RETIRED DUE TO AGE (NOT DUE TO DISABILITY):

1. Fulfills usual and customary tasks and roles, other than earning an income, in the household or community.
2. Fulfills usual and customary tasks and roles, other than earning an income, in the household or community in a limited way.
3. Not able to fulfill usual and customary tasks and roles, other than earning an income, in the household or community.

If disabled or unemployed a score of 4 is assigned

PULSES Profile*†

P—Physical condition including diseases of the viscera (cardiovascular, gastrointestinal, urologic, and endocrine) and neurologic disorders:

1. Medical problems sufficiently stable that medical or nursing monitoring is not required more often than 3 month intervals.
2. Medical or nurse monitoring is needed more often than 3 month intervals but not each week.
3. Medical problems are sufficiently unstable as to require regular medical and/or nursing attention at least weekly.
4. Medical problems require intensive medical and/or nursing attention at least daily (excluding personal care assistance only).

U—Self care activities (drink/feed, dress upper/lower, brace/prosthesis, groom, wash/bathe, perineal care) dependent mainly upon upper limb function:

1. Independent in self care without impairment of upper limbs.
2. Independent in self care with some impairment of upper limbs.
3. Dependent upon assistance or supervision in self care with or without impairment of upper limbs.
4. Dependent totally in self care with marked impairment of upper limbs.

L—Mobility activities (transfer chair/toilet/tub or shower, walk, stairs, wheelchair) dependent mainly upon lower limb function:

1. Independent in mobility without impairment of lower limbs.
2. Independent in mobility with some impairment in lower limbs; such as needing ambulatory aids, a brace or prosthesis, or else fully independent in a wheelchair without significant architectural or environmental barriers.
3. Dependent upon assistance or supervision in mobility with or without impairment of lower limbs, or else partly independent in a wheelchair or else there are significant architectural or environmental barriers.
4. Dependent totally in mobility with marked impairment of lower limbs.

---

*The PULSES profile is a scale reflecting independence in life functioning.
†Reprinted with permission of Carl V Granger, MD, Professor, Family Medicine and Community Health, Brown University; Director, Physical Medicine and Rehabilitation, The Memorial Hospital, Nantuckett, RI. Material adapted from Moskowitz E, McCann C: Classification of disability in the chronically ill and aging. *J Chr Dis* **5:** 342–346, 1957.

S—Sensory components relating to communication (speech and hearing) and vision:

1. Independent in communication and vision without impairment.
2. Independent in communication and vision with some impairment such as mild dysarthria, mild aphasia, or need for eyeglasses or hearing aid, or needing regular medication.
3. Dependent upon assistance, an interpreter or supervision in communication or vision.
4. Dependent totally in communication or vision.

E—Excretory functions (bladder and bowel):

1. Complete voluntary control of bladder and bowel sphincters.
2. Control of sphincters allows normal social activities despite urgency or need for catheter, appliance, suppositories, etc. Able to care for needs without assistance.
3. Dependent upon assistance in sphincter management or else has accidents occasionally.
4. Frequent wetting or soiling from incontinence of bladder or bowel sphincters.

S—Consider intellectual and emotional adaptability (O of ESCROW), support from family unit (C of ESCROW), financial ability (R of ESCROW), and social interactions (S of ESCROW):

1. Fulfills usual role(s) and performs customary tasks.
2. Must make some modification in usual role(s) or performance of customary tasks.
3. Dependent upon assistance, supervision, encouragement or assistance from a public or private agency due to any of the above considerations.
4. Dependent upon long-term institutional care (chronic hospital, nursing home, etc.) excluding time-limited hospitalization for specific evaluation, treatment or active rehabilitation.

PULSES TOTAL—BEST SCORE IS 6/6. WORST SCORE IS 6/24.

INSTITUTE FOR REHABILITATION AND RESTORATIVE CARE
LONG-RANGE EVALUATION SYSTEM OUTPATIENT ASSESSMENT*

Name: _____, _____ Number: _____ Facility: _____
     Last   First

Intake date: _____ Admission date: _____ Interval date: _____

Date of birth: _____ Discharge date: _____ Followup date: _____

Marital Status: ☐ Male   ☐ Female
- ☐ Single
- ☐ Married   *Mode of Evaluation:*
- ☐ Widowed   ☐ Outpatient visit
- ☐ Divorced   ☐ Rehab home visit
- ☐ Separated   ☐ Telephone with patient

Educational Level: ☐ VNA home visit
- ☐ Grammar school or less   ☐ Telephone with _____
- ☐ Some high school   ☐ Medical record review
- ☐ High school diploma   ☐ Hospital visit
- ☐ Some college
- ☐ College degree   Address: _____
- ☐ Some graduate school   Number & Street
- ☐ Graduate/professional degree   _____
               Town & State   Zip

Major Handicapping Condition: Telephone No: _____/_____
(RT-7 Code)   _ _ _ _   Census Tract: _ _ _ _
               Date of Onset: _____

Limbs:	Good	Fair	Poor	Null	Communication:	Intact	Limited	Helper	Null
R Upper	☐	☐	☐	☐	Verbal	☐	☐	☐	☐
L Upper	☐	☐	☐	☐	Hearing	☐	☐	☐	☐
R Lower	☐	☐	☐	☐	Vision	☐	☐	☐	☐
L Lower	☐	☐	☐	☐					

Activities of Self-Care and Mobility:

	Independent		Dependent	
	Intact	Limited	Helper	Null
Drink/Feed	☐	☐	☐	☐
Dress upper body	☐	☐	☐	☐
Dress lower body	☐	☐	☐	☐
Don brace or prosthesis	☐	☐	☐	☐ None
Groom	☐	☐	☐	☐
Wash or bathe	☐	☐	☐	☐
Bladder continence	☐	☐	☐ Accidents	☐ Incontinent
Bowel continence	☐	☐	☐ Accidents	☐ Incontinent
Perineal care (at toilet)	☐	☐	☐	☐
Other hand skills	☐	☐	☐	☐
Transfer, chair	☐	☐	☐	☐
Transfer, toilet	☐	☐	☐	☐
Transfer, tub or shower	☐	☐	☐	☐
Transfer, automobile	☐	☐	☐	☐
Walk 50 yards on level	☐	☐	☐	☐
Stairs, Up/down 1 flight	☐	☐	☐	☐
Walk outdoors 50 yards	☐	☐	☐	☐
Wheelchair, 50 yards	☐	☐	☐	☐ None

Figure C-1. Institute for Rehabilitation and Restorative Care—Long-Range Evaluation System Out-patient Assessment (Reprinted with permission of Carl V Granger, MD, Professor, Family Medicine and Community Health, Brown University; Director, Physical Medicine and Rehabilitation, The Memorial Hospital, Nantuckett, RI.)

—2—

Evaluate the Degree of Physician or Nurse (RN or LPN) Care Required (P of PULSES): (Do not include visits for physical or occupational therapy.)

1 ☐ Medical problem is sufficiently stable that physician or nurse monitoring is not required more often than 3-month intervals.
2 ☐ Medical problem requires physician or nurse monitoring more often that 3-month intervals, but not each week.
3 ☐ Medical problem is sufficiently unstable as to require regular physician and/or nurse attention at least weekly.
4 ☐ Medical problem requires intensive physician and/or nurse attention at least daily (excl. personal care assistance).

Diagnoses: (Only add diagnoses not previously recorded) ICDA-8

_____ ___ ___ ___ ___
_____ ___ ___ ___ ___
_____ ___ ___ ___ ___
_____ ___ ___ ___ ___
_____ ___ ___ ___ ___

Malignancy Status: ___ ___ ___

Complications: ___ ___ ___ ___ ___ ___

List proven or suspected complications (other than the major handicapping condition) that significantly interfered with the rehabilitation effort.

Architectural Barriers:

☐ Irrelevant—Has access into and out of home, to all levels if multi-story, and to all rooms without safety hazard or requiring assistance, or else not relevant to the problem.

☐ Minor—Has access into and out of home and to all essential levels if multi-story and to all rooms essential to well-being and participation in family activities. Some non-essential rooms may not be accessible, or else inconvenience may be imposed by thresholds, narrow passages, or awkward arrangement of furniture. However, able to manage without assistance.

☐ Major—Not able to manage without assistance in getting into or out of home or in gaining access to rooms essential to well-being and/or participation in family activities.

Environment (E of ESCROW):

1 ☐ Lives in quarters that are adequate for size of family, without major architectural barriers, accessible to convenient forms of transportation and other necessary facilities, in a safe neighborhood, and free of significant major problems.
2 ☐ Lives in quarters that are either inadequate for size of family, with minor architectural barriers, inaccessible to convenient forms of transportation or necessary facilities, in a marginal neighborhood, or else has other minor problems.
3 ☐ Lives in housing with major problems, but does not desire to move because of them.
4 ☐ Lives in housing with major problems and desires to move because of them.

Social Supports (S of ESCROW):

1 ☐ Maintains a balance of social contacts by way of visiting, phone calls, hobbies, and interests, etc. Able to solve problems without undue reliance on others outside the family unit. Has one or more close or dependable friendships.
2 ☐ Social contacts are restrictive. May frequently rely on others outside the family unit to solve problems. May not readily identify a close or dependable friendship.
3 ☐ The patient or someone else in the family unit occasionally requires assistance at home from a person or agency from the outside such as the Visiting Nurse Association, home care, counseling services, etc.
4 ☐ The patient or someone else in the family unit is consistently dependent upon assistance at home from a community agency at least weekly.

Figure C-1. *(continued)*

—3—

Household Constellation:
- ☐ Alone
- ☐ Spouse
- ☐ Children
- ☐ Spouse and children
- ☐ Parent(s)
- ☐ Other relative(s)
- ☐ Friend(s)
- ☐ Institution
- ☐ Other _____

Community Agency(ies) Involved:
- ☐ Visiting Nurse Association
- ☐ State vocational agency
- ☐ Welfare
- ☐ Meals-on-Wheels
- ☐ Homemaker/home health aide
- ☐ Transportation support
- ☐ Outreach worker
- ☐ Other _____

Cluster of Family Members (C of ESCROW):
(Do not answer if patient lives alone.)
1. ☐ The family unit consists of at least one member besides the patient related by marriage, kinship, or else a close personal companion; as a unit the family is sufficiently competent physically and mentally to provide adequate support to the patient at home at this time and under forseeable circumstances.
2. ☐ The family unit is as above, but under particular conditions of stress they may not be able to support the patient either physically or mentally, or else particular circumstances such as a job require a crucial family member to be away from the home part of the day.
3. ☐ The impact of the condition has been such to change either the work effort, pattern of socialization, interests and hobbies, or other important activities of some family member.
4. ☐ The impact of the condition has been such as to produce severe strain or produce disruptions of relationships between family members.

Source of Referral:
- ☐ Rehab inpatient
- ☐ In-house acute care
- ☐ In-house outpatient dept.
- ☐ Other hospital _____
- ☐ Other physician _____
- ☐ Vocational rehabilitation agency
- ☐ Welfare/Medicaid
- ☐ LTCF (nursing home, chronic hospital)
- ☐ Other _____

Source of Payment:
- ☐ Self/family
- ☐ Insurance plan (BC/BS, etc.)
- ☐ Worker's compensation
- ☐ Vocational rehabilitation agency
- ☐ Welfare/Medicaid
- ☐ Medicare
- ☐ Association/fund
- ☐ Other _____

New Action Taken (Referrals Made):
- ☐ Visiting Nurse Association
- ☐ Vocational rehabilitation agency
- ☐ Welfare/Medicaid
- ☐ Private physician
- ☐ Hospital _____
- ☐ Meals-on-Wheels
- ☐ Transportation support
- ☐ Outreach worker
- ☐ Podiatrist
- ☐ Mental health clinic
- ☐ Other _____

Resources (R of ESCROW):
1. ☐ The family is able to absorb the costs of the disability without increased indebtedness.
2. ☐ The family is required to incur debts to handle costs of the disability.
3. ☐ The family requires some form of public assistance to cover medically related costs (Medicaid or Medical Assistance).
4. ☐ The family requires public assistance to cover medical and subsistence costs (Welfare or SSI—Supplemental Security Income).

Figure C-1. *(continued)*

—4—
This Page is Optional

Intellectual Ability/Problem Solving:
1. ☐ Intact—Able to comprehend meaning, retain instructions and follow through a sequence of steps, particularly in a novel situation. Makes use of previously learned information. Able to self correct if errors are made. Sustains attention until task is completed.
2. ☐ Limited—Has minimal limitations in problem-solving; modification of environment may be required.
3. ☐ Helper—Limitations in problem-solving require a structured environment and/or another person is involved for supervision, cuing, coaxing, or assistance.
4. ☐ Null—Unable to function appropriately due to limitations despite assistance.

Perceptual-Motor Ability/Gnosis-Praxis:
1. ☐ Intact—Able to discriminate between differences in the environment by hearing, sight, touch, and visuospatial orientation. Able to reproduce a requested motion or activity.
2. ☐ Limited—Limitation in perceptual-motor minimal; modification of environment may be required.
3. ☐ Helper—Another person is involved for assistance, supervision, cuing, coaxing; and/or a structured environment is required for adequate function.
4. ☐ Null—Unable to function due to limitations despite assistance.

Self-Esteem/Regard for Self (Hopefulness):
1. ☐ Intact—Able to feel hopeful about situation with sense of purpose and worthwhileness preserved. No evidence of inappropriate discouragement or anxiety, hypochondriasis, misuse of drugs or alcohol. Able to go through grief reaction to real loss without undue denial, indifference, or hysteria.
2. ☐ Limited—Minimal limitations in self-esteem; a modified environment may be required.
3. ☐ Helper—Manifest depression requires another person to be involved for assistance, supervision, or cuing. A structured environment is required.
4. ☐ Null—Manifest depression severely limits function despite assistance.

Emotional Stability/Regard for Others:
1. ☐ Intact—Able to remain cooperative without being demanding or overly dependent upon others. Evidence of satisfying interactions with staff, other patients and family members.
2. ☐ Limited—Minimal limitations in emotional stability; modifications of environment may be required.
3. ☐ Helper—Anti-social behavior requires a structured environment; and/or another person is involved for assistance, supervision, cuing, or coaxing.
4. ☐ Null—Anti-social behavior severely limits function despite assistance.

Judgment-Reliability/Insight (Realism):
1. ☐ Intact—Aware of and understands limitations or disability problems. Able to plan, work out, or incorporate compensations or substitutions, or else asks for appropriate assistance while working toward solutions and while using sound judgment.
2. ☐ Limited—Minimal limitations in insight; may require environmental modification.
3. ☐ Helper—Poor insight, judgment, or reliability require a structured setting and/or another person involved for assistance, supervision, cuing, or coaxing.
4. ☐ Null—Insight, judgment, or reliability is not appreciably helped by assistance.

Figure C-1. *(continued)*

—5—

Limiting Conditions:
☐ Weakness
☐ Pain
☐ Inflammation
☐ Contracture
☐ Skin ulcer
☐ Ataxia
☐ Spasticity
☐ Rigidity
☐ Sensory loss
☐ Abnormal length (Amp)
☐ Other _____

Aids and Appliances:
☐ Uses any orthosis
☐ Uses limb prosthesis
☐ Has any kind of ostomy
☐ Has bladder device
☐ Uses 1 cane/crutch
☐ Uses 2 canes/crutches
☐ Uses walkerette
☐ Uses wheelchair
☐ Uses lift device
☐ Uses grab bars
☐ Other _____

Weight Status:
☐ Normal
☐ Underweight
☐ Slightly to moderately overweight
☐ Significantly overweight

Falls Within Last Year:
☐ None
☐ One to three
☐ Four to seven
☐ Eight or more

Outlook (O of ESCROW):
1 ☐ The individual functions independently without impairment in the following areas: problem-solving, regard for others, perceptual-motor ability, judgment, reliability, and self-esteem. The individual feels *able to make decisions easily.*
2 ☐ The individual functions independently with mild impairment in some area(s) mentioned above or else has *moderate difficulty making decisions.*
3 ☐ The individual is observed to function appreciably better with assistance, supervision, cuing, coaxing, or a structured environment due to one or more of the problems mentioned above or else *has great difficulty making decisions.*
4 ☐ The individual is not particularly benefited by assistance with problems mentioned above or else actually *makes very few, if any, decisions.*

Vocational Status:
☐ Homemaker
☐ Student
☐ Competitive employment
3 ☐ Non-competitive employment (Sheltered workshop, etc.)
4 ☐ Unemployed, but employable and unable to find work
☐ Retired due to age
4 ☐ Too disabled to work, to be a homemaker, to be a student; or is retired due to disability

For Competitive Employment, Homemaker or Student:
1 ☐ There are no work or educational or homemaking restrictions. Essentially devotes full time to major activity(ies). Time lost does not exceed one day per month on the average.
2 ☐ The individual may have a work or educational or homemaking restriction, or may require some modification such as part-time, light work, etc. Time lost does not exceed more than 2 to 5 days per month on the average.
3 ☐ Work or education is attended in a special facility adapted for the handicapped, *or else* time lost may exceed one week per month on the average. If a homemaker, assistance is needed from outside the home to perform household tasks.

For Retired Due to Age: (Do not answer if patient is retired due to disability.)
1 ☐ Fulfills usual and customary tasks and roles, other than earning an income, in the household and/or community.
2 ☐ Fulfills usual and customary tasks and roles, other than earning an income, in the household and/or community in a limited way.
3 ☐ Does not fulfill usual and customary tasks and roles, other than earning an income, in the household or community.

Figure C-1. *(continued)*

Systematic Functional Assessment Tool / 407

—6—

Remarks:

Discharged To:
☐ Home
☐ Acute hospital _____
☐ Chronic hospital _____
☐ Nursing home
☐ Other _____

Evaluator: _____

Figure C-1. *(continued)*

APPENDIX D

A Community Needs Survey for Adult Day Care*

REPORT SUMMARY

The following report from the Department of Human Services is an attempt to determine the need for Adult Day Care Services for elderly residents who live with other household members and cannot be left alone during the day.

Figures D-1 and D-2 on the following pages show the postcard and covering letter mailed to 400 pre-selected, carefully unnamed residents at City addresses. The first 200 cards went to households whose residents were more than 60 years of age (Group A). The next 200 cards were sent to the homes of younger persons who had living with them at least one person more than 60 years old (Group B). Of the 400 questionnaires that were mailed, replies were received from 116: 55 from Group A and 61 from Group B.

Summary of results, based on % of 116 responses, unless otherwise noted:

1. *Have you ever before heard of Adult Day Care?*
   52% have heard of Adult Day Care, 48% have not.

*From Department of Human Services, Newton, Mass, 1979

2. *If an Adult Day Care Center were available in Newton, is there anyone in your household who presently would be in need of such service?*
   11% replied with present need; if responses are considered en bloc (all 400), the figure becomes 3¼%.
3. *Do you have any other family members living in Newton who presently would be in need of Adult Day Care?*
   3.5% acknowledge family members in Newton apart from them who need care; the en bloc percentage is 1%.
4. *Present age of person(s) needing Adult Day Care?*
   18% are between 60 and 69; 41% are between 70 and 79; and 41% are 80 and older.
5. *Is person(s) needing Adult Day Care male or female?*
   24% are male; 76% are female.
6. *Do you see any future need for this service by someone living in your household?*
   32% of the replies signified "yes."
7. *If yes, in what year?*
   Future dates ranged from "any time now" through the year 2010.
8. *At the rate of $20 per day, could you or the senior citizen living in your household afford to pay for the services?*
   29.5% of the replies were "yes": 59% were "no": 11.5% did not answer.
9. *Please indicate any other unmet needs of senior citizens living in your household.*
   7.75% of the returns answered this; of them, 33% specified "lower real estate taxes": the remainder were diffused, singular.

From the Questionnaire:

1. Have you ever before heard of Adult Day Care?

   116 replies were received from the 400 mailed questionnaires—a substantial 29% return. It is somewhat surprising that only 23 of the A Group—the senior citizen householders—answered that they had previously heard of Adult Day Care. Returns from Group B, householders with older persons living in their homes, showed that 37 had heard of Adult Day Care. Altogether, 60 of 116 (52%) were aware of its existence.

The figures:

Group A	**Group A**
Have heard	Have not heard
23 (42%)	32 (58%)

QUESTIONNAIRE
THE NEED FOR ADULT DAY-CARE SERVICES IN NEWTON

1. Have you ever before heard of Adult Day Care?
   Yes ☐   No ☐

2. If an Adult Day Care Center were available in Newton, is there anyone in your household who presently would be in need of such service?
   Yes ☐   No ☐

3. Do you have any other family members living in Newton who presently would be in need of Adult Day Care?
   Yes ☐   No ☐

4. Present age of person(s) needing Adult Care?
   Person 1. _____   Person 2. _____

5. Is person(s) needing Adult Day Care male or female?
   Person 1. _____   Person 2. _____

6. Do you see any future need for this service by someone living in your household?
   Yes ☐   No ☐

7. If yes, in what year? _____

8. At the rate of $20 per day, could you or the senior citizen living in your household afford to pay for the services?
   Yes ☐   No ☐

9. Please indicate any other unmet needs of senior citizens living in your household.

For office use only.

BUSINESS REPLY MAIL
FIRST CLASS   PERMIT NO. 44865   NEWTON, MA.

POSTAGE WILL BE PAID BY ADDRESSEE

NO POSTAGE
NECESSARY
IF MAILED IN THE
UNITED STATES

Department of Human Services
City Hall
1000 Commonwealth Avenue
Newton, Centre, Ma. 02159

Figure D-1. Questionnaire Postcard Sent to Selected Residents

Group B	Group B
Have heard	Have not heard
37 (61%)	24 (39%)

Totals: 60 (52%) have heard of Adult Day Care
<u>56</u> (48%) have not heard of Adult Day Care
116

2. If an Adult Day Care Center were available in Newton, is there anyone in your household who presently would be in need of such service?

   Among 55 replies from senior citizen householders in Group A were 9 stating that Adult Day Care would be needed by at least one member of the household. Younger residents in Group B felt that 4 in their homes should have it.
   Statistically:

Group A	Group B	Total
9/55 (16%)	4/61 (7%)	13/116 (11%)

But: If the postcard mailings are considered en bloc, then the resulting percentage of "yes" answers to the questions becomes very small indeed. So: to question 2 we should have

Group A	Group B
9/200 (4½%)	4/200 (2%)

And, overall, the total would read: 13/400, or 3¼%.

3. Do you have any other family members living in Newton who presently would be in need of Adult Day Care?

   Those polled in Group A reported only 1 among them with a family member in Newton who might need Adult Day Care; Group B returns indicated only 3 in similar circumstance.
   Statistically:

Group A	Group B	Total
1/55 (2%)	3/61 (5%)	4/116 (3.5%)

As with question 2 above, the "yes" returns were also numbered against the total mailings; predictably, the percentage of affirmative answers is much smaller:

Group A   **Group B**

1/200 (½%)   3/200 (1½%)

And the total would read 4/400, or 1%.

The following is a breakdown of residential areas of Newton in which live those persons who answered "yes" to questions 2 and 3 of the questionnaire.

Residence by ward and precinct numbers Newton

Ages	1/1	1/2	1/3	2/2	2/3	3/2	3/3	4/1	5/1	6/1	6/3	8/1	8/2
60–64	1									1	1		
65–69		1											
70–74				1			1	1	1				
75–79					1			2					
80 +			1			1			1			1	2

Ward 1 Precincts 1,2,3	Newton Nonantum Newton Corner	Total:	3	17.647%
Ward 2 Precincts 2,3	Newtonville		2	11.764%
Ward 3 Precincts 2,3	West Newton		2	11.764%
Ward 4 Precinct 1	Auburndale		3	17.647%
Ward 5 Precinct 1	Newton Upper Falls		2	11.764%
Ward 6 Precincts 1,3	Newton Centre		2	11.764%
Ward 8 Precincts 1,2	Newton Centre		3	17.647%
			17	99.997%

4. Present age of person(s) needing Adult Day Care?

From the replies to questions 2 and 3 there appears to be no unusual pattern of age differential among those listed in need of Adult Day Care:
Statistically:

Group A

Ages	#	%
60–69	3	30%
70–79	3	30%
80 +	4	40%

Group B

Ages	#	%
70–79	4	57%
80 +	3	43%

Combined Total

Ages	#	%
60–69	3	18%
70–79	7	41%
80 +	7	41%
	17	100%

5. Is person(s) needing Adult Day Care male or female?

Group A	Group B	Total
M—1 (10%)	M—3 (43%)	M— 4 (24%)
F—9 (90%)	F—4 (57%)	F—13 (76%)
10	7	17

6. Do you see any future need for this service by someone living in your houshould?
7. If yes, in what year?

Questions 6 and 7, which must be considered jointly, drew a large response from those answering the questionnaire:

From Group A 18 persons (33%) disclosed a probable future need for Adult Day Care and Group B residents were similarly concerned: 19 (31%) expected some future need of such help.

Affirmative answers to Questions 6 totaled 37 of 116 returns: 32%.

It is in the answers to the question "when?" that most interest lies. The "yes" replies, separated by Groups, follow below. One note: the replies are given exactly as written on the postcards, including question marks.

Group A		Group B	
"maybe"	1	"good question"	1
"any time now"	1	"who knows"	1
(not immediately)		"do not know"	1
"possibly 1980"	1	"possibly"	1
1980	1	1980–1981	1
1981	1	1985	1
1983 +	1	1988–1990	1
1984?	1	"possibly 1989"	1
"possibly 1984"	1	1989	1

	Group A			Group B	
	"5–10 years"	1		1999	1
	1990	1		2000	1
	2000	1		2010	1
	"perhaps, year unknown"	1		"?"	7
	"possibly, when unknown"	1			19
	"?"	5			
		18			

8. At the rate of $20 per day, could you or the senior citizen living in your household afford to pay for the services?

	Group A				Group B		
	Yes	No	No answer		Yes	No	No answer
Of 55:	16	22	17	Of 61:	12	27	22
	29%	40%	31%		20%	44%	36%

Totals:

	Yes	No	No answer
Of 116:	28	49	39
	24%	34%	42%

There is an additional subtotal of interest: of the 17 householders who replied to questions 2 and 3 that their homes contained, or that their families in Newton included other members who presently needed Adult Day Care help, the following are their answers to question 8 concerning ability to pay for A.D.C. services.

	Group A				Group B		
	Yes	No	No answer		Yes	No	No answer
	1	7	2		4	3	–
	10%	70%	20%		57%	43%	0%

Totals:

	Yes	No	No answer
Of 17:	5	10	2
	29.5%	59%	11.5%

9. Please indicate any other unmet needs of senior citizens living in your household.

This is a totally open-ended question; it is disconcerting that of 116 persons returning the questionnaire only 9 indicated that senior citizens in their household had any unmet needs—a figure of 8% of the returns. All of them are reproduced below exactly as written.

From Group A

1. "*Good* paying jobs for *able* senior citizens"
2. "Discontinued, but still desirable, visits from the V.N.A."
3. "Nursing homes charge too much; no wonder our taxes are so high"
4. "Property tax reduction; grocery store for Newton Center"
5. "Need for person(s) who can stay in home providing care for senior citizens when family must be away weekends"

From Group B

1. "Keep them clean so they can be healthy"
2. "More realistic deduction of R.E. tax for elderly"
3. "R.E. tax relief on school tax for all citizens over 70"
4. "Work"

Totals: 5/55   (9%)   4/61   (6.5%)

All: 9/116   (7.75%)

A final note: three respondents wrote "none" in answer to this query, and one said, "we appreciate all Newton does for senior citizens. It makes life much pleasanter."

Table D-1
The Need for Adult Day Care in the City of Newton

Returns of Questionnaires to 400 Pre-Selected Newton Residents
Chronological number is the Department of Human Service's arbitrary listing; x indicates a returned questionnaire

1	51	101	151	201	251 x	301	351 x
2	52	102	152	202	252 x	302	352
3	53	103 x	153	203 x	253 x	303	353
4	54 x	104	154	204	254 x	304	354
5 x	55	105	155 x	205	255 x	305 x	355
6	56	106 x	156 x	206 x	256	306	356
7 x	57	107	157 x	207 x	257	307	357 x
8 x	58	108	158	208	258	308	358 x
9	59 x	109 x	159 x	209	259	309	359
10	60	110	160 x	210	260	310 x	360 x
11	61	111 x	161	211	261	311	361 x
12	62 x	112 x	162	212	262 x	312	362
13	63	113	163 x	213	263 x	313 x	363
14 x	64	114 x	164	214 x	264	314	364
15	65	115	165	215 x	265	315	365 x
16 x	66	116	166 x	216	266	316	366
17	67	117	167	217	267	317 x	367
18	68 x	118	168	218	268 x	318	368
19	69	119	169 x	219	269	319 x	369
20	70	120	170	220	270 x	320	370
21	71 x	121 x	171	221	271 x	321 x	371 x
22	72 x	122 x	172 x	222 x	272	322	372
23 x	73	123	173 x	223	273	323	373
24	74	124 x	174	224	274	324	374
25	75	125	175	225 x	275	325 x	375
26	76 x	126 x	176	226	276	326	376
27	77 x	127	177	227	277 x	327 x	377
28	78	128	178 x	228	278 x	328	378
29	79	129	179	229	279	329	379
30	80	130 x	180	230	280 x	330	380
31	81 x	131	181	231	281 x	331	381 x
32	82	132	182	232	282	332	382 x
33	83	133 x	183	233 x	283	333	383 x
34	84	134	184	234	284	334	384
35 x	85 x	135	185	235	285	335 x	385
36	86	136	186	236	286	336	386
37	87	137	187	237	287	337 x	387
38	88 x	138	188	238	288 x	338 x	388 x
39	89 x	139	189 x	239 x	289	339 x	389 x
40	90	140	190	240	290	340 x	390
41	91 x	141	191	241	291 x	341	391
42	92	142	192	242	292	342	293 x
43	93 x	143	193	243	293	343	393
44	94 x	144 x	194	244 x	294	344	394
45 x	95	145 x	195	245 x	295	345	395 x
46	96	146	196 x	246 x	296 x	346	396
47	97	147 x	197	247	297	347 x	397
48 x	98	148	198	248 x	298 x	348	398
49 x	99	149	199	249	299	349	399
50 x	100	150 x	200	250 x	300	350	400

Group A   55   Group B   61

Total: 116

```
EXECUTIVE DEPARTMENT                                          TELEPHONE
                                                              552-7100

                    City of Newton, Massachusetts
                             Incorporated 1873
                              CITY HALL
                  COMMONWEALTH AVENUE AND WALNUT STREET
                         NEWTON CENTRE  02159
THEODORE D. MANN
    MAYOR
```

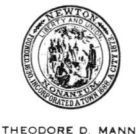

May 1979

Dear Resident,

    Your household has been selected to assist the Newton Council on Aging in determining the need for a new service in our community. The Council is presently studying the need for ADULT DAY CARE services for elderly residents who live with other household members and cannot be left alone during the day.

    ADULT DAY CARE is essentially a program designed to serve the elderly who do not require 24 hour institutional care, but who can benefit by a therapeutic program of social activity, physical rehabilitation, counseling and recreation. A typical ADULT DAY CARE center is open Monday through Friday between the hours of 9 a.m. and 5 p.m. A senior citizen can utilize this service for five days or less per week. Transportation can be provided to an ADULT DAY CARE center for those who require this service. For those eligible, ADULT DAY CARE can be paid for by the Medicaid program; otherwise, participants or their families must pay for this service.

    Your answers to the enclosed questionnaire will be greatly appreciated. All answers will be utilized strictly for statistical purposes. Please note that no postage is necessary to return the enclosed postcard.

    If you have any questions or desire more information, please contact the Department of Human Services at 552-7170. Please return the questionnaire within two weeks.

    Thank you in advance for your cooperation.

Sincerely,

Theodore D. Mann
Mayor

Enclosure

Figure D-2. Cover letter from the Mayor of Newton sent with questionnaire

Index

Active-problem-list sheet, 326–327
  example of (figure), 333
Activities. *See* Program activities
Administration on Aging, 56–57, 60, 135, 157, 161–162, 222–223
Administrative staff, 252–255
Admission agreement, 323
  example of (figure), 326
Admission criteria
  establishing, 284–288
  in Florida, 199
  forms for, 285, 286, 287, 289, 290, 291, 292, 293, 294
Adult day care
  clients for (*see* Elderly; Population at risk, identifying)
  defined, 3, 238, 239
  funding of (*see* Funding)
  future research in, 374–377
  hypotheses of, 4
  as long-term care, 3–4

Adult day care *(continued)*
  planning for (*see* Adult day-care planning)
  programs in (*see* Adult day-care programs)
  state standards for, 167–168, 168–171, 196–197
  see also Long-term care
Adult day-care planning
  community services, continuum of, in, 38–52
    figure, 39
    see also Community services for elderly, continuum of
  community services, coordinating, in, 54–61
    model projects for, 61–64 (*see also names of individual projects*)
    theoretical model for, 64–67
  outreach in, 52–53
  principles of, 36–38

419

Adult day-care planning *(continued)*
  see also Long-term-care planning
Adult day-care programs
  evaluating *(see* Evaluation)
  in Florida, 195–201 *(see also* Florida, adult day-care programs in)
  history of, 145, 173
    in Britain, 146–148, 181, 183–184, 188–189 *(see also* Britain, geriatric day hospitals in)
    in Canada, 146–150
    in Denmark and Sweden, 150–151
    in Israel, 148
    in Russia, 146
    in US, 146, 151–173, 174–178 *(see also* US day-care movement)
  implementing *(see* Implementation)
  medical-rehabilitative model of *(see* Medical-rehabilitative model)
  objectives of *(see* Objectives)
  planning *(see* Adult day-care planning)
  psychiatric day-treatment programs vs, 243
  psychosocial model of, 154, 266
    medical-rehabilitative model vs, 266–267
  Robins's four models of, 172, 239–242, 252
    tables, 173, 241, 253
  staffing *(see* Staffing)
Adult Protective Services of San Diego, 348, 349–350
Aides, role of, 263
Alternatives, examining, in long-term-care planning, 27, 28, 32
American College of Nursing Home Administrators, surveys by, 168–169
  tables, 169, 170–171
American Nurses Association, 55
Anderson, J., study by, 12
Anderson, N.N., Stone L.B., quoted, 125
Annual report, 307–308
  example of (figure), 309–315
Appropriateness, a criterion in data collection, 88
Archer, S.E., Fleshman, R., study by, 31
Assessment, 25, 28
  evaluation and, 345, 348
    figure, 345
  functional, of disability *(see* Disability, functional assessment of)

Assessment *(continued)*
  of needs *(see* Needs assessment)
  of participant *(see* Admission criteria)
Audit in problem-oriented record system, 308, 319–321
Authorization and release sheet, 334–335
  example of (figure), 337

Bagnall, M.K., quoted, 183
Barthel index, 116–117
Baseline data, 70, 72–75
Baycrest Jewish Adult Day-Care Center, 149, 150
"Block grant" proposal, 203, 205
Blum, H., 24
Boucher, study by, 182
Boundary of a system, 18
Brierer, J., 146
Britain
  day centers in, 147–148, 181, 182, 188
  geriatric day hospitals in
    functions of, 184–185, 188–189
    funding of, 189–190
    history of, 146–147, 181, 183–184, 188–189
    objectives of, 182
    operational problems in, 187–188
    reasons for attending, 185–186
    size of, optimal, 186
    in social-service system, 190–192
    vs U.S., 182, 187, 190, 191, 192–193
Brocklehurst, J.C.
  quoted, 146–147, 183–184
  studies by, 183, 185–186, 187
Brocklehurst, J.C., Tucker, J.S., study by, 185
Budget
  establishing, 268–270
  forms for, 269, 271, 272
Burton approach, 117–118
  table, 119
Burton D., Granger C., Greer D., et al, study by, 117–118, 119

California Department of Health Services, 348
  cost-analysis study by, 367–373
    tables, 368, 369, 370, 371
  quoted, 350

California Department of Health
Services *(continued)*
  Requirements of Living Scales of, 344
    table, 346–347
  California Medi-Cal study, 367–373
    tables, 368, 369, 370, 371
Cameron, D.E., 146
Canada, day care in, 146–150
Carman, Representative, 167
Carp, F.M., quoted, 46
Carter, J., quoted, 182
Carter, M.D., quoted, 152
Chronic disease. *See* Disability
Clerical staff, role of, 263–264
Cleveland Study, 107–108, 115, 126
Closed-ended questions, 84, 88, 89
  example of (figure), 85
Community
  elderly in, depend on relatives, 109, 126–129
  institution vs, studies on, 108–111, 129–133, 134
  role of, in developing philosophy, 235–237
Community Care for the Elderly, 196
Community-forum approach, 90, 94–95
Community organizations, a funding source, 226, 228
Community outreach plan, establishing, 282–284
Community referral sheet, 338–339
  example of (figure), 340
Community Services Act of 1974, 224
Community services for elderly
  continuum of, 38–40
    congregate housing in, 39, 45–46
    elderly social services in, 39, 40–42
    Foster Care for Elders in, 39, 46–47
    health maintenance organizations in, 39, 43–44
    home health care in, 39, 42–43
    hospice as, 39, 51–52
    hospitals in, 39, 50–51
    independent housing in, 39, 44–45
    neighborhood health centers in, 39, 44
    nursing homes in, 39, 48–50
    respite care in, 39, 47–48
  coordinating, in adult day-care planning, 54–61
  model projects for, 61–64 *(see also names of individual projects)*

Community services for elderly *(continued)*
  theoretical model for, 64–67
Comprehensive Assessment System for Seniors, 118, 119–122
  figure, 123
  table, 121
Computer, used in record system, 307
Congregate housing, 39, 45–46
Congressional Budget Office, study by, quoted, 133
Congressional hearing of 1980, 154–166. *See also names of individual participants*
Conly, S.
  quoted, 135
  study by, 134–135
Constraints in long-term-care planning, 19, 20–21, 27, 28, 31–32
Cosin, L., quoted, 188
Cost-benefit analysis, 249, 363–366
  figures, 365, 366
  see also California Medi-Cal study
Cost-effectiveness analysis, 367
  table, 367
  see also California Medi-Cal study; Evaluation, Weissert study as
Costs, health-care, among elderly, 5–6
Council on Aging, 1976 report from, quoted, 104
Crawford, C.O., Leadly, S.M., quoted, 37
Criteria, defined, 248–249

Daily attendance and transportation sheet, 335–336
  example of (figure), 338
Data
  baseline, 70, 72–75
  collecting, 27, 28, 29–30
    methods of *(see* Data-collection methods)
  defined, 72
  examining and applying, 99–101
  sources of *(see* Data sources used in needs assessment)
  see also Record; Record system
Data base
  of problem-oriented record, 316, 317
    example of (figure), 320
  see also names of individual data-collection forms

Data-collection methods
  criteria for, 86–88
  observation and measurement, 82–83
  questioning, 83–86, 88–99 (*see also* Questioning method)
  survey illustrating, 408–417
Data sources used in needs assessment, 76
  figure, 83
  by health-need indicators, 80–81
  major, 76–79
  for population counts, 80
  professional organizations as, 82, 83
  tables, 76–79, 80–81
Day care
  adult (*see* Adult day care)
  defined, 238–239
Day center, British, 147–148, 181, 182, 188
  day hospital vs, defined, 148
Day hospital
  day center vs, defined, 148
  geriatric
    British (*see* Britain, geriatric day hospitals in)
    history of, 146–147, 149–150, 181, 183–184, 188–189 (*see also* Adult day-care programs, history of)
  psychiatric, history of, 146
Delphi technique, 96–98
Demands
  defined, 7
  of elderly, for long-term care, 9, 12
Demographic indicators, outline, 74
Denmark, day care in, 150
Denniston, O.L., study by, 354
Disability
  community maintenance and, 127
  functional assessment of, 111–112
    methods of, 113–120, 397–407 (*see also names of individual methods*)
    purposes of, 112–113
  institutionalization and, 110–111
  percentages of, among elderly, 4–5, 105–108
    tables, 106, 107
Discharge sheet, 331
  example of (figure), 336
Douglas, L.M., 342
Driscoll, D., testimony of, quoted, 158–160
Drucker, P.F., quoted, 27
Dzhagrov, 146

Effectiveness Performance Objectives, 349–350
Effectiveness Performance Update, 350
  example of (figure), 351
Elderly
  in community
    depend on relatives, 109, 126–129
    vs institution, 108–111, 129–133, 134
  community services for (*see* Community services for elderly)
  demands of, for long-term care, 9, 12
  disabilities of (*see* Disability)
  income and health-care costs of, 5–6
  institutionalized, 5, 13, 108–111, 151 (*see also* Elderly, in community vs institution)
  life expectancy of, 5
    table, 6
  needs of, for long-term care, 7–9 (*see also* Needs assessment)
  population shifts and, 6, 7–9, 104–105, 195
    figures, 7, 8
    tables, 9, 10–11
  see also Population at risk, identifying
Elderly social services, 39, 40–42
Elder-services network, 56–58
  figure, 57
Environmental indicators, outline, 74–75
Environment of a system, 18
ESCROW profile, 116, 397–400
Ethics in philosophy, 234
Evaluation, 25, 26, 28, 34, 35
  assessment and, 345, 348
  figure, 345
  California Medi-Cal study as, 367–373
    tables, 368, 369, 370, 371
  cost-benefit analysis, 363–366
    figures, 365, 366
    see also Evaluation, California Medi-Cal study as
  cost-effectiveness analysis, 367
    table, 367
    see also Evaluation, California Medi-Cal study as; Evaluation, Weissert study as
  defined, 342–344
  flow sheet used in, 358–359
    table, 358, 359, 360, 361
  future research and, 374–377
  method of, choosing, 359–361

Evaluation *(continued)*
  objectives and, 246–249, 345, 348
    figures, 248, 345
  planning for, 351–352
    table, 352
  structure, process, and outcome, 362–363
    figures, 363, 364
  summative and formative, 362
  terms used in, defined (figure), 353
  tools used in, 352–358
    figures, 355, 356–357
  uses of, 348–351
    figure, 349
  Weissert study as, 373–374

Face and admission referral sheet, 322–323
  example of (figure), 324–325
Facility requirements, establishing, 270, 271, 272
Family
  elderly depend on, in community, 109, 126–129
  involvement of, in program, 295–296
Farndale, J., study by, 187, 188
Federal-State Cooperative Program for Local Population Estimates, 80, 391
Federal studies on adult day care, 1974–1978, 152–154
Feedback, 19, 20
Field-survey approach, 90, 93–94
First National Conference on Congregate Housing for Older People, 45–46
Fisher, G., quoted, 366
Fleming, A., quoted, 126
Florida
  adult day-care programs in
    facilities and staff of, 198–199
    funding and administration of, 196
    goals of, 197
    licensing of, 196–197
    models of, 197
    participants in, 197–198
    participants in, assessing, 199
    services provided by, 199–201
  elderly population in, 195
Flow sheet, evaluation, 358–359
  table, 358, 359, 360, 361
Ford, Representative, 167
Forms, examples of
  active-problem-list sheet, 333

Forms, examples of *(continued)*
  admission agreement, 326
  admission criteria, 285, 286
  assessment form, 289, 290, 291, 292, 293, 294
  assessment guide, 287
  authorization and release sheet, 337
  budget, 269, 271, 272
  calendar of activities, 301, 302
  community referral sheet, 340
  daily attendance and transportation sheet, 338
  discharge sheet, 336
  effectiveness performance update, 351
  emergency plan, 280–281
  face and admission referral sheet, 324–325
  medical preadmission sheet, 327, 328
  participant profile, 330, 331, 332–333
  participants' interests survey, 297, 298
  participants' rights sheet, 337
  physician's order sheet, 329
  plan of care and flow sheet, 334
  program-activities outline, 299, 300
  program director job description, 278
  progress sheet, 335
  referring social worker's statement, 329
  service contract, 279
  volunteer job application, 275
  volunteer job description, 274
Foster Care for Elders, 39, 46–47
Foster Grandparent Program, 41
Foundation for Health Care Evaluation, 130
Foundations, a funding source, 226
  figure, 227
Friendship Center of New York, 64
Funding
  "block grant" proposal and, 203, 205
  in Britain, 189–190
  distribution of, 202–203
    figure, 203
    table, 204
  in Florida, 196
  sources of, government
    Community Services Act of 1974, 223
    National Health Insurance, 13, 224
    Older Americans Act, 171, 202, 204, 210–223 (*see also* Older Americans Act)
    Revenue Sharing, 202, 224

Funding *(continued)*
    Social Security Act, 171, 202,
        206–210, 228 (*see also* Social
        Security Act)
    sources of, private
        community organizations, 226, 228
        foundations, 226, 227
        private insurance, 13, 224–226
Future orientation in long-term-care
    planning, 24

Georgia Alternative Health Service
    Project, 134, 135
Geriatric Authority of Holyoke, 63
Gerontology centers as data source, 82
Goal-attainment outline, 247
    figure, 248
    use of, 358–359
    table, 358, 359, 360, 361
Goals in long-term-care planning, 23–24,
    27, 28–29
Gottesman, L.E., Brody, E., quoted,
    109
Granger, C.V., study by, 115–117,
    397–401
    figure, 402–407
Grant proposal, Title III, example of
    (figure), 212–221
Greer, D., Sherwood, S., Morris, J.N., et
    al, 111

Hall, A.D., Fagan, R.E., 16
Hammerman, J., Friedsam, H.H., Shore,
    H., quoted, 109
Health-care team. *See* Staffing
Health problems. *See* Disability
Health-status indicators, outline, 75
Health Systems Agencies, 58–60
    figure, 59
Hebrew Rehabilitation Center for the
    Aged, 110, 112, 117, 118, 126
    passim
Home Care Corporation, 290–295
Home health care, 39, 42–43
    defined, 54–55
Hospice, 39, 51–52
Hospitals, 12, 39, 50–51
House Select Committee on Aging,
    154–155
Housing and Urban Development Act of
    1970, quoted, 45

Implementation, 25, 26, 28, 33,
    266–268, 304
    admission process in, 284–288, 289,
        290, 291, 292, 293, 294
    budget in, 268–270, 271, 272
    community outreach in, 282–284
    facility requirements in, 270, 271, 272
    family involvement in, 295–296
    policies and procedures in, 277–281
    program activities in, 296–302
    staffing in, 272–273
    transportation system in, 288, 289,
        290, 291, 292, 293, 294–295
    volunteers in, 273–277
Independent housing for the elderly, 39,
    44–45
Information/communication system in
    long-term-care planning, 19–20
    figure, 19
Inputs, 19–20
Institution
    community vs, studies on, 108–111,
        129–133, 134
    elderly in, characterized, 5, 13,
        108–111, 151
    role of, in early US day-care movement,
        146, 151–152
    *see also names of individual kinds of
        institutions*
Insurance
    private, 13, 224–226
        table, 225
    public (*see* Medicaid; Medi-Cal;
        Medicare; National Health
        Insurance)
Interdisciplinary participant approach,
    example of (figure), 252
Interviews, 83, 84, 85–86
Israel, geriatric day hospitals in, 148

James, G., study by, 354–355
Johnson, President L., quoted, 56

Kahana, E., Coe, R.M., quoted, 134
Kaiser Foundation, 43
Karafiath, D., study by, 12
Kent/Hirsch Survey, 128
Kerlinger, F., study by, 88
Key-informant approach, 90, 91–92
Klapfish, A., testimony of, quoted,
    164–166
Kovar, M.G., 13

LaVor, J., 108
Levindale Hebrew Geriatric Center and Hospital, 153, 207, 255, 256
Long-Range Evaluation System, 115–117, 397–401
  figure, 402–407
Long-term care
  adult day care as, 3–4
  clients for (*see* Elderly; Population at risk, identifying)
  fragmentation of services in, 125–126
  future research in, 124–125
  health-insurance reimbursement for, 13 (*see also* Insurance)
  needs and demands for, of elderly, 7–9, 12 (*see also* Needs assessment)
  planning for (*see* Long-term-care planning)
  population shifts affect, 6, 7–9, 104–105, 195
    figures, 7, 8
    tables, 9, 10–11
  residential (*see* Institution)
  see also Adult day care
Long-term-care planning
  importance of, 13–14
  systems theory and, 16–34 (*see also* Planning function; Planning system, long-term-care, subsystems in; Process; System)
  see also Adult day-care planning; Assessment; Evaluation; Implementation; Philosophy
Long-term-care-system indicators, outline, 75
Lowenthal, M.F., Robinson, B., study by, 128

Maddox, G.L., 192
Maimonides Day Hospital, 149–150
Martin, A., Millard, P.H.
  study by (1978), quoted, 189
  study by (1975), 186, 190
Massachusetts Association of Adult Day Care Centers, 303
Medicaid, 5, 13, 153, 225
  assessment form for, 289, 290, 291, 292, 293, 294
  in California (*see* Medi-Cal)
  in Massachusetts, 54, 157, 164–166, 167–168, 207
  see also Title XIX (Medicaid)

Medicaid Community Care Act of 1980, 166–167
  text of, 387–390
Medicaid waiver studies, 132–133
Medi-Cal, 168, 207–209, 348
  cost-analysis studies for, 367–373
  tables, 368, 369, 370, 371
Medical preadmission sheet, 323
  example of (figure), 327, 328
Medical-rehabilitative model, 154, 197
  implementing, 266–304 (*see also* Implementation)
  psychosocial model vs, 266
  table, 267
Medicare, 5, 13, 42, 48–49, 62, 153, 154, 206, 225. *See also* Title XVIII (Medicare)
Medicare Amendments of 1980, 167
Michigan Association of Senior Day Care Centers, 303
Mitchell, J., study by, 134
Models. *See* Medical-rehabilitative model; Psychosocial model; Robins E.G., four models of
Monroe County Long-Term-Care Program, 132–133, 134, 135
Morris, J.N., Mor, V., study by, 118–122
Morrison, K., testimony of, quoted, 161–162

Nagi, S.Z., studies by, 107, 108, 111
National Association of Community Health Centers, 205
National Association of State Units on Aging, as data source, 82
National Center for Health Services Research, 132, 154, 157, 162–163, 373
National Commission on Community Services, 100
National Conference on Aging, 3
National Council on Aging, 157, 158, 172
  quoted, 239
National Health Insurance, 13, 224
National Health Planning and Resources Development Act, 58–60
National Institute on Adult Day Care, 158–160, 172, 173
  rules of operation of (figure), 174–178
National League for Nursing, 55

Needs
  defined, 6–7
  of elderly, for long-term care, 7–9
  assessing (*see* Needs assessment)
Needs assessment, 69–70
  concepts in, defined, 71–73
  data, baseline, for, defined, 70, 72–75
  data, collecting, in, 82–99, 408–417
    (*see also* Data-collection methods)
  data, examining and applying, in,
    99–101
  data sources used in, 76–82, 83 (*see also* Data sources used in needs assessment)
  defined, 71–72
  functional assessment of disability in,
    112–113 (*see also* Disability, functional assessment of)
  future research in, 124–125
  population at risk, identifying, in,
    104–108
  survey used in, 408–417
Neighborhood health centers, 39, 44
Norm, defined, 249
Nurse, role of, 256–257
Nurse-practitioner, role of, 60
Nursing homes, 5, 13, 39, 48–50, 151, 152. See *also* Institution
Nutrition, Title VII program for, 202, 222–223
  tables, 204, 223
Nutritionist, role of, 260–261

Objectives
  defining, 27, 28, 32–33, 244–246
  evaluation and, 246–249, 345, 348
  figures, 248, 345
  example of (figure), 246, 247
Objectivity, a criterion in data collection, 87
Occupational therapist, role of, 258–259
Older Americans Act, 41, 56
  Title V, 202, 222
    table, 204
  Title IV, 202, 211, 222
  Title VII, 202, 222–223
    tables, 204, 223
  Title III, 171, 202, 210–211, 223
    grand proposal for, example of (figure), 212–221
    table, 204

Older Americans Resources and Services, 115
On Lok Senior Health Services, 206, 228, 348
Organizational chart, example of (figure), 254
Organization of a system in long-term-care planning, 21–22
Orkand Corporation, study by, 126
Outputs, 19, 20
Outreach in adult day-care planning, 52–53
Outreach plan, community, establishing, 282–284

Palmore, E., study by, 109
Participant profile sheets, 323
  examples of (figures), 330, 331, 332–333
Participants'-rights sheet, 335
  example of (figure), 337
Parts of a system, 18
Pathy, M.S., 189
Pathy, M.S., Peach H., study by, 190
Pepper, Representative C., 154, 166, 167
  statements by, quoted, 155–157
Philosophy
  community's role in developing,
    235–237
  components of, 234–235
  defined, 233
  examples of, 237, 242
    figures, 238, 243
  importance of, 233, 235
  program definition based on, 238–239
  program objectives based on, 244–246
Physical therapist, role of, 257–258
Physician, role of, 12, 60, 262–263
Physician's order sheet, 323
  example of (figure), 329
Planning, adult day-care. *See* Adult day-care planning
Planning, long-term-care. *See* Long-term-care planning
Planning for evaluation, 351–352
  table, 352
Planning function
  characteristics of, 22–24
  defined, 22, 26–27
Planning subsystem in planning system,
  25–26, 28

Planning system, long-term-care,
    subsystems in, 17, 25–26
  figure, 25
  see also Assessment; Evaluation;
    Implementation; Planning subsystem
    in planning system
Plan of action, formulating, in long-term-
    care planning, 27, 28, 33
Plan of care and flow sheet, 328, 330
  example of (figure), 334
Plan of care in problem-oriented record,
    316, 317–318
  example of (figure), 322
  see also Plan of care and flow sheet
Policies and procedures
  establishing, 277
  forms for, 278–281
Population at risk, identifying, 76, 79,
    104–108
Population estimates, sources of, 80
  list, 391–396
Population shifts, 6, 7–9, 104–105, 195
  figures, 7, 8
  tables, 9, 10–11
Prevention, three levels of, 244–245
  table, 245
Problem list of problem-oriented record,
    316, 317
  example of (figure), 321
  see also Active-problem-list sheet
Problem-oriented record system. *See*
    Record system, problem-oriented
Problems, identifying, in long-term-care
    planning, 27, 28, 30–31
Process
  defined, 26
  planning, long-term-care as, 26–34
  figures, 28, 35
Professional organizations as data source,
    82
  figure, 83
Professional staff, 255–256, 256–263.
    See also names of individual professions
Program activities
  determining, 296, 298–300
  in Florida, 200
  forms for, 297, 298, 299, 300, 301,
    302
Progress sheet, 331
  example of (figure), 335
Project Find, 63–64

Project Triage, 61–63, 125, 134, 135
Psychiatric day-treatment programs,
    242–243
  philosophy of, example of (figure), 243
Psychosocial model, 197
  medical-rehabilitative model vs, 266
  table, 267
Public Law 92-603, 153
PULSES profile, 116, 400–401
Purposes of long-term-care planning, 24

Quality assurance, 247–249
Questioning method, 83–84
  application of, 90–99 (*see also names of
    individual approaches*)
  developing questions for use in, 88–90
  interviews used in, 83, 84, 85–86
  questionnaires used in, 83, 84–85, 86
Questionnaires, 83, 84–85, 86
Quinn, J., quoted, 66

Rates-under-treatment approach, 90,
    92–93
Rathbone-McCuan, E., Rose, M., Bland,
    J., study by, 153
Raugel, Representative, 167
Record
  problem-oriented, 308
    components of, 316–318
    format of, examples of, 318–319,
      320, 321, 322
    forms used in composing, 322–339
      (*see also names of individual forms*)
    team approach and (figure), 319
  see also Record system
Record system
  annual report in, 307–308
    example of (figure), 309–315
  computer in, 307
  criteria for, 307
  functions of, 305–306
  problem-oriented, 306, 341
    advantages of, 339, 341
    audit in, 308, 319–321
    correction of deficiencies and, 308,
      320–321
    overview of, 308
    problem-oriented record in (*see*
      Record, problem-oriented)
    scientific method and (figure), 316
  types of, 306

Record system *(continued)*
  see also Record
Recreational therapist, role of, 259–260
Referring social worker's statement sheet, 323
  example of (figure), 329
Relatives. *See* Family
Reliability, a criterion in data collection, 86
Requirements of Living Scales, 344
  table, 346–347
Resource, 304
Resources and constraints, examining, in long-term-care planning, 27, 28, 31–32
Respite care, 39, 47–48
Retired Senior Volunteer Program, 41
Revenue Sharing, 202, 224
Robins, E.G., four models of, 172, 239–242, 252
  tables, 173, 241, 253
Russia, first day hospital in, 146
Ryder, C.F., quoted, 105

Sacramento Senior Day Care Center, 348
San Diego Senior Adult Day Program, 256
Schaefer, M., quoted, 21, 26–27
Schweiker, R., quoted, 205
Scientific method, problem-oriented record system and (figure), 316
Selig, A., study by, 358
Service-population approach, 90, 95–96
Sherwood, S., quoted, 107
Siegel, L., Atkinson, C., Cohen, A., study by, 90
Silberstein, Dr., quoted, 148
SOAP progress notes in problem-oriented record, 316, 318
  examples of (figure), 322
  see also Progress sheet
Social-indicators approach, 90, 91
Social Security Act
  Title XVIII, 202, 206
  Title XIX, 171, 202, 206–209, 228
  Title XX, 171, 202, 209–210, 228
Social worker, role of, 60–61, 261–262
Socioeconomic indicators, outline, 74
Sorenson, J., study by, 367
Speech therapist, role of, 260

Staffing, 251, 264–265
  administrative, 252–255
  in Britain, 184, 185, 186, 187
  in Florida, 198–199
  interdisciplinary approach to, 251 passim
  figure, 252
  needs for, establishing, 272–273
  organizational chart for, example of (figure), 254
  professional, 255–256, 256–263 (*see also names of individual professions*)
  for Robins's four models of services, 252
  table, 253
  support, 256, 263–264 (*see also names of individual positions*)
Standards, defined, 248
State associations, role of, 302–304
Structure, process, and outcome, 362–363
  figures, 363, 364
Suchman, E., study by, 354
  figure, 355
Support staff, 256, 263–264. *See also names of individual positions*
Sweden, day care in, 150–151
System
  characteristics of, 18–22
  defined, 16–17
  long-term-care planning as, 17
Systems theory, long-term-care planning and, 16–34. *See also* Planning function; Planning system, long-term-care, subsystems in; Process; System

Technicians, role of, 263
Throughputs, 19, 20
Time perspective, used in examining data, 99–100
Title XVIII (Medicare), 202, 206
Title V, 202, 222
  table, 204
Title IV, 202, 211, 222
Title XIX (Medicaid), 171, 202, 206–209, 228
Title VII, 202, 222–223
  tables, 204, 223
Title III, 171, 202, 210–211, 223

Title III *(continued)*
  grant proposal for, example of (figure), 212–221
  table, 204
Title XX, 171, 202, 209–210, 228
Townsend, P., Gottesman, L.E., quoted, 109
Trager, B., quoted, 239
Transcentury Report, 153–154
Transportation, 264
  in Britain, 187
  in Florida, 199–200
  system of, establishing, 288, 289, 290, 291, 292, 293, 294–295
Truth in philosophy, 234–235

U.S. day-care movement
  American College of Nursing Home Administrators surveys on, 168–169
    tables, 169, 170–171
  congressional hearing on, 1980, 154–66 *(see also names of individual participants)*
  federal studies on, 1974–1978, 152–154
  institutional background of, 146, 151–152
  Medicaid Community Care Act of 1980 and, 166–167
  Medicare Amendments of 1980 and, 167
  National Institute on Adult Day Care in, 172, 173
    rules of operation of (figure), 174–178
  programs in, current models of, 171–172
    table, 173

U.S. day-care movement *(continued)*
  see also Medical-rehabilitative model; Psychosocial model; Robins, E.G., four models of
  state standards in, 167–168, 168–171, 196–197

Validity, a criterion in data collection, 87
Values, role of, 100–101, 234
Van driver, role of, 264
Vanik, Representative, 167
Vermont Peer Standards Review Organization, 110, 131
Volunteers
  forms for, 274, 275
  policies concerning and recruitment of, 198, 273–277
Volunteers for Services to Older Persons, 118 passim, 135
VonBertalanffy, L., 16

Warheit, G., Bell, R., Schwab, J., study by, 90
Waxman, Senator H., 166
Weed, L., 114, 308, 318
Weiler, P., Rathbone-McCuan, E., 114
Weissert, W.
  quoted, 124, 132, 162–163, 239
  studies by, 154, 373–374
Wertlieb, H., Dee, M., quoted, 168
Williams, C., quoted, 46
Woodford-Williams, E., Alvarez, A., study by, 184, 189
Woods, H., testimony of, quoted, 157–158
Worcester Home Care Study, 132